THE
CARDIAC RHYTHMS

A Systematic Approach to Interpretation

RAYMOND E. PHILLIPS, M.D., F.A.C.P.

Senior Attending Physician, Phelps Memorial Hospital,
North Tarrytown, New York; Instructor and Attending
Physician to Outpatients, The New York Hospital—Cornell
Medical Center, New York City; Exercise Cardiologist, Work
Physiology Unit, Montefiore Hospital and Medical Center, New York

MARY K. FEENEY, R.N., B.S.N.

Clinical Instructor, ICU/CCU, Columbia Hospital School of Nursing,
and Staff Member, Coronary Surveillance Unit, St. Luke's Hospital,
Milwaukee, Wisconsin. Formerly Supervisor, Critical Care Areas,
and Coordinator, Electrocardiography Courses for Nurses,
Phelps Memorial Hospital, North Tarrytown, New York

W. B. SAUNDERS COMPANY / PHILADELPHIA / LONDON / TORONTO

W. B. Saunders Company: West Washington Square
Philadelphia, Pa. 19105

12 Dyott Street
London, WC1A 1DB

833 Oxford Street
Toronto, Ontario M8Z 5T9, Canada

The Cardiac Rhythms: A Systematic Approach to Interpretation   ISBN   0-7216-7220-5

Print No.:   9   8   7   6   5   4

PREFACE

The Cardiac Rhythms presents a plan for acquiring skill in the electrocardiographic interpretation of the heartbeat. The subject is introduced on an elementary level and developed to an intermediate degree of complexity. The orientation is directed in particular to preparing the reader for the Cardiac Care Unit experience.

The book has been designed as a primer for self-study and is intended to help the student recognize and describe the common disorders of the cardiac rhythm. The reader who is already familiar with the fundamentals of the subject can gain further proficiency in analysis through the numerous examples of arrhythmias and clinical rhythm sequences. The book is also useful as an illustrative outline and exercise supplement for a formal course or for group instruction. For the cardiac care team, the system of presentation may serve as a guide for standardizing clinical description and for organizing a unit logbook of arrhythmias.

The text has been integrated into a stylized pictorial frame of reference with a step-by-step exposition of the basic determinants of heart rate and rhythm. The dynamics of the normal heartbeat are given considerable attention to establish a sound working knowledge of physiological principles before proceeding to the more difficult abnormal rhythms. Pertinent effects of the autonomic nervous system and the cardiac drugs are introduced early in the text and are expanded within the schematic framework. Anatomical and electrophysiological details are included only to that depth which is essential for the interpretation of the cardiac rhythms.

While all disturbances of the heartbeat fall within a relatively few basic types, they appear in endless variations of a given pattern and in combinations of patterns. Because of this, multiple examples of each class are provided. A workbook format has been followed so that the reader may actively participate in problem solving while developing the practice of careful search and accurate diagnosis. Emphasis is placed on the use of descriptive terminology and comprehensive interpretation. At various stages in the book, test electrocardiograms are presented to give the reader an opportunity to evaluate his progress.

We wish to thank the staff of the Coronary Care Unit at Phelps Memorial Hospital, North Tarrytown, New York, where many ideas for this presentation were formulated.

Raymond E. Phillips

Mary K. Feeney

CONTENTS

Chapter 1

THE HEARTBEAT

The heart is a compact muscular organ which performs solely as a pump. Functionally, it is composed of two flow circuits, each made up of two chambers. Normally these circuits operate synchronously and rhythmically. The basic structure of the heart and its patterns of flow can be explained through simplified sketches of the embryological development of the organ.

A DEVELOPMENTAL ANATOMY

The first heartbeat in the human being appears during the fourth week of embryonic life. At this stage of development, the heart is a thickened muscular bulb along a midline circulatory tube. The heartbeat is a simple peristaltic wave which begins at the hind end of the cardiac bulb and moves forward. This contractile motion propels the fluid content of the circulatory tube. (See figure top of following page.)

The early heartbeat consists of three fundamental actions:

1. *Automaticity:* generation of an electrical stimulus.
2. *Conduction:* spread of this stimulus through the cardiac mass.
3. *Contraction:* mechanical response of cardiac muscle to the stimulus.

This sequence will repeat itself with each subsequent beat and, in the average person, will occur 3,000,000,000 times.

The pulsating bulb at this stage elongates rapidly, becoming bent upon itself into an abrupt S-shape. The thickened midchamber is the primitive ventricle, which leads into the arterial trunk. The lower venous channels (the future atria) will be repositioned forward. The contractile wave and circulatory flow continue to follow the contortions and convolutions of the cardiac tube. (See figure bottom of following page.)

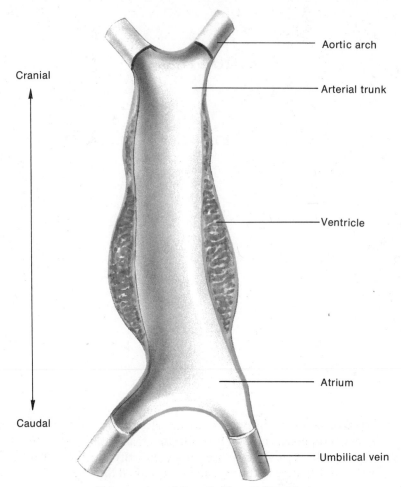

Cranial

Caudal

Aortic arch

Arterial trunk

Ventricle

Atrium

Umbilical vein

Cutaway view of the primitive cardiac tube.

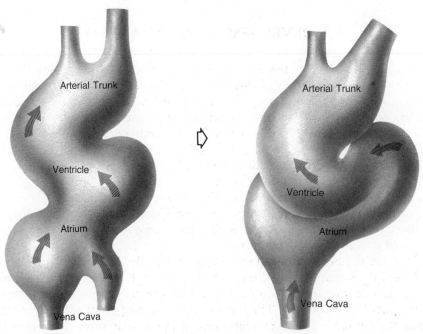

Arterial Trunk

Ventricle

Atrium

Vena Cava

Arterial Trunk

Ventricle

Atrium

Vena Cava

Convolutions of the cardiac tube.

The ventricular chamber develops a thick muscular wall, while the thinner-walled atrial chamber balloons out around the stem of the ventricles. Venous channels lead into the atrium. The ventricular outflow tract, which is directed forward, is the arterial trunk.

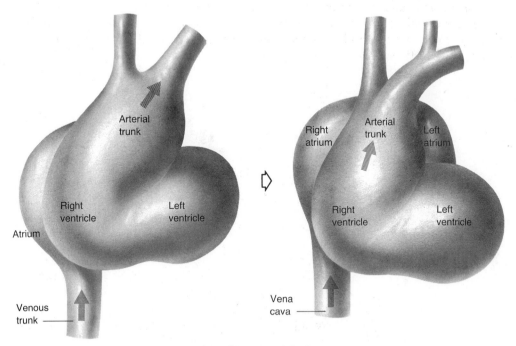

Basic architecture of the heart.

By the seventh week of development, the atrium and the ventricle have become divided into right and left chambers by vertical partitions of muscular and fibrous tissue called septa. In addition, another vertical division splits the arterial trunk longitudinally, creating the pulmonary artery and the aorta. These vessels criss-cross near their origin, where they are separated by the spiral septum.

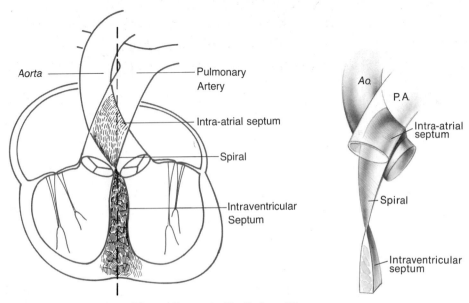

The cardiac septa: Vertical partitions.

   Horizontal partitions of the heart are provided by four valves which permit
flow of blood in one direction only. The tricuspid and bicuspid (or mitral) valves
are interposed between the atrial and ventricular chambers. They are thin, fibrous,
funnel-shaped structures with inner, moveable edges which are attached to the
floor of the ventricles by fibrous strands, the chordae tendineae. Two valves at the
origin of the pulmonary artery and the aorta are each composed of three leaflets
or cusps. These are referred to as the semilunar valves or, individually, as the pulmonary and aortic valves.

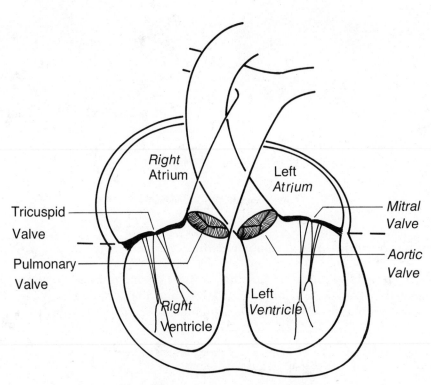

The cardiac valves: horizontal partitions.

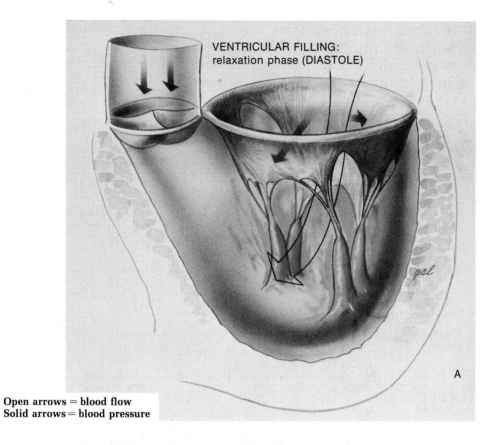

VENTRICULAR FILLING:
relaxation phase (DIASTOLE)

A

Open arrows = blood flow
Solid arrows = blood pressure

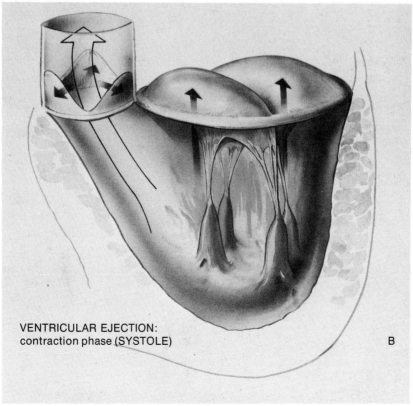

VENTRICULAR EJECTION:
contraction phase (SYSTOLE)

B

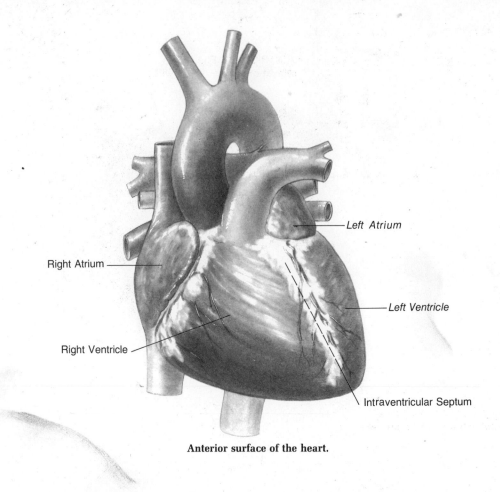

Right Atrium

Left Atrium

Right Ventricle

Left Ventricle

Intraventricular Septum

Anterior surface of the heart.

The heart lies in the chest so that the right atrium and ventricle are more toward the anterior than the left atrium and ventricle. The interventricular septum occupies a position oblique to the surface of the anterior chest.

POSTERIOR

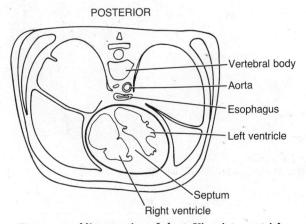

Vertebral body

Aorta

Esophagus

Left ventricle

Septum

Right ventricle

Transverse oblique section of chest: View into ventricles.

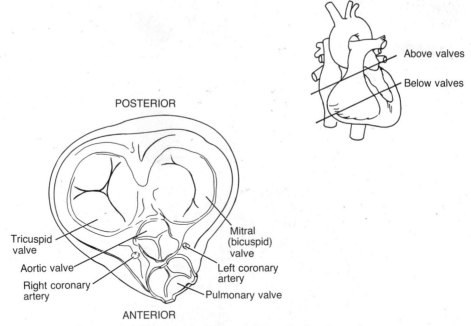

POSTERIOR

Tricuspid
valve

Mitral
(bicuspid)
valve

Aortic valve

Left coronary
artery

Right coronary
artery

Pulmonary valve

ANTERIOR

Transverse oblique section of heart: View of valves from above.

Above valves

Below valves

After birth, the right-sided chambers relay systemic venous blood toward the lungs.

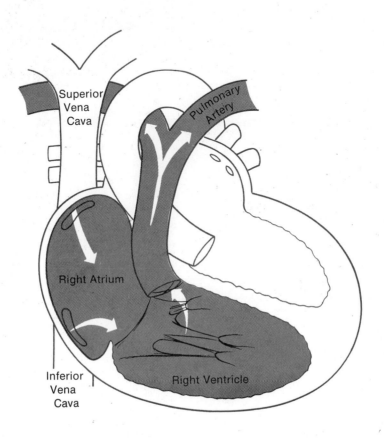

Superior
Vena
Cava

Pulmonary
Artery

Right Atrium

Inferior
Vena
Cava

Right Ventricle

The pair of chambers on the left receive blood oxygenated in the lungs and propel it into the vessels of the general circulation.

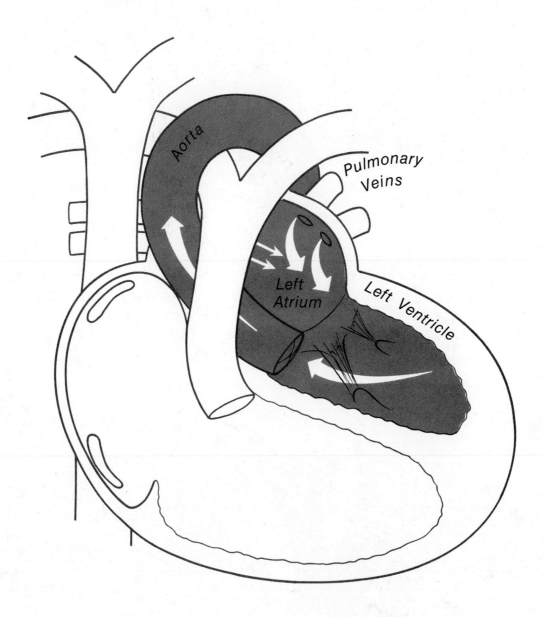

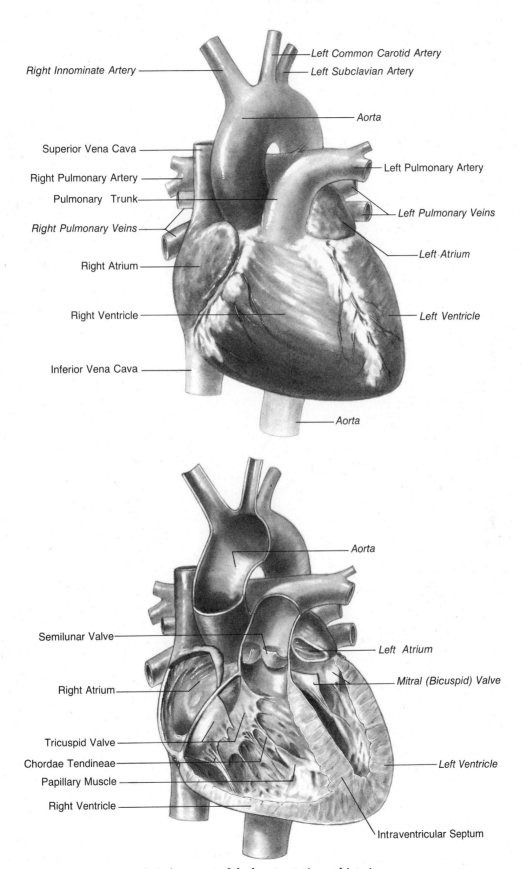

Right Innominate Artery

Left Common Carotid Artery

Left Subclavian Artery

Aorta

Superior Vena Cava

Left Pulmonary Artery

Right Pulmonary Artery

Pulmonary Trunk

Left Pulmonary Veins

Right Pulmonary Veins

Right Atrium

Left Atrium

Right Ventricle

Left Ventricle

Inferior Vena Cava

Aorta

Aorta

Semilunar Valve

Left Atrium

Mitral (Bicuspid) Valve

Right Atrium

Tricuspid Valve

Chordae Tendineae

Left Ventricle

Papillary Muscle

Right Ventricle

Intraventricular Septum

Anterior aspect of the heart, exterior and interior.

The forward flow of blood in each normal heartbeat is determined by the simultaneous contractions of the atria, which are almost immediately followed by those of the ventricles. Thus the sequence established in the simple cardiac tube during embryonic life is maintained in maturity despite great changes in the architecture of the heart.

The basic functioning unit of the heart is a contractile strand of muscle composed of many cells. Such units of fibers interconnect throughout the myocardium and, contracting harmoniously, force the movement of blood.

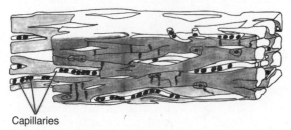

Capillaries

Myocardial fibers. (Reproduced with modification from Fox, C. C., and Hutchins, G. M.: Johns Hopkins Med. J., 130:291, 1972).

A schematic view of the heart will be used throughout this book to illustrate the electrical system. All four chambers are shown with the atrial and ventricular septa cut in cross section. The sites of impulse formation and the conduction pathways will be presented sequentially, using this diagram as a basis.

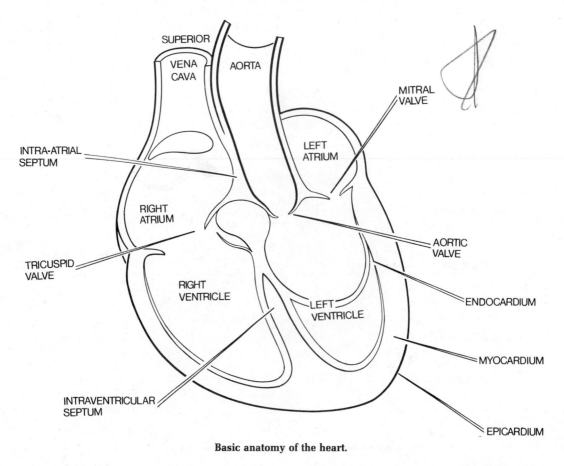

Basic anatomy of the heart.

ELECTROPHYSIOLOGY

While the basic mechanical events of the heartbeat are rather simple to explain, control of the pumping action is more complex. This regulating system is composed of clusters of specialized muscle cells which generate electrical currents and of tracts which convey them to the myocardial mass. Normally rhythmic impulses produce coordinated chamber contractions. The intricate sequences of excitation, however, are susceptible to structural and biochemical interference at many points, resulting in a wide variety of electrical abnormalities. These disorders make up the cardiac arrhythmias.

Living cells are packages of aqueous fluids containing the units of metabolism — oxygen and the derivatives of glucose, amino acids, and fatty acids. The wrapper of each cell is a complex membrane of protein and lipid material which has a highly selective permeability and can perform energy-requiring work. The cells themselves are bathed in fluid to which the cell membranes are constantly exposed. The circulatory fluids, those contained within the blood vessels, continually refresh the cellular bath so that exchanges of gases, electrolytes, metabolites, and water can take place between the intracellular and the extracellular fluids. In this exchange, the cell membrane plays a crucial role.

Much of the energy expended by the cell membrane is used to create an unequal distribution of electrolytes between the intracellular and extracellular fluids. For example, sodium ions are forced out of the cell so that the extracellular fluid is about 14 times as concentrated as the intracellular fluid. Potassium ions, on the other hand, are pumped into the cell to maintain a concentration of 30 times that of the fluid outside the cell. The intracellular and extracellular distribution of these and other cations (positively charged ionic substances) are represented in the illustration at the top of the following page.

In the active cell, more anions (negatively charged ionic substances) than cations tend to accumulate on the inner surface of the membrane. This produces an electrical charge or potential of the membrane itself, having an electrically negative interior surface and a positive exterior surface. It is a form of stored energy known as the **transmembrane potential.** The amount of this electrical force can be measured in the single cell using extremely fine electrodes, one outside and one inside the cell, each connected to a highly sensitive instrument, the galvanometer. The transmembrane potential of the average cell is −85 thousandths of a volt, or −85 millivolts.

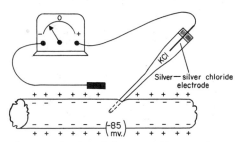

Measurement of the membrane potential of the nerve fiber using a microelectrode. (Reproduced from Guyton, A. C.: *Basic Human Physiology: Normal Function and Mechanisms of Disease.* **Philadelphia: W.B. Saunders Company, 1971).**

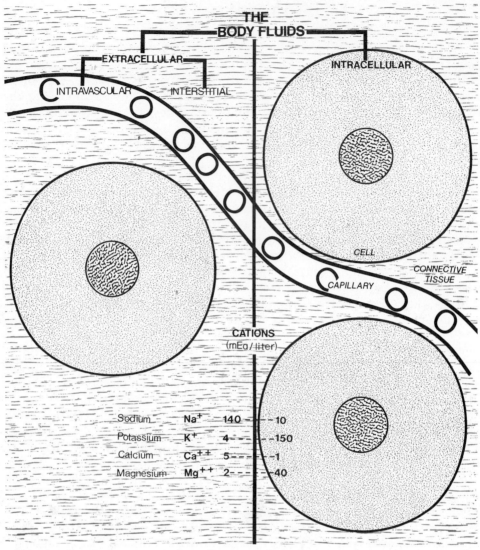

		CATIONS (mEq/liter)	
Sodium	Na$^+$	140	10
Potassium	K$^+$	4	150
Calcium	Ca^{++}	5	1
Magnesium	Mg^{++}	2	40

Distribution of the body fluids in tissue, with concentrations of the major cations in the extracellular and intracellular compartments.

When the cell has attained its maximum transmembrane potential and is in a steadily charged or **polarized** state, it is referred to, curiously, as the **resting cell.** This biological package can be thought of at this stage as a radio which is turned on, its tubes warmed up, but not actually playing. The radio will broadcast when it receives transmissions of a certain wavelength from a station to which it has been tuned. The resting cell will be activated when it receives a signal to which it is sensitive.

Activation of cells can be initiated by a variety of physical and chemical stimuli. In the case of nerves and muscles, the cells respond to electrical stimuli and are said to be excitable tissues. Immediately upon receiving such stimuli, the cell membrane undergoes a sudden change in polarity in which the transmembrane potential is neutralized, a process called **depolarization.** Sodium pours into the cells while potassium flows out. The electrical disturbance thus created is referred to as an **impulse.**

Most excitable cells maintain a steady, fully polarized state unless stimulated or unless adverse physiological conditions (such as hypoxia, cold, drug toxicity, or electrolyte imbalance) interfere with the electrical work of the cell membrane. Other cells are relatively unstable when their maximum transmembrane potential has been developed and tend to undergo depolarization without any outside stimulation. This self-generated or spontaneous impulse formation occurs in certain areas of the heart and is known as **automaticity.** A cell or group of cells with sustained automatic action, producing a series of impulses which control the heartbeat, is known as a cardiac **pacemaker.**

An impulse tends to spread from the cell (or cells) of origin to adjacent excitable cells, causing a wave of depolarization through the tissue. Impulses generally travel rapidly in nerve fibers, and the function of nerve cells is that of conducting impulses. In muscle, depolarizing waves spread at a much slower rate. The myofibril, in addition to conveying the impulse to adjacent fibers, also contracts as a response to depolarization.

The rate at which an impulse travels is termed the **conduction velocity.** This determines the sequence of activation of various parts of the myocardium from an impulse arising in the cardiac pacemaker.

Soon after depolarization, the cell membrane begins to restore the resting polarity of the cell. This process is called **repolarization.** It requires expenditure of energy by the membrane, which pumps sodium out of the cell and potassium into it. Calcium ions line the pores of the cell membrane and have a crucial function in the transport of these electrolytes. The entire process proceeds rapidly, but not quite as rapidly as depolarization, and ends when the original transmembrane potential has been established once again. At this point, the cell is ready to respond to another stimulus or, in the case of automatic cells, to undergo self-excitation.

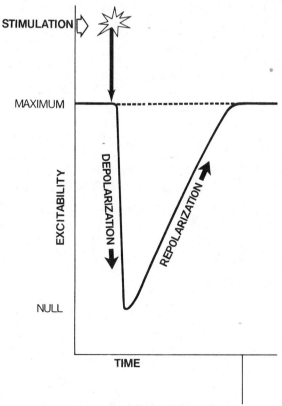

Activation of the excitable cell.

The intricately complex physical and chemical events of depolarization and repolarization involve millions of cells in the heart and occur with each beat. We will now examine the action of the heart in terms of normal **impulse formation** and **conduction,** as recorded by the electrocardiogram.

TABLE OF SYMBOLS USED IN THIS TEXT

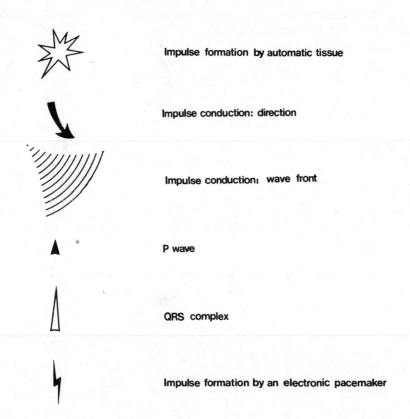

Impulse formation by automatic tissue

Impulse conduction: direction

Impulse conduction: wave front

P wave

QRS complex

Impulse formation by an electronic pacemaker

Chapter 2

THE ELECTROCARDIOGRAM

The **electrocardiograph** is an instrument which is sensitive to small electrical currents emitted by the body. The instrument is basically a galvanometer with a recording device which transcribes electrical activity onto paper. The current on the body surface is derived almost entirely from the heart.

The direction of deflection of the writing device is determined by the relative electrical state of electrodes placed at various locations on the body surface. An upward deflection is designated **positive**, a downward deflection, **negative**. The extent of the vertical deviation depends upon the magnitude of the electrical charge. Thus the greater the electrical potential, the wider the vertical excursion or amplitude.

As the writer oscillates vertically in response to changing body surface potentials, graph paper is rolled past at a constant speed towards the left. This transcribes the vertical movement over a horizontal plane, recording the oscillations in relation to time and creating the form of the **electrocardiogram.**

To restate, vertical dimension or amplitude represents the amount of electrical potential between electrodes at a given instant. Horizontal measurements give the factor of time over which a deflection occurs, and sequential events are read from left to right. From the figures so recorded, an enormous amount of information can be deduced about the activity of the heart.

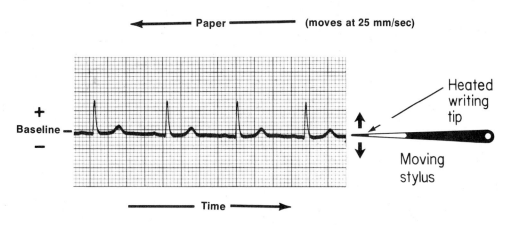

Representation of the activity of an electrocardiograph.

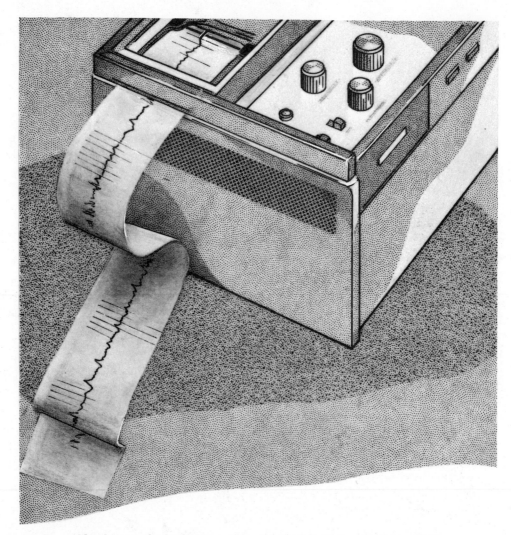

The electrocardiograph. Paper rolls out to the left. Stylus vibrates vertically.

COMPONENTS OF THE CARDIAC CYCLE

The dominating pacemaker of the heart lies in a cluster of cells located in the wall of the right atrium between the inlets of the superior and inferior vena cava. These cells are modified myocardial fibers which have lost contractile activity and which together serve as a center of automaticity known as the **sinus node.** Impulses originating from the sinus node spread to adjacent myocardial cells and propagate as a wave of depolarization through the atria.

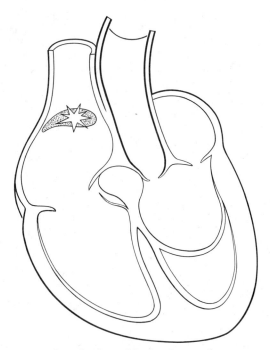

Impulse formed in the sinus node.

The amount of electrical current released from the sinus node is too small to cause a deflection in the standard electrocardiogram. The first recorded event in the cardiac cycle is depolarization of the atrial muscle as the impulse from the sinus node spreads through it. This figure is termed the **P wave.** Contraction of the atrial muscle immediately follows its depolarization. (The electrocardiogram records only electrical activity, not the mechanical events of muscular contraction.)

The sinus node and atrial muscle then begin to recharge energy, a process called **repolarization,** in preparation for the next beat. This process of depolarization and repolarization is a fundamental property of nerve and muscle cells in general. The electrocardiographic recording of atrial repolarization is sometimes observed, but it is usually very small or obscured by electrical events of much greater magnitude which occur simultaneously.

A dense cluster of conducting fibrils is present within the lower intra-atrial septum. This is the **atrioventricular (A-V) node,** which acts as a relay station for impulses from the atria to the ventricles. It, in turn, depolarizes from impulses which have coursed through the atria. This is a relatively slow activity with small electrical potentials in a small anatomical area. On the standard electrocardiogram,

The Electrocardiogram

Atrial Depolarization

Electrocardiographic Representation

BASELINE

BEGINNING OF ATRIAL DEPOLARIZATION

P WAVE

COMPLETION OF ATRIAL DEPOLARIZATION

not enough electrical energy is discharged to produce a visible deflection. This period is therefore electrically silent on the electrocardiogram and is represented by a straight or *isoelectric* line which immediately follows the P wave.

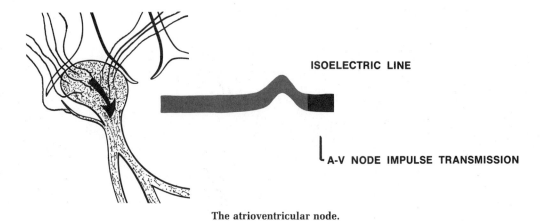

The atrioventricular node.

The impulse, after passing through the A-V node, enters a compact tract of conductile fibers known as the **common bundle** or the **bundle of His.** This pathway of modified muscle cells divides at the upper ventricular septum into **right** and **left bundle branches.** The impulse is conducted rapidly along these fibers in the

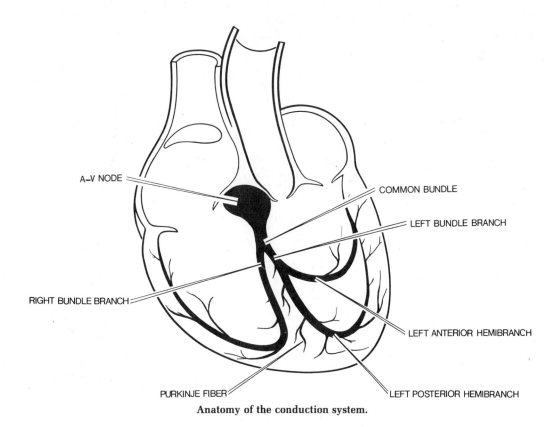

Anatomy of the conduction system.

endocardial layer of the right and left ventricles. Their smallest branches, the Purkinje fibers, are distributed throughout the muscular septum, the inner ventricular wall, and the papillary muscles.

The branches of the conduction tract end in twigs which are intimately associated with the contractile fibers of the myocardium. This tract, from the branching of the common bundle to the terminal ramifications in the ventricular muscle, is called the **Purkinje system.**

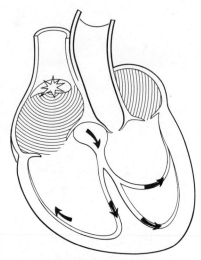

Pathways of conduction.

After being dispersed throughout the inner surface of the ventricles (the endocardium), the impulse traverses the ventricular mass itself as a wave of depolarization moving toward the outer surface (the epicardium).

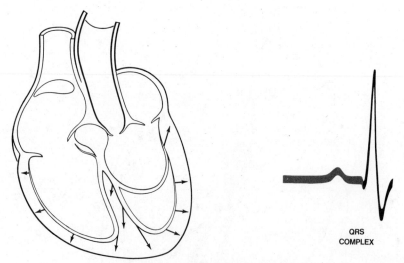

QRS
COMPLEX

Electrical activation of the ventricles.

Ventricular depolarization normally occurs first in the interventricular septum, forming the initial portion of the ventricular ECG complex. The remainder of the complex is derived from the summation of all electrical forces as the right and left ventricles depolarize. This figure in the electrocardiogram is designated the **QRS complex.**

The QRS complex is followed by a short period of apparent electrical inactivity, called the **ST segment.** This is usually isoelectric but may be somewhat sloping.

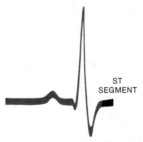

Following depolarization, the ventricles repolarize. The restoration of electrical potential is represented on the electrocardiogram by the **T wave.**

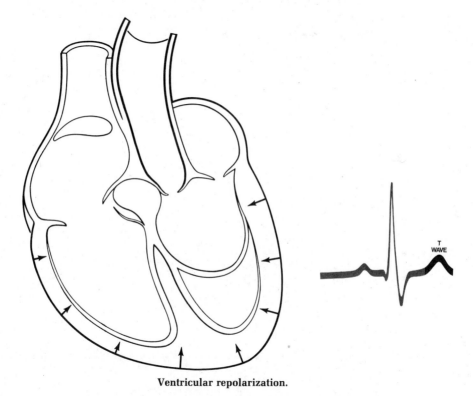

Ventricular repolarization.

A small smooth hump is sometimes seen after the T wave. It is called the **U wave.** Its origin relates to complex events of late repolarization.

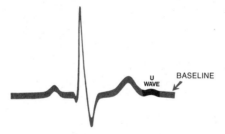

When repolarization has been completed, the stylus of the electrocardiograph returns to a flat, resting state or **baseline.** The cardiac cycle has been completed and will begin again with another impulse from the sinus node. In the normal adult, these impulses are set by the sinus node at a rate of 60 to 100 beats per minute.

ELECTROCARDIOGRAPHIC REPRESENTATION

To correctly designate components of the cardiac cycle, it is easiest to look first for the QRS complex. This is, of course, not the first event of the cardiac sequence, but it is the most readily identifiable. The QRS complex represents a brief and intense electrical event in a large muscle mass (the ventricles). The rapid inscription of the component results in a thin line which has sharply angular characteristics.

Practice in *first* recognizing the QRS complex in these easy tracings will be rewarding in terms of later interpretation of more difficult arrhythmias.

The reader should complete the labeling of the QRS complexes in the accompanying strip.

Identification of the P wave before the QRS complex and the T wave after can be made next. Amplitude alone is an unreliable differentiating feature, since the QRS complex may be smaller than the P or T wave.

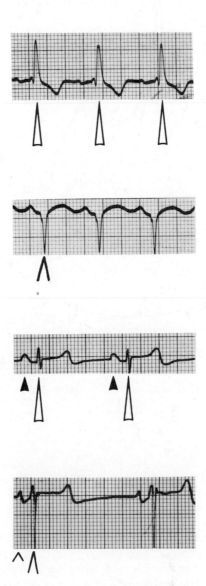

After the QRS complex has been clearly identified, look for the P wave just before it. The contour is more rounded than that of the QRS complex. Its configuration may be:

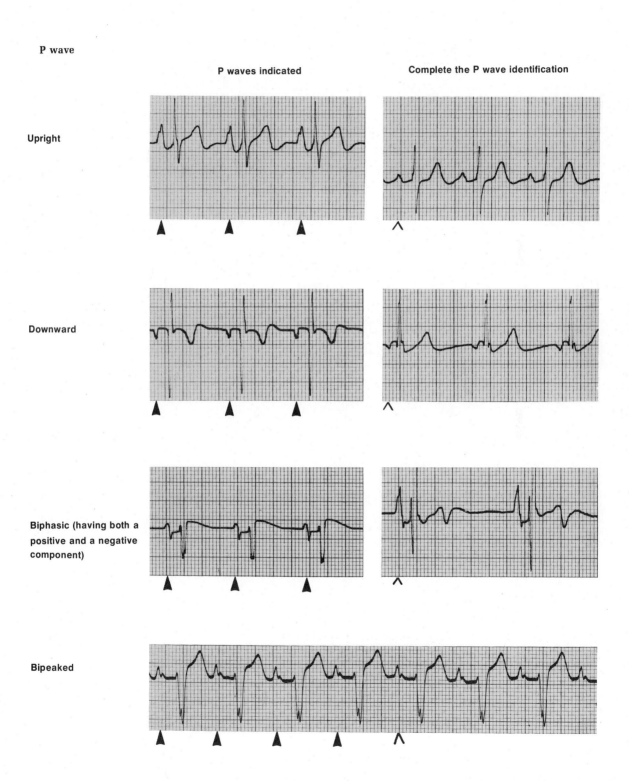

P wave

P waves indicated   **Complete the P wave identification**

Upright

Downward

Biphasic (having both a
positive and a negative
component)

Bipeaked

Components within the QRS complex follow standardized nomenclature.

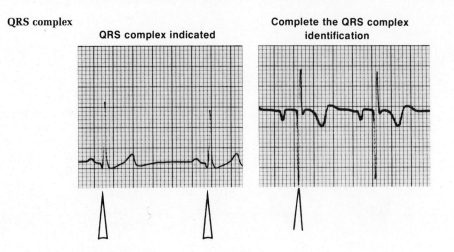

The *initial* downward deflection of a recording is termed the **Q wave.**

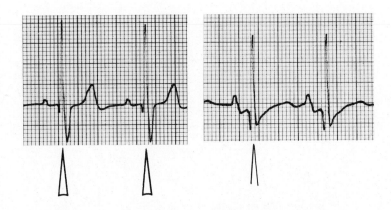

The **R wave** is the first *upward* component. It may follow the downward Q wave, or the R wave may be the initial component of the complex. Even though

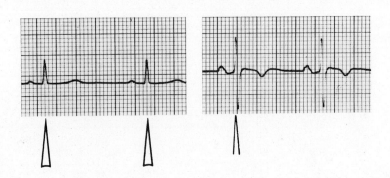

an R wave is the only component of the ventricular beat present in the first example, the figure is referred to as the **QRS complex.**

Illustration continued on opposite page.

QRS complex continued

QRS complex indicated   Complete the QRS complex identification

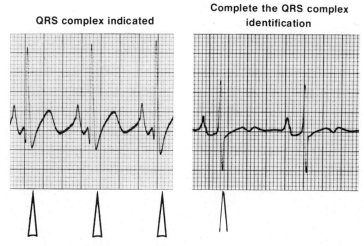

A downward deflection directly after the R is called the **S wave.**

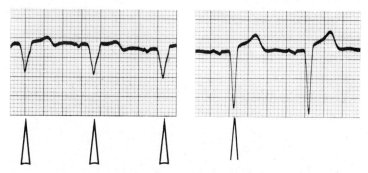

To further complicate terminology, a QRS complex which is completely down-ward (negative) is commonly called a QS form.

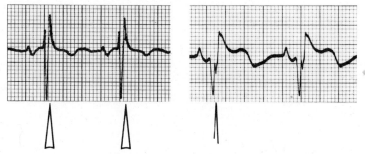

Sometimes a second upright deflection is present. It is termed **R prime (R′).**

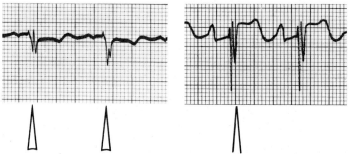

A downward deflection after R′ is called **S prime (S′).**

The **T wave,** corresponding to repolarization of the ventricles, is usually gently curved and may appear in a great variety of contours.

T wave

Complete the T wave identification.

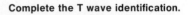

Simple upright

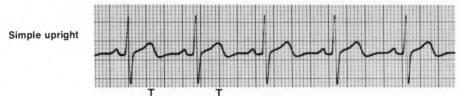

Simple downward

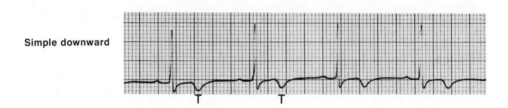

Double peaked

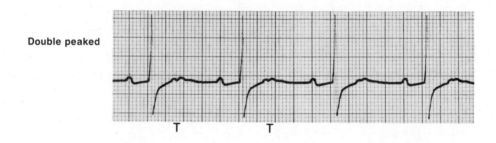

Tall and peaked

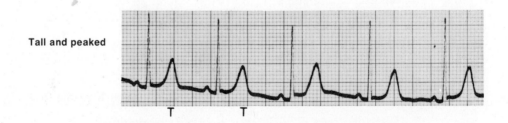

Flat

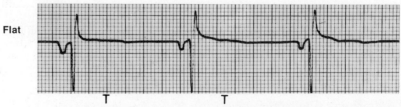

Illustration continued on opposite page.

T wave continued

Biphasic

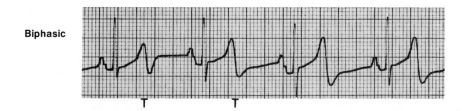

The **U wave** is seldom of help in interpreting arrhythmias, but the reader must be able to identify it to avoid confusing it with other components.

U Wave

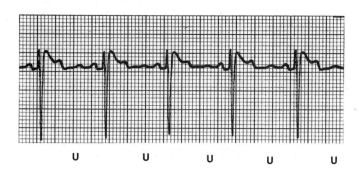

Identify the U wave in each cardiac cycle.

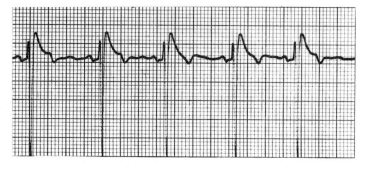

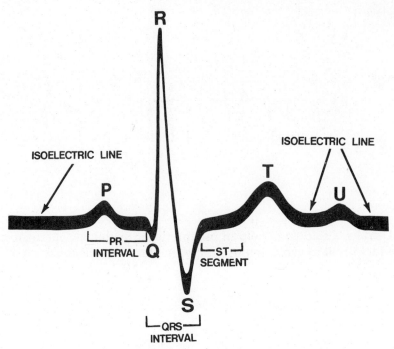

Electrocardiographic components of the cardiac cycle.

These electrocardiograms are from normal adults. Note the succession of beats, each representing a complete cardiac cycle. Each contains a P wave, a QRS complex, and a T wave. Each component is similar in *shape, height,* and *width* to its corresponding component in another beat.

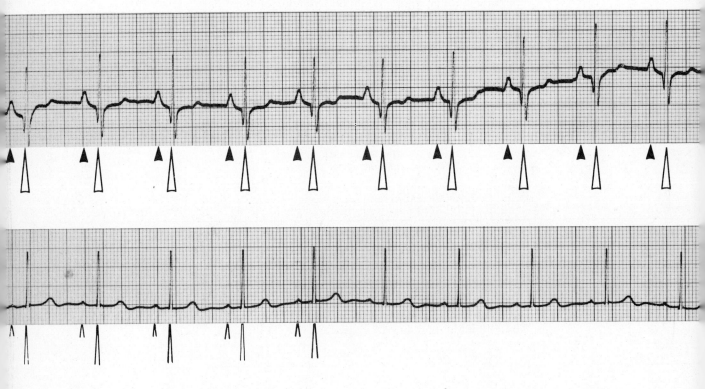

Finish designating the P waves and QRS complexes in each cardiac cycle.

Mark all P waves and QRS complexes with the appropriate symbols.

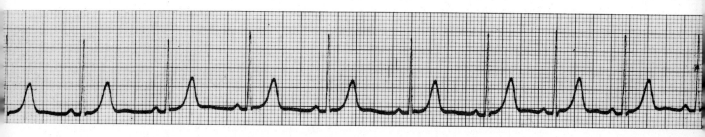

REVIEW

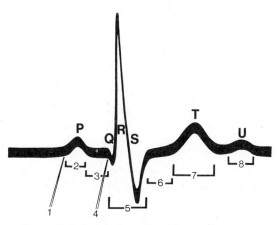

Sequential electrical events of the cardiac cycle.

TABLE 1.

Sequential Electrical Events of the Cardiac Cycle	Electrocardiographic Representation
1. Impulse from the sinus node	Not visible
2. Depolarization of the atria	P wave
3. Depolarization of the A-V node	Isoelectric
4. Repolarization of the atria	Usually obscured by the QRS complex
5. Depolarization of the ventricles	QRS complex
a. intraventricular septum	a. initial portion
b. right and left ventricles	b. central and terminal portions
6. Activated state of the ventricles immediately after depolarization	ST segment: isoelectric
7. Repolarization of the ventricles	T wave
8. After-potentials following repolarization of the ventricles	U wave

ELECTROCARDIOGRAPHIC PAPER

Conventional electrocardiographic paper is crosshatched with a grid of stand-ardized dimensions. Its vertical and horizontal lines are exactly one millimeter apart. For convenience in visual reference, every fifth line both vertically and horizontally is in heavier print.

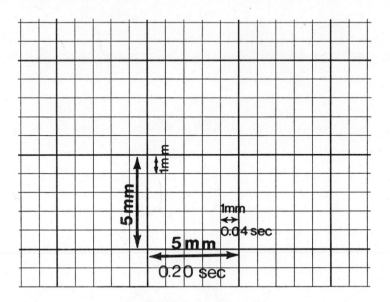

The horizontal axis represents *time*, reading from left to right. Each 1 mm grid interval, at a standard recording speed of 25 millimeters per second, represents 0.04 second. The vertical axis corresponds to the *amplitude* of the electrocardiographic components.

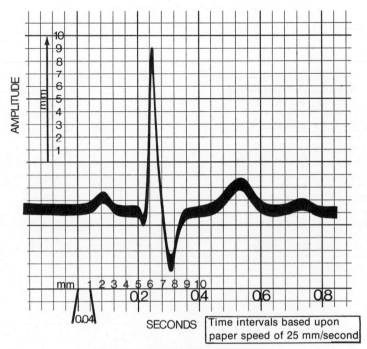

The electrocardiographic grid system.

DETERMINATION OF RATE

The heart rate may be determined by several methods using the electrocardiogram. The following methods are based upon a standard electrocardiographic paper speed of 25 mm per second.

The Ruler Method

The One Beat Ruler

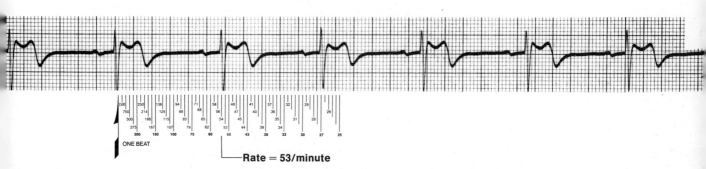

A ruler for rate, millimeters, and seconds is provided on the endsheet at the back of the book. This may be cut out and used throughout the text. A clear plastic version of this ruler is also available (see p. 341).

Place the reference arrow on a distinct point of one cardiac cycle. Usually a peak within the QRS complex is most convenient. Identify the corresponding point in the next cardiac cycle. The rate in cycles per minute is indicated at this location on the scale.

Rate = 53/minute

This ruler gives rapid and fairly accurate measurements, particularly at slower rates. It must be understood that only the interval from one beat to another is used to determine the number of cardiac cycles occurring in a full minute. This presupposes that each interval is the same. With nearly regular rhythms, the method is accurate enough for most clinical work.

The Three Beat Ruler

Line the reference arrow up with a portion of one cardiac cycle. Count the subsequent three cycles and read off the rate at the corresponding site of the third beat. This is again given in cycles per minute.

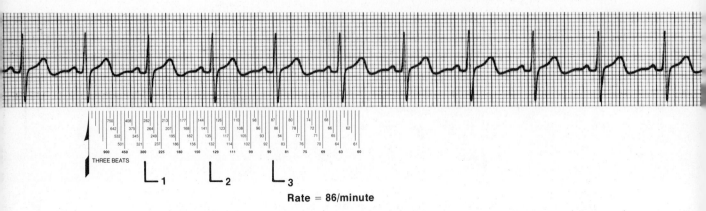

Rate = 86/minute

At rapid rates, this ruler is more useful than the one beat scale, since markings have more gradual rate changes. Note that as the rate gets faster, the interval between a given rate difference gets shorter (e.g., the actual distance between rate markings 90 and 100 is much less than that between 60 and 70). This spacing follows a logarithmic progression.

The three beat ruler automatically averages the intervals of three cardiac cycles. This decreases some of the variability in rate per minute determination inherent in the one beat ruler.

The Grid Method

A rapid and useful method for estimating heart rate involves comparing two adjacent beats on the grid system with 0.2-second (dark line) interval marks. If corresponding points of two consecutive beats fall exactly 0.2 second apart, the heart rate is 300 per minute.

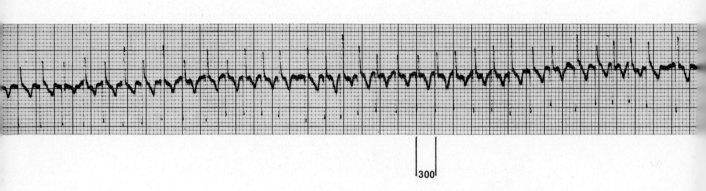

300

Beats occurring at 0.4-second intervals (two heavy grid lines apart) denote a rate of 150 per minute.

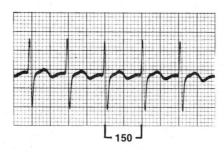

When the cardiac cycle repeats itself three heavy grid lines apart, the interval is then 0.6 second. In one minute, 100 such cycles occur (60 seconds ÷ 0.6 second = 100 per minute).

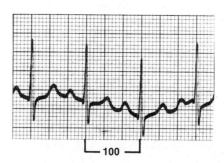

Corresponding points of adjacent cardiac cycles which are exactly 0.8 second (or 20 mm) apart indicate a rate of 75 per minute. This represents an interval of four heavy grid lines.

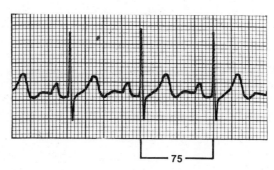

When adjacent beats are 1.0 second or five heavy grid lines apart, the rate is 60 per minute. This interval is 25 mm.

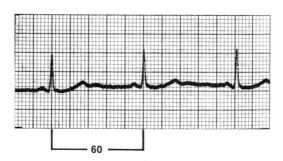

Since sinus tachycardia is defined as a sinus rate greater than 100 and sinus bradycardia as a rate less than 60, the three and five heavy grid line intervals serve as handy reference guides for quickly determining if the cardiac rate is within normal limits.

TABLE 2.   The Grid Method.

Number of Large Squares	Interval Between Beats	Rate Per Minute	
1	0.2 sec	300	
2	0.4 sec	150	
3	0.6 sec	100	
4	0.8 sec	75	normal sinus rhythm
5	1.0 sec	60	
6	1.2 sec	50	
7	1.4 sec	43	
8	1.6 sec	37	
9	1.8 sec	33	
10	2.0 sec	30	

When difficulty is encountered because no beats fall on the grid line, you may find it helpful to use calipers (mechanical dividers). The points of the dividers are placed on similar areas of two adjacent beats, then moved (without altering their relative position) so that one of the points is placed on a dark grid line. The rate can then be determined by the interval between the caliper points. Estimation is made if the second point falls between two dark lines.

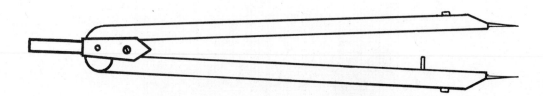

Calipers for determination of electrocardiographic intervals.

The Scan Method

A third method for rate determination makes use of the **three-second markers** found on most standard electrocardiographic paper (some manufacturers use one second markers). The number of complexes between markers are counted. Since there are 20 three-second intervals in a minute (60 sec ÷ 3 sec = 20 per minute), simply multiplying by 20 will give the number of beats in each minute.

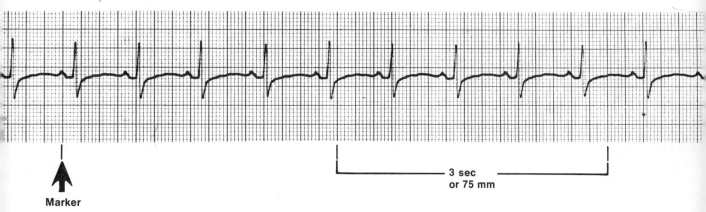

Marker

3 sec
or 75 mm

Calculations

Number of beats in 3 seconds: 4.5
Number of three-second intervals in 1 minute: $\times 20$
Beats per minute: 90.0

This method is fairly accurate. It is especially advantageous in very irregular rhythms and in extremely rapid or slow rates. In very slow rates, greater accuracy will be achieved by counting the beats in two of the three-second intervals (six seconds) and multiplying by ten.

THE STANDARD ELECTROCARDIOGRAM

The standard electrocardiogram is composed of twelve tracings or leads, each recording the electrical potentials between a specific set of electrodes placed at different points on the subject's body. Each tracing represents the same cardiac events, but from different electrical points of view.

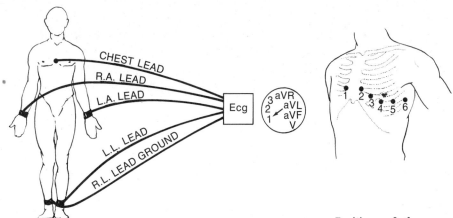

Lead arrangement of the standard electro-cardiogram.

Positions of the precordial (V) leads in the standard electro-cardiogram.

(From Goldman, M. J.: Principles of Clinical Electrocardiography, 7th ed., Los Altos, California, Lange Medical Publications, 1970.)

For reference, a table of the standard ECG leads is included, matched with the sets of electrodes from which potentials are measured. In all lead systems, the right leg serves as the **electric ground** in order to minimize interference from extraneous electrical sources.

TABLE 3.   Standard ECG Leads.

		Leads	Positive Electrode	Negative Electrode
Bipolar	1.	I	Left arm	+ Right arm
	2.	II	Left leg	+ Right arm
	3.	III	Left leg	+ Left arm
Unipolar	4.	aVR	Right arm	
	5.	aVL	Left arm	Central terminal*
	6.	aVF	Left leg	
Precordial	7.	V_1	Right of sternum in 4th intercostal space (4th ICS)	
	8.	V_2	Left of sternum in 4th ICS	
	9.	V_3	Midway between V_2 and V_4	Central terminal*
	10.	V_4	Midclavicular line in 5th ICS	
	11.	V_5	Midway between V_4 and V_6	
	12.	V_6	Lateral chest in 5th ICS	

*The *central terminal* is a combination of electrode potentials, producing a summation effect. This serves as the single negative or *indifferent* electrode. The specific combination of electrodes for each lead is automatically determined in the lead selector switch.

In the following example, all tracings were taken from the same patient within a few minutes. Note how the forms of the complexes vary from lead to lead.

EXTREMITY LEADS

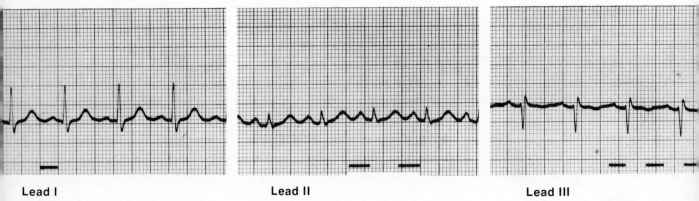

Lead I   Lead II   Lead III

Illustration continues on opposite page.

Illustration continued

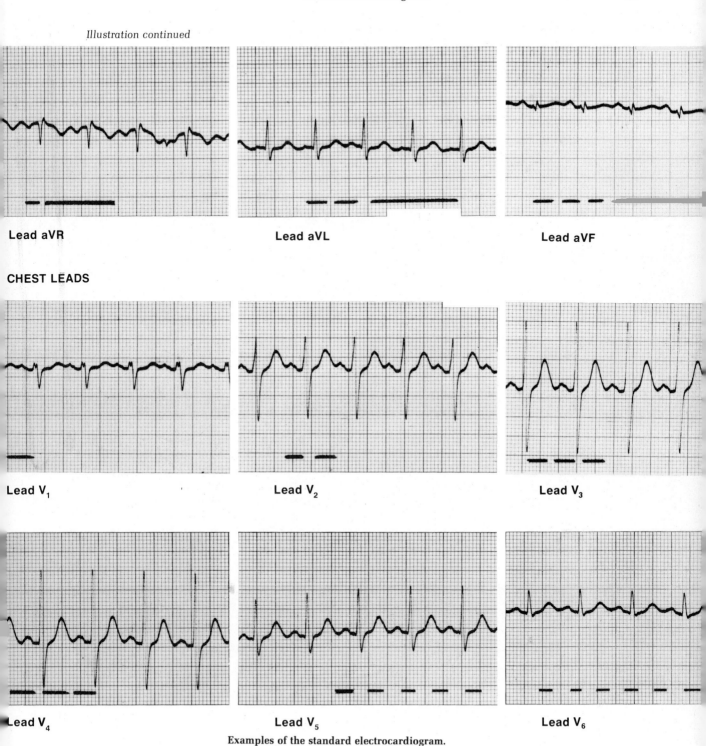

Examples of the standard electrocardiogram.

The electrocardiographer uses all 12 leads to synthesize the electrical events emanating from the heart in order to determine and localize certain details of dynamics. For interpretation of arrhythmias, however, a single lead in which each component of the cardiac cycle is clearly discernible is usually adequate. Therefore in continuous cardiac monitoring, one well-selected lead is serviceable. If given a standard 12-lead electrocardiogram, scan *all* leads for the most readable one, particularly one in which the P waves are quite distinct.

ARTIFACTS

Many factors may interfere with electrocardiographic recording. These can often be identified by characteristic features known as **artifacts.** Examples of such artifacts follow.

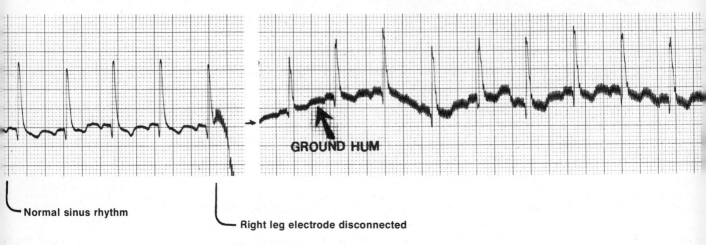

Normal sinus rhythm

Right leg electrode disconnected

Electrical hum produced by 60-cycle ground interference.

This tracing was recorded from lead I. Electrical ground interference can be observed upon disconnection of the right leg electrode. The inscription then wanders off the paper but returns a few seconds later when the second portion of the tracing is recorded.

With ideal electrical grounding, the recording will not change when the right leg electrode is detached. Some instruments are protected from electrical interference by automatically shutting off electrical input to the writer when the right leg electrode is disconnected.

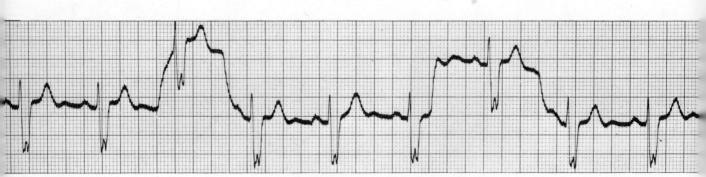

Baseline drifting from patient movement.

During the recording, the patient raised her right arm on which was taped an electrode. Note also a mild degree of 60-cycle electrical interference from improper grounding.

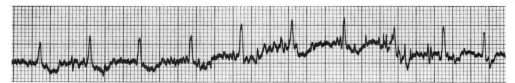

Artifact from muscle tremor.

The patient had Parkinson's disease. An electrocardiogram taken during sleep revealed normal sinus rhythm without recording interference from tremulousness.

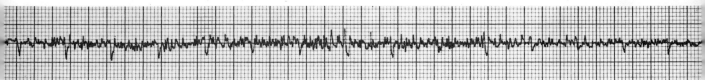

Continuous electrical interference from faulty lead attachment.

The left arm electrode was found to be loosely attached to the lead wire, and insufficient electrode jelly was used in the electrode plate well.

A good recording depends upon good electrode contact with the skin. To minimize electrical resistance, the skin should be prepared by rubbing briskly with gauze and alcohol or acetone. This removes surface oils and the most superficial layer of cornified epidermis, both of which impede electrical flow between the electrode and the body. The well-type electrode is preferred to the plate electrode because it contains a jellylike interphase between the electrode metal and the skin. Thus a more stable, artifact-free tracing can be obtained.

STANDARDIZATION MARKERS

To insure that the amplifier of the electrocardiograph provides a standard amount of energy to the recorder, a reference marker is provided on the instrument. Activation of a standardization key causes a deflection of the writer. By convention, a vertical deflection of 10 mm indicates 1 millivolt, which is the accepted standard for clinical electrocardiography, and the deflection is adjusted to this distance. The adjustment affects the amplitude of all components on the electrocardiogram, and it is important in making deductions related to chamber enlargement and other abnormalities. However, it is not necessary to standardize amplitude if the cardiac rhythm is the only focus of attention. Standardization markings must be recognized and not confused with components of the cardiac cycle.

Identify standardization markers

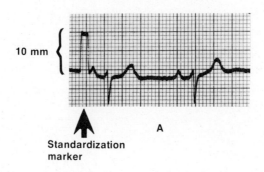

10 mm

Standardization
marker

A

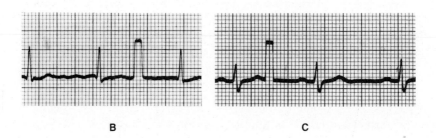

B   C

MONITORING THE CARDIAC RHYTHM

Adaptation of the **oscilloscope** to electrocardiography has provided the technical means for observing the cardiac rhythm continuously over an extended period of time at the bedside and during exercise. From continuous cardiac monitoring has come a greatly increased understanding of the significance of arrhythmias and a much earlier recognition of important rhythm changes in the high-risk patient.

The oscilloscope is basically a **cathode-ray tube** which receives electrical potentials from the subject. It differs from the electrocardiogram in that it fires the electrical signal with an electron gun toward the opposite end of the tube. A beam of electrons is formed which is focused by deflection plates onto the tube face or screen. Fluorescent material in the screen glows because of the electrical excitation, forming a visual image.

An amplifier regulates the vertical oscillations of the spot of light, and a sweep circuit controls its movement horizontally across the screen from the viewer's left to his right. The pattern is momentarily fixed by fluorescence, permitting easier inspection of each sweep.

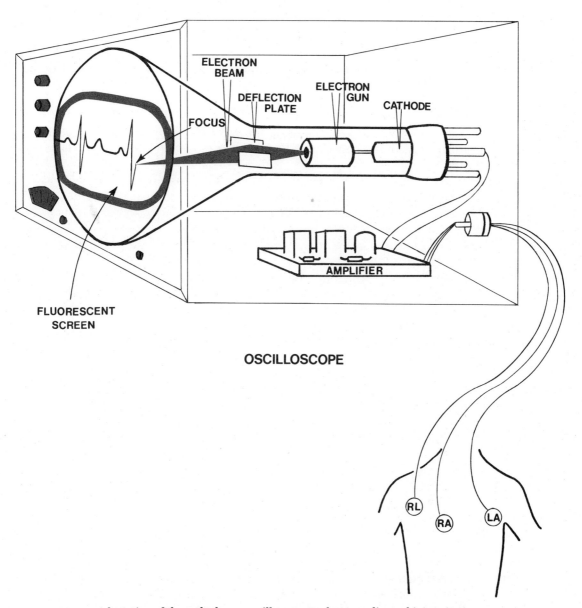

Adaptation of the cathode ray oscilloscope to electrocardiographic monitoring.

INDIVIDUALIZED ELECTRODE PLACEMENT

A single, clearly discernible lead can be used which requires only three electrodes. These may be placed directly on the chest where they are less confining over long periods than on the extremities.

Many systems for positioning electrodes have been devised. For simplicity and ease in remembering, we prefer using bipolar **lead I,** which requires **right arm** and **left arm** electrodes. A third electrode, **right leg,** is necessary for an electrical ground. Electrode positions which give an ideal monitoring pattern can be located in a systematic way on each patient.

Several features should be present in the ideal rhythm monitoring pattern:

1. The baseline is stable. Electrodes placed on the chest tend to minimize distortion from the patient's movements. If significant baseline wandering from respiratory excursions occurs, improvement is usually obtained by moving the LA electrode closer to the sternum.
2. P waves and QRS complexes are clearly seen for rapid and precise identification.
3. For instruments which indicate heart rate and have tachycardia-bradycardia alarm systems, the R spike is of high amplitude relative to P and T wave amplitude.
4. Electrical interference is negligible. Monitoring instruments, as well as adjacent electrical equipment and the bed itself, must be thoroughly grounded. An electrically powered bed is often a source of pattern interference, and its plug should usually be disconnected.
5. Chest electrodes are wide enough apart to allow placement of the electrocardioversion paddle.
6. Electrodes are securely affixed to the skin (shaving may be indicated). The movement of patient and rescuer during cardiac emergencies may result in an electrode being pulled off at the very moment when it is most needed.

This one-lead (three electrodes) arrangement is convenient and precise enough for interpretation of cardiac rhythms. It is, however, not comparable to any of the standard ECG leads; the P wave, QRS complex, and T wave shapes and amplitudes, as well as the ST segment positions, are not identical. Therefore, this special monitoring lead should not be used to identify patterns of hypertrophy, ischemia, infarction, or metabolic disturbances which can be diagnosed from the conventional 12-lead system.

Suggested Lead Placement

1. Select **lead I** on the cardiac monitor.
2. Attach the **right leg** electrode securely to a convenient place on the right upper anterior chest or to the lateral wall (either side). This is an electrical **ground** electrode and *not* a recording electrode. Its position is not critical.
3. Attach the **right arm** electrode securely to the right of the lower sternum.
4. The **left arm** electrode is now applied to several positions over the left anterior chest to locate a satisfactory rhythm pattern. If semipermanent electrodes are routinely used, first use a detachable metal plate for the LA electrode until the best location is selected. Observe the rhythm pattern as the LA electrode is repositioned along indicated axes. Try moving it upwards, then leftward. There are great pattern variations among individuals, and a few moments' experimenting with lead placement for an easily readable tracing is well worth the effort. When a satisfactory position is found, the detachable metal plate on the LA electrode can be replaced with the semipermanent electrode. (This substitution prevents wasting the disposable electrodes, since they lose adhesiveness if moved from place to place.)

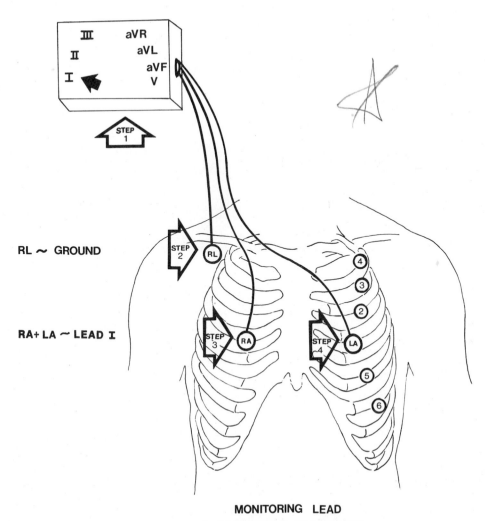

MONITORING LEAD
ELECTRODE PLACEMENT
Steps for placement of electrodes on chest to obtain the ideal monitoring lead.

A visual or auditory alarm is incorporated into many cardiac monitoring oscilloscopes and is activated by heart rates above or below a set limit. The instrument senses any vertical oscillation beyond a certain amplitude, and its sensitivity is adjusted so that one, and only one, deflection of each cardiac cycle is of this magnitude. Thus each beat should provide one signal to the pulse sensor.

A positive deflection on the oscilloscope can be detected with the sensor mechanism set for positive polarity. A single, tall, upright QRS component (R spike) is the most suitable element of the cardiac cycle to fall within the sensitivity range of the instrument. All other components should be well below this amplitude. If the sensitivity is set too low, some or all of the cardiac cycles will not be counted, and a slower than true heart rate will be registered. If the sensitivity is too high, more than one component of each cycle may provide a detected signal, and a greater than true rate will be counted. False counting in either direction, when sufficiently great, will activate the alarm. Proper selection of the cardiac cycle pattern and setting of tolerable rate limits will minimize miscounting by the instrument.

Some oscilloscope monitoring units have an adjustment which reverses polarity, creating a vertical inversion and a mirror image of the cardiac pattern. This is sometimes helpful in obtaining a good monitoring pattern when the QRS complex has an isolated deep, downward spike.

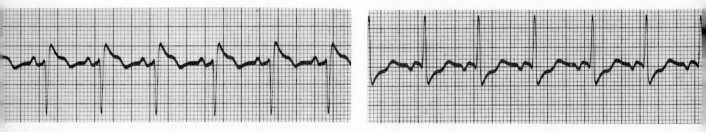

First position of suggested cardiac monitoring lead. Same electrode position, reversed polarity.

In attempting to establish the electrode positions for obtaining an ideal monitoring pattern, observe the characteristics of the following examples:

1. Distinct P wave.
2. Single, tall, upright spike in QRS complex.
3. P and T waves of small amplitude relative to amplitude of upright spike of QRS complex.

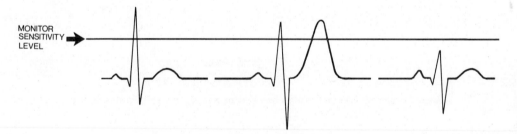

Monitoring lead patterns.

TABLE 4.

	Ideal	T Wave Too High	R Spike Too Low
	R well above sensitivity level	Double rate will be indicated	No signal will be sensed
	No interference likely from relatively small P and T waves	Tachycardia by alarm warning system	Bradycardia by alarm warning system
Corrective Maneuvers		Reposition **left arm** electrode or reverse polarity of instrument	Increase **gain** on instrument

Which of the following are good monitoring leads? Suggest changes when indicated. **(All numbered electrocardiograms require answers which may be found in a special section beginning on page 343.)**

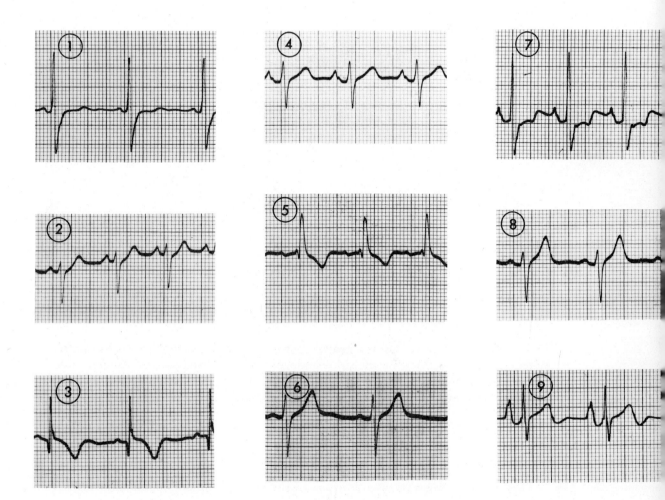

The pulse rate limits can be set so that a considerable margin is left to allow for extraneous signals such as patient movement. As a rule, the upper limit can be set about 30 beats per minute above the average heart rate of the individual. The lower limit may be routinely set at 50 per minute. However, if the average heart rate is close to this, the limit should be set lower, perhaps ten beats per minute below the average rate. These limits will usually permit instant indications of significant changes in rate without producing excessive false alarms.

Chapter 3

THE SINUS NODE

IMPULSE FORMATION

Normal Sinus Rhythm

The rhythmic action of the heart is normally controlled by electrical impulses which are generated within the sinus node and are conveyed to the muscular mass, causing coordinated contraction of paired chambers. In the adult, this series of electrical and mechanical events ordinarily recurs 60 to 100 times a minute.

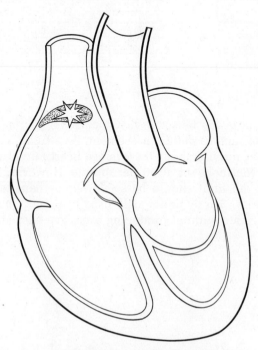

The sinus node: Impulse formation.

This electrocardiogram is a cardiac monitoring lead taken from a normal, recumbent individual.

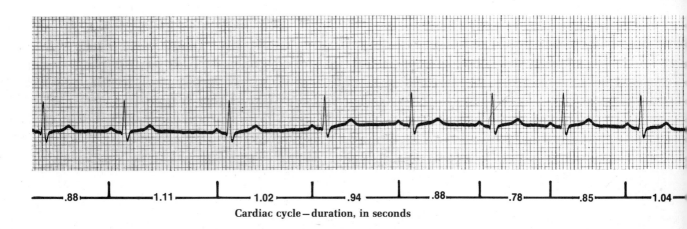

Cardiac cycle—duration, in seconds

Note that one cardiac cycle is similar to another regarding P waves, QRS complexes, and T waves in both form and duration between components.

Also note that the intervals between each cardiac cycle change slightly from beat to beat so that the rate varies continually to a minor degree. This is a normal periodic irregularity which is coincident with the phases of respiration and is a characteristic feature of **normal sinus rhythm.** (The term *regular* is reserved for rhythms in which no variations in rate occur.)

In quiet breathing, the heart rate speeds up during inspiration. This speedup is caused by hemodynamic reflexes in which the blood volume of the lungs expands while the volume in the right heart chambers falls. Pulse slowing occurs in exhalation.

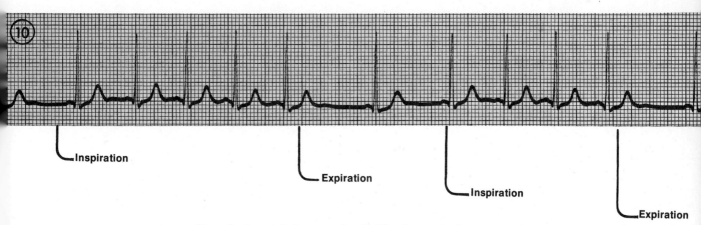

Inspiration

Expiration

Inspiration

Expiration

Sinus rhythm variations associated with quiet respirations.

This example represents an exaggeration of the normal phasic rate changes but is presented to demonstrate the phenomenon clearly.

Measure the slowest rate _____.

the fastest rate _____.

Use the one beat ruler and express each rate in beats per minute.

The following tracings illustrate normal sinus rhythm. In each tracing label all components of one cycle. Also determine the intervals between cycles; this may be expressed as rate, using the one beat ruler.

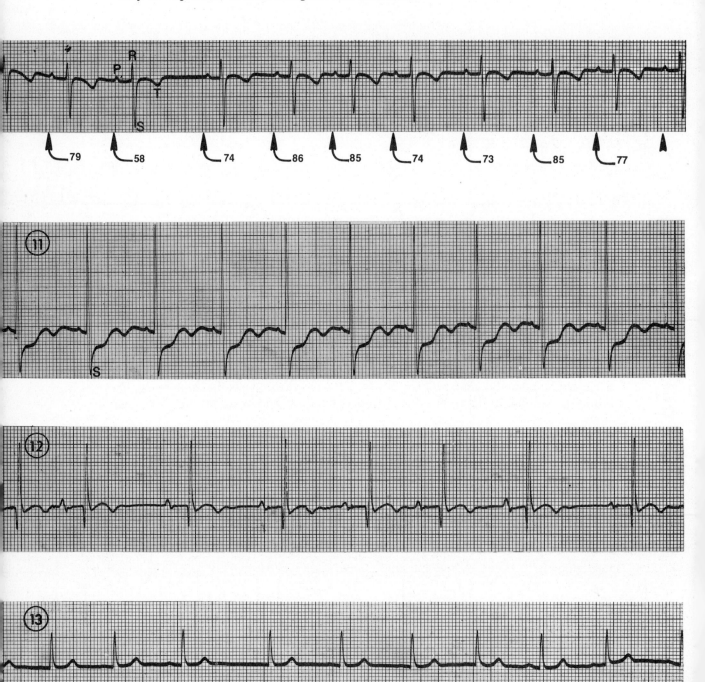

Sometimes components can be difficult to recognize. In this tracing, some complexes have P waves with extremely low amplitude, but they can be positively identified on close inspection.

Sinus Arrhythmia

When the phasic variations in sinus rate due to respiration are unusually prominent the term **sinus arrhythmia** is applied. This is *not* really an abnormal rhythm. It is generally more pronounced in young adults. This slowing-speeding pattern can be striking in some persons.

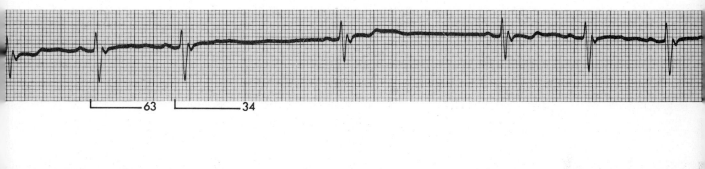

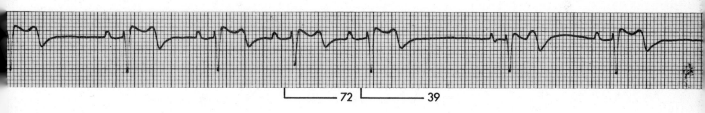

In the following examples of sinus arrhythmia, mark off each cardiac cycle and determine the fastest and slowest rates, using the one beat ruler.

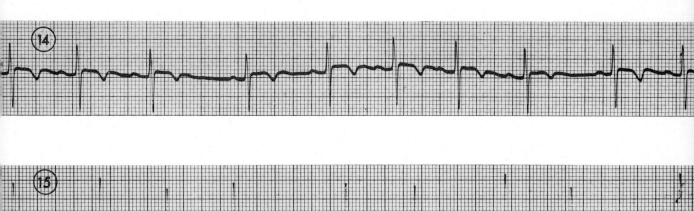

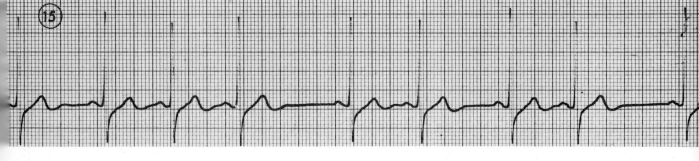

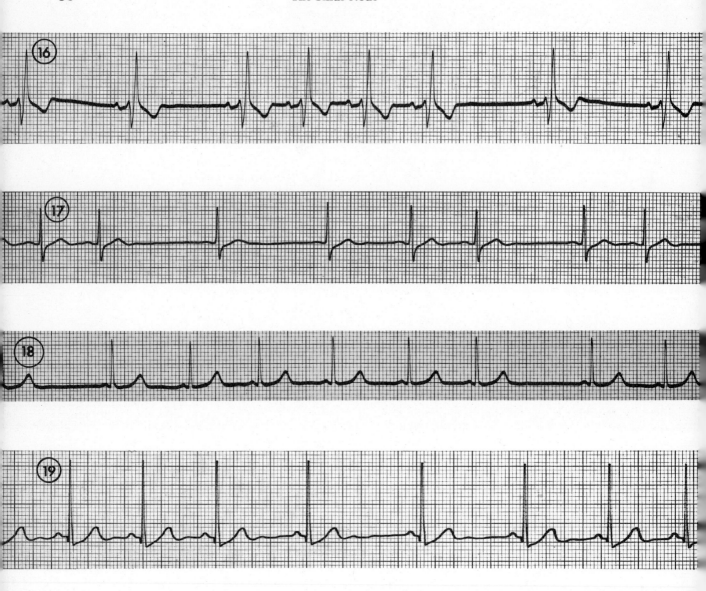

Deep, forced breath holding will intensify the phasic variations in rate of the sinus node pacemaker. This physiological response depends upon reflexes which involve pressure-volume sensory receptors in the heart, blood vessels, and autonomic nervous system, and upon chemical factors of the blood.

This rhythm strip series is taken from a healthy 40-year-old man during prolonged breath holding in deep inspiration.

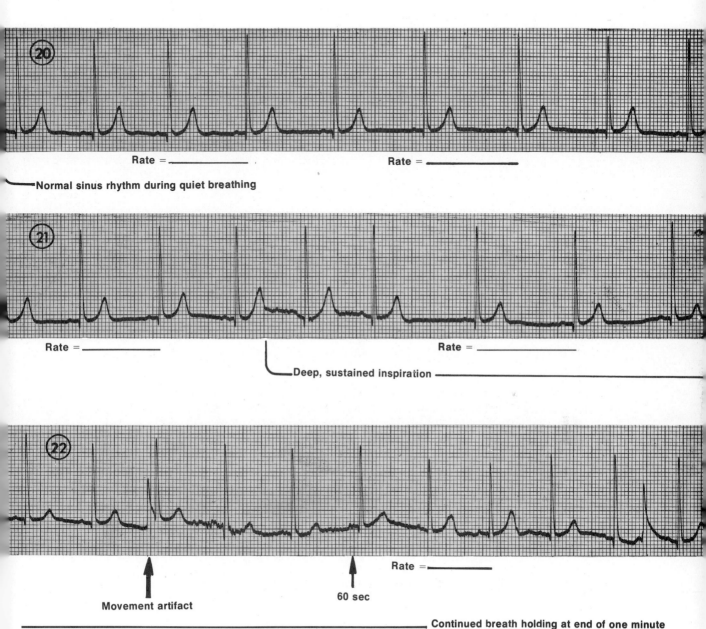

Rate = _____   Rate = _____

—Normal sinus rhythm during quiet breathing

Rate = _____   Rate = _____

└—Deep, sustained inspiration _____

↑ Movement artifact   ↑ 60 sec   Rate = _____

_____ Continued breath holding at end of one minute

The first few beats are often accelerated on deep inspiration from sudden expansion of total lung capacity. This results in an increased blood volume in the lungs, and a decrease in the blood volume in the right heart chambers, reflexly producing a more rapid sinus beat. Following this, autonomic nervous system forces become dominant, causing significant slowing of impulse formation. When breath holding is continued, the carbon dioxide level in the blood rises, causing gradual speeding of the rate.

Sinus Irregularity

Sinus irregularity is a term which denotes variations in the cadence of impulse formation within the sinus node that have no relationship to the phases of breathing. The rhythm is erratic, reflecting an unevenness in the processes of automaticity of the sinus pacemaker. This irregularity occurs in diseases which affect the sinus node but also may often be present in healthy individuals.

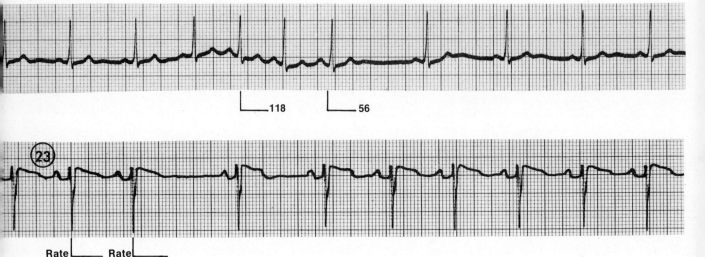

These variations in rate of impulse formation are determined in part by a complex neural mechanism known as the **autonomic nervous system.** This network affects smooth muscle and glands throughout the body, continually adjusting the involuntary functions of organs to the physiological demands of the organism. In the heart, the autonomic nervous system serves a prominent role in regulating the rate as well as the velocity of impulse conduction and the strength of contractions.

Autonomic control is divided into two highly integrated functional entities, the **sympathetic** and **parasympathetic** nervous systems. This subject is introduced at this point to provide a basic understanding of cardiac dynamics which can then be developed throughout the text.

AUTONOMIC NERVOUS SYSTEM

The heart rate is continually adjusted by a complex and sensitive regulatory mechanism responding to extracardiac stimuli. Body position, physical activity, respiration, temperature, blood volume, peripheral vascular tone, and emotional reactions all modify the frequency of impulse formation. Thus, the pulse is modulated to the demands of cardiac output. This finely tuned mechanism is also affected by many drugs and may be deranged by various diseases.

A major influence in cardiac reflex activity is exerted by the **autonomic nervous system,** composed of two counterbalancing forces: the sympathetic and the parasympathetic divisions. Their opposing effects tend to maintain a delicate balance which can be tipped in favor of one or the other by any of innumerable physiological and pathological factors.

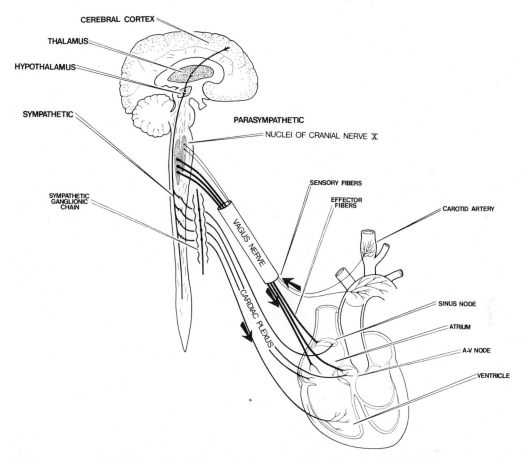

Composite diagram of the autonomic nervous system divisions innervating the heart.

Note in particular:
1. The ventricles have only sympathetic innervation.
2. Sympathetic reflexes may originate at many levels of the nervous system, from the spinal cord to the cerebral cortex.
3. The parasympathetic fibers in the vagus nerve are both effector and sensory fibers.

TABLE 5. Divisions of the Autonomic Nervous System Innervating the Heart.

	The Autonomic Nervous System		
	Sympathetic	*Parasympathetic*	
Peripheral nerves	Cardiac plexus	Vagus nerve	
Types of fibers	Effector	Effector	Sensory
Source	Cerebral cortex Thalamus Hypothalamus Spinal cord	Brain stem nuclei	Aortic root and arch Carotid sinus
Distribution	Sinus node Atria A-V node Ventricles	Sinus node Atria A-V node	Brain stem nuclei

Structure of the Sympathetic Nervous System

This complex network originates in cells of the brain stem. Its neurons course downward in the spinal cord, and branches emerge from the upper thoracic region to form the cardiac plexus. These branches terminate at the sinus node and the A-V node and in the muscle of the atria and ventricles.

Structure of the Parasympathetic Nervous System

This system includes the cranial nerves, of which the tenth is distributed to the heart. The system's nuclear center is in the brain stem, and the effector fibers make up the **vagus nerve,** terminating at the sinus and atrioventricular nodes. These fibers are also distributed to atrial musculature but not usually to ventricular.

The vagus nerve contains sensory neurons which convey impulses from vascular structures near the heart to the central nervous system. These neurons arise from the arch of the aorta and the internal carotid arteries and end in the tenth cranial nerve nucleus. Changes in pressure and chemistry within these vessels are transmitted to the nuclear center by these sensory fibers and may evoke reflexes by the effector fibers of the vagus nerve.

A chemical substance known as a **neurohumoral transmitter** is stored in the nerve endings of the sympathetic and parasympathetic nervous systems. Impulses coursing through the autonomic nerves cause release of this substance which in turn initiates a response of effector cells in the immediate vicinity. The difference between a sympathetic and parasympathetic response depends on the chemical nature of the transmitter substance.

Physiology of the Sympathetic Nervous System

The neurohumeral transmitter at postganglionic sympathetic nerve endings is **norepinephrine** (or noradrenalin). When this agent is discharged from sympathetic nerve terminal branches, responsive effector cells are stimulated, resulting in a *sympathetic action.* In the heart, sympathetic stimulation tends to increase the rate of impulse formation in automatic tissue. The velocity of cardiac impulse propagation in the conductile fibers is accelerated and the force of contractile fibers increased.

The adrenal gland synthesizes and stores *norepinephrine* and *epinephrine* (adrenalin). When stimulated, the gland secretes these hormones into the blood stream, which carries them to the various receptor organs. Their direct action on the heart, through a hormonal mechanism, is similar to that of neurally transmitted norepinephrine.

These agents are referred to as *sympathetic* or *adrenergic hormones* and the effects elicited by them as *sympathetic* or *adrenergic responses.* These terms are applied interchangeably regardless of the origin (neural or adrenal) of the stimulating transmitter. The sympathetic nervous system affects the heart by *excitation* of automaticity, conductivity, and contractility.

Physiology of the Parasympathetic Nervous System

Stimulation of parasympathetic fibers causes release of **acetylcholine** at the system's nerve endings. The vagus nerve, subserving parasympathetic function to the heart, has a general inhibitory influence on the rate of cardiac impulse formation and on the velocity of conduction. The force of myocardial contractility is not altered substantially by vagal stimulation. Acetylcholine and its analogues are known as *cholinergic agents,* and the effects of vagal stimulation are known as *cholinergic responses* which tend to *depress* automaticity and conductility within the heart.

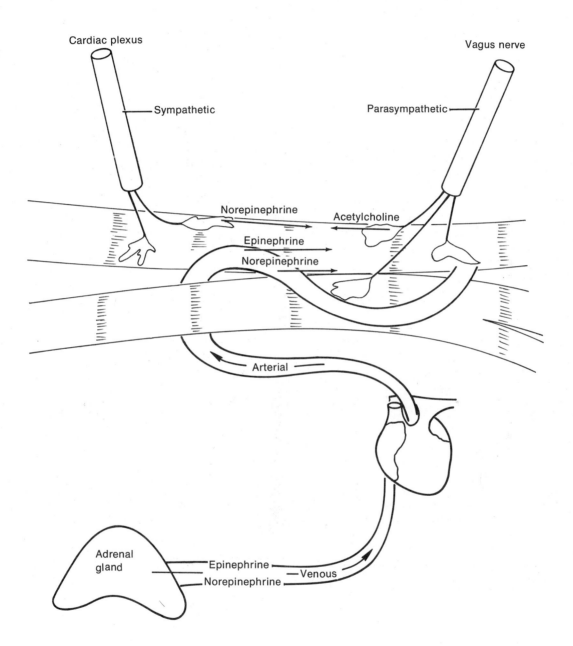

Regulatory Mechanism of the Autonomic Nervous System

The sympathetic and parasympathetic nervous systems maintain a delicate balance of opposing forces — excitation and depression — on the electrical sequences of cardiac activity. A great number of variables may affect the stability of this regulatory mechanism, by either stimulating or inhibiting either system, causing a shift in the relative influence in favor of one or the other.

This dynamic equilibrium of the autonomic nervous system is analogous to a car moving at a steady speed with continuous pressure **(tone)** applied to both the accelerator **(sympathetic)** and brake **(parasympathetic)** pedals. The driver may go faster by increasing the accelerator pressure **(adrenergic stimuli)** or slower by pushing harder on the brake **(cholinergic stimuli).**

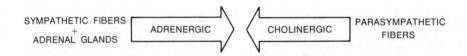

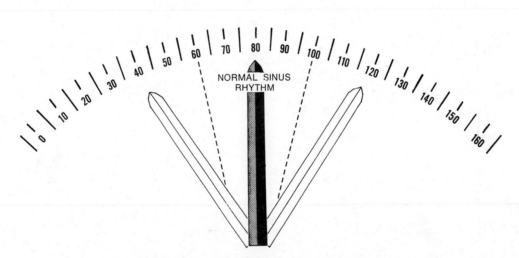

Balance of sympathetic and parasympathetic forces.

The driver can also change his rate of motion by letting up on either controlling pedal. Decreased pressure on the accelerator leaves a predominating braking influence and the car slows **(adrenergic inhibition).** If, during the steady state, braking action is reduced and accelerator tone held constant, the car's velocity increases **(cholinergic inhibition).**

We shall now apply these principles of autonomic nervous system control in the study of normal sinus rhythm and the variations of sinus impulse formation.

SINUS NODE: IMPULSE FORMATION

Excitation

When the sinus node is driven or excited to discharge at rates over 100 per minute, the term **sinus tachycardia (ST)** is applied.

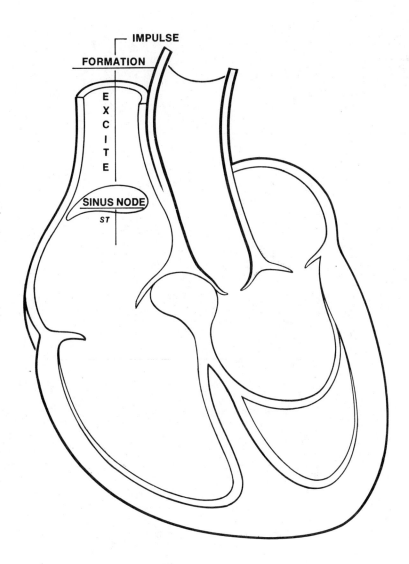

The term **excitation** is hereafter used in this text to denote intensification of activity in automatic or conductive tissues. Excitation of these tissues produces an increase or acceleration of pacemaker rate or conduction velocity. Factors which cause changes in this direction in impulse formation and conduction are referred to as excitatory or stimulatory. Such factors may be of a physiological, pharmacological, or pathological nature.

Sinus Tachycardia

As the sinus rate speeds, the P wave of a cycle appears closer to the T wave of the previous beat, and, at very rapid rates, it becomes harder to distinguish. (This emphasizes the importance of selecting a clear, diagnostic lead on monitored patients.)

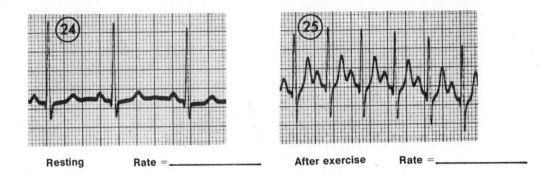

Referring to our driving analogy, the accelerator is pressed harder by adrenergic stimuli, and the sinus node responds by increasing its rate of impulse formation.

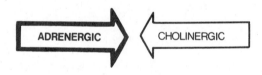

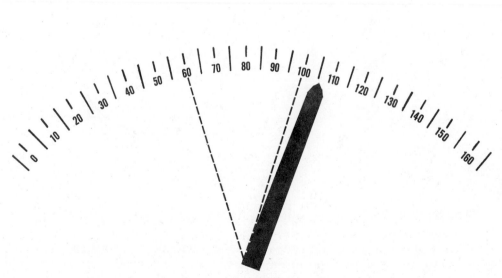

Sympathetic tone increases, producing speeding of rate.

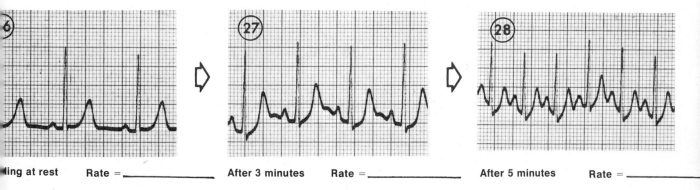

ing at rest   Rate = _____   After 3 minutes   Rate = _____   After 5 minutes   Rate = _____

Physiological response to exercise.

Note the acceleration of sinus rate in response to climbing stairs.

Sinus tachycardia is a natural response to certain physiological and pathological factors and is not actually an arrhythmia. It may be induced by conditions affecting the myocardium (ventricular failure, myocarditis) or by extracardiac disorders. The clinician should identify the basis of sinus tachycardia and not accept it as a primary disorder of the cardiac rhythm.

Sinus tachycardia may occur from increased metabolic demand (fever, hyperthyroidism) and elevated circulatory flow (heat exposure, anemia, arteriovenous communications). Shock, congestive heart failure, acute myocardial infarction, and pulmonary embolism accelerate the heart rate, tending to compensate for diminished blood flow. Hypoxia and hypercapnea are physiochemical conditions leading to sinus tachycardia. Sinus impulse formation is stimulated by sympathetic nervous system forces (emotional excitation, pain reflexes, adrenal gland responses, and adrenergic drugs) and by suppression of parasympathetic nervous system tone (cholinergic inhibitor drugs).

The following tracings are taken from a 21-year-old woman with viral gastroenteritis, who has a temperature of 100.8° and experiences lightheadedness on standing. Notice the change in rate and blood pressure that follows the change from a recumbent to a sitting position.

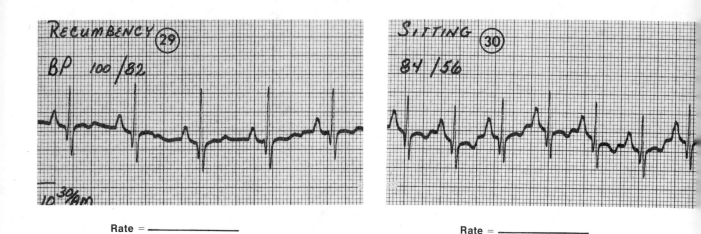

Rate = _____   Rate = _____

The acute viral illness with fever and the prolonged bed rest contribute to this symptomatic postural response.

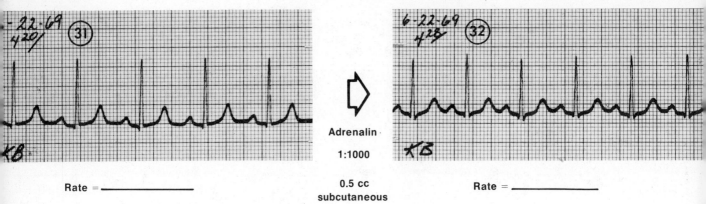

Rate = _____   0.5 cc   Rate = _____
                          subcutaneous

Sympathetic stimulation with pharmacologic agent.

An increase in heart rate follows subcutaneous administration of adrenalin for bronchial asthma.

By decreasing forces (releasing brake pressure), sinus tachycardia may result. Atropine, an **anticholinergic** agent, causes such a parasympathetic nervous system block. It is noted that many mixed proprietary drugs contain derivatives of atropine, especially the sedatives, analgesics, and medications used for gastrointestinal disturbances.

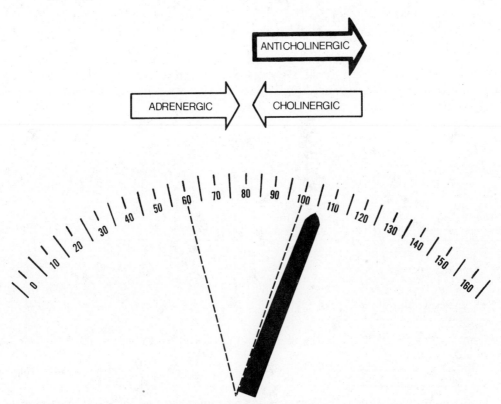

Inhibition of parasympathetic tone, producing speeding of rate. Sympathetic forces now dominate.

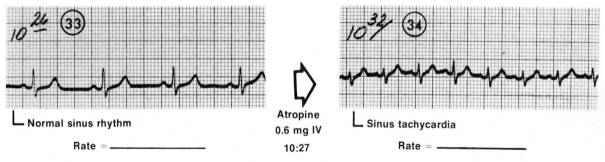

Normal sinus rhythm

Atropine
0.6 mg IV
10:27

Sinus tachycardia

Rate = _____   Rate = _____

Excitation of sinus node impulse formation by pharmacologic block of parasympathetic control.

Atropine inhibits the steady stimulation of the vagus nerve by its anticholinergic effect. The normally present braking action of vagal tone is released, and the sinus rate speeds up.

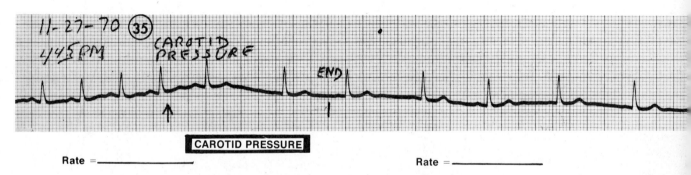

CAROTID PRESSURE

Rate = _____   Rate = _____

Transition from sinus tachycardia to normal sinus rhythm by parasympathetic stimulation.

Increased vagal tone, by reflexes from external pressure applied over the carotid artery, produces an abrupt slowing in the sinus rate.

Digitalis is used primarily to treat myocardial insufficiency because of its salutary effect on the contractile force of the myocardial fiber. In addition, digitalis affects the heart by increasing parasympathetic activity to the atrial and A-V nodal structures. The clinician can use this property of digitalis for accentuating vagal tone to advantage in certain arrhythmias. The following tracings were taken from a 65-year-old man with congestive heart failure.

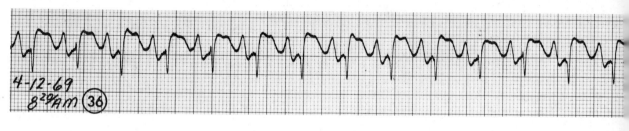

Interpretation = _____   Rate = _____

Interpretation = _____

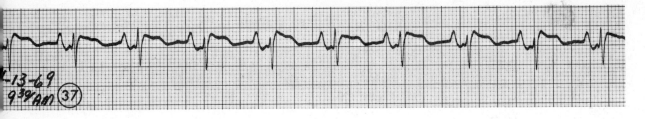

Interpretation = _____   Rate = _____

Treatment with Digitalis started.

Sinus rhythm slows, congestive heart failure improves, and vagal tone increases after digitalis is administered.

Examples of Sinus Tachycardia

Label representative P, QRS, and T. Denote rate by all three methods.

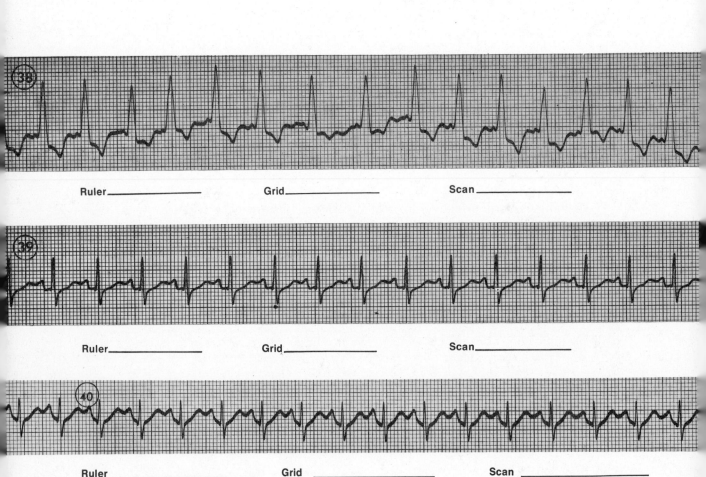

Ruler_____   Grid_____   Scan_____

Ruler_____   Grid_____   Scan_____

Ruler _____   Grid _____   Scan _____

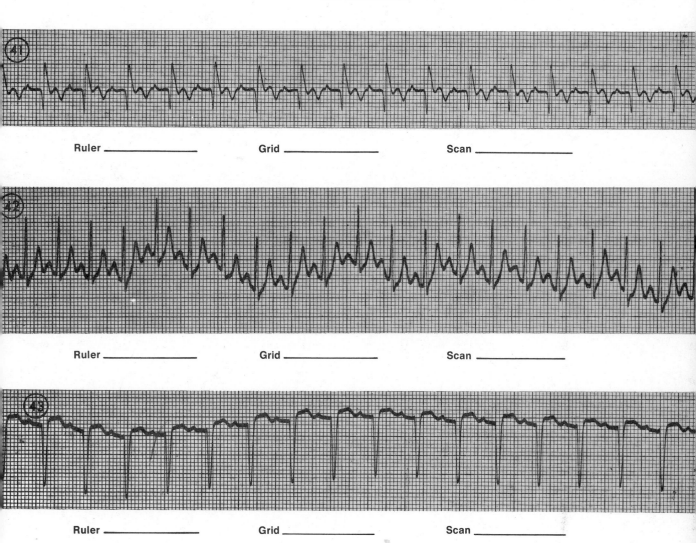

41

Ruler _____   Grid _____   Scan _____

42

Ruler _____   Grid _____   Scan _____

43

Ruler _____   Grid _____   Scan _____

SINUS NODE : IMPULSE FORMATION

Depression

SB = Sinus Bradycardia
SP = Sinus pause
SA = Sinus arrest

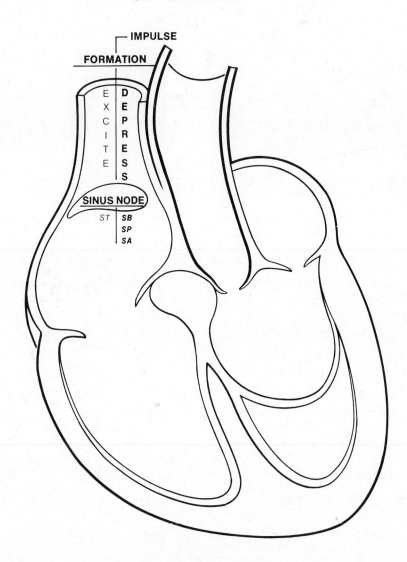

Sinus Bradycardia

A sinus node pacemaker rate less than 60 per minute is termed **sinus bradycardia** (SB).

Depression is used herein as the converse of excitation. Factors which depress impulse forming or conducting tissues cause slowing of pacemaker rate or conduction velocity. Inhibition of these determinants may be produced by physiological, pharmacological, or pathological factors.

Normal individuals with a strong degree of parasympathetic tone often have sinus bradycardia. This rhythm is most commonly found in young adults, especially those conditioned by vigorous athletics.

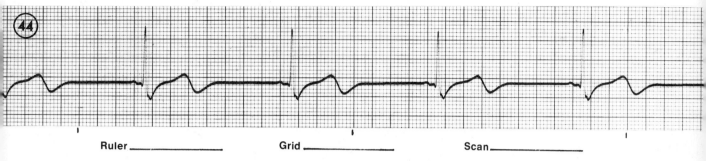

Ruler_____ Grid_____ Scan_____

Sinus bradycardia may occur when the metabolic rate is reduced, as during sleep, and in myxedematous or hypothermic states. Increased intracranial pressure may cause an abnormally slow pulse. Sudden appearance of sinus bradycardia in a patient with cerebral edema or subdural hematoma is an important clinical observation.

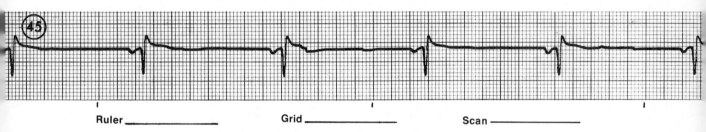

Ruler_____ Grid_____ Scan _____

Examples of Sinus Bradycardia

Identify components; determine rate.

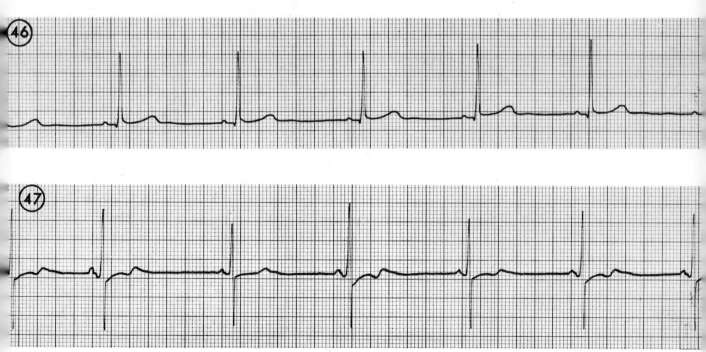

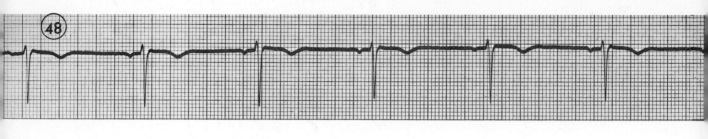

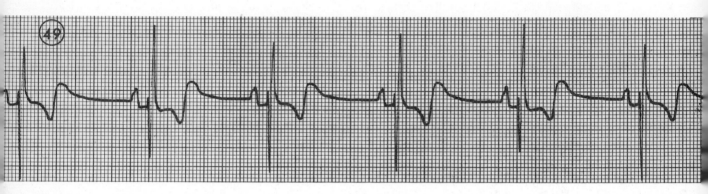

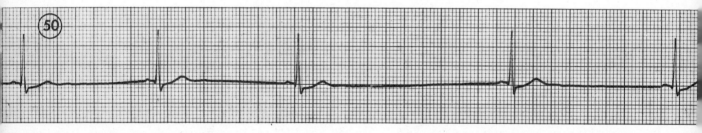

Rate: for shortest interval = _____   for longest interval = _____

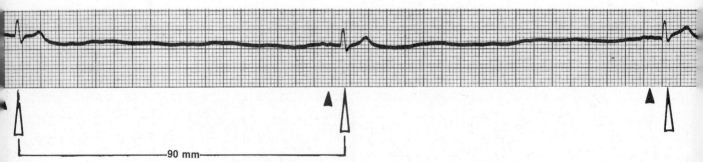

Examples of severe pathologic depression of sinus node impulse formation.

This extremely slow rate falls beyond the one beat ruler scale (less than 25 beats per minute). An accurate rate can be obtained by determining the distance between beats. There are 90 mm between the first and second cardiac cycles. Since each millimeter represents 0.04 second, the interval represents 3.6 seconds (90 × 0.04). Divide the seconds in one minute (60) by the interval in seconds (3.6) to obtain the rate in minutes: 60 ÷ 3.6 = 17 beats per minute.

Depressed rhythms of sinus node impulse formation may be produced by:

1. *Decreasing sympathetic tone:* Reserpine depletes stored adrenergic substances in sympathetic nerve endings, while propranolol inhibits their neurotransmission. Slowing of the pulse rate is produced by both agents.

Example: Propranolol

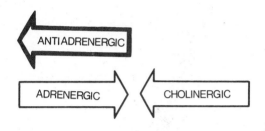

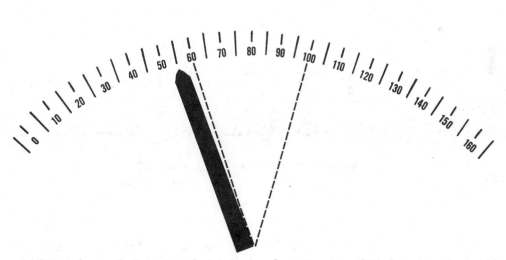

Inhibition of sympathetic tone, producing slowing of rate. Parasympathetic forces now dominate.

2. *Increasing parasympathetic tone:* Vagal stimulation characteristically leads to reflex slowing of sinus node impulses. This may be produced by manual pressure over a carotid artery or by vomiting, forced voiding, and straining at stool (forms of the Valsalva maneuver).

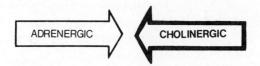

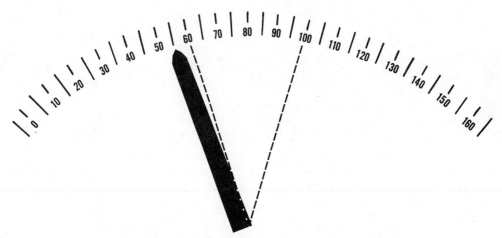

Parasympathetic tone increases, producing slowing of rate.

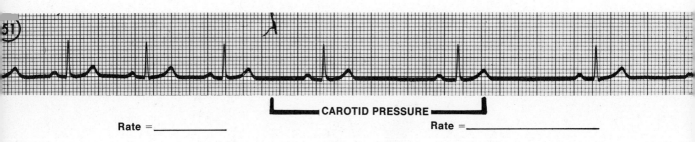

Rate =_____   Rate =_____

Carotid pressure is a convenient way of increasing vagal tone, and much can be learned of an individual's cardiac autonomic nervous system with this maneuver. Certain precautions are required, however. The pressure should be light and of brief duration; the patient must be recumbent and continuous monitoring of the cardiac activity must be utilized. Known carotid artery or cerebrovascular disease is a contraindication for its usage. It is prudent to be prepared for arrhythmias which may require immediate therapy.

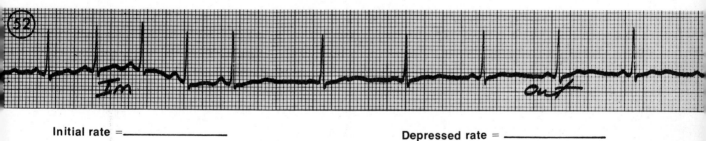

Initial rate =_____   Depressed rate = _____

Sinus slowing during full inspiration.

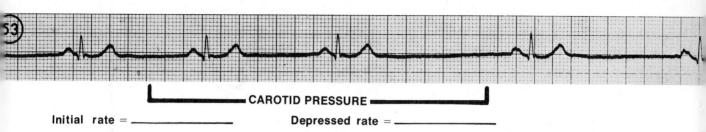

CAROTID PRESSURE

Initial rate = _____   Depressed rate = _____

Sinus rate change with carotid pressure.

What is the change in rate?

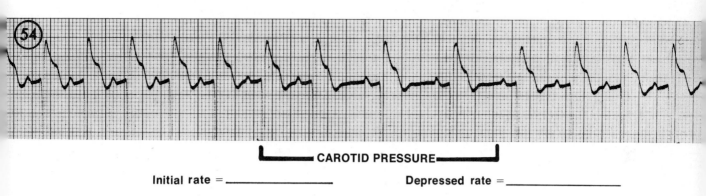

CAROTID PRESSURE

Initial rate = _____   Depressed rate = _____

Sinus tachycardia shows pronounced slowing of rate with carotid pressure.
Note that the deceleration is gradual.

Sinus Pause

A momentary cessation of sinus impulse formation followed by spontaneous resumption of cadence is referred to as **sinus pause**.

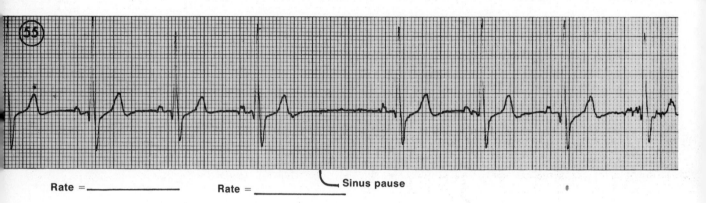

Rate =_____   Rate =_____   Sinus pause

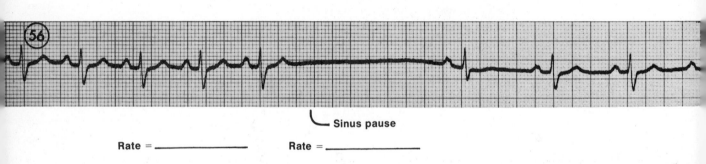

Sinus pause

Rate =_____   Rate =_____

Examples of the Sinus Pause

Compare the basic with the delayed rate.

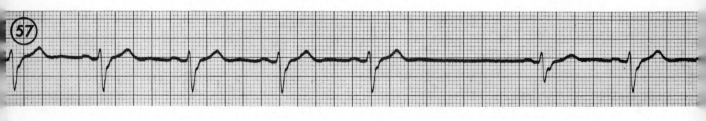

Basic rate =_____   **Delayed rate** =_____

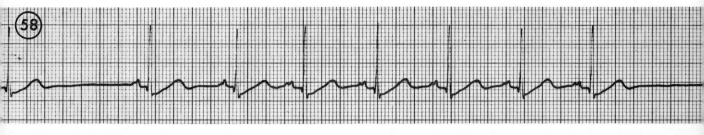

Basic rate = _____   Delayed rate = _____

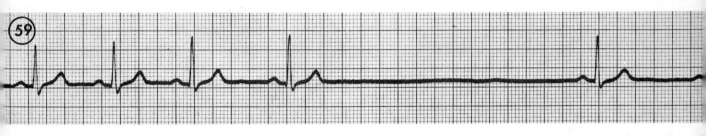

Basic rate = _____   Delayed rate = _____

Sinus Arrest

Sinus arrest is the prolonged failure of the sinus node to initiate impulses. Usually an alternate or secondary impulse-forming tissue outside the sinus node will maintain the heartbeat, but at a rate slower than the normal sinus rate. (This mechanism will be discussed under escape rhythms.)

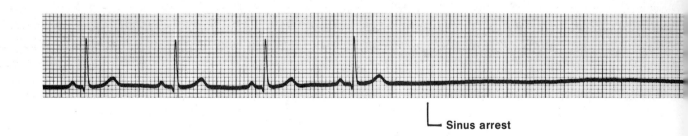

└ Sinus arrest

Sinus Arrest Sequence

A 68-year-old man incurred a sudden brief period of syncopy of uncertain cause. He was admitted to the Cardiac Care Unit where he was found to have sinus bradycardia. Continuous tracings obtained a few hours after admission revealed sudden failure of sinus impulse formation. (**Horizontal arrows at end of one tracing and beginning of another indicate a continuous recording.**)

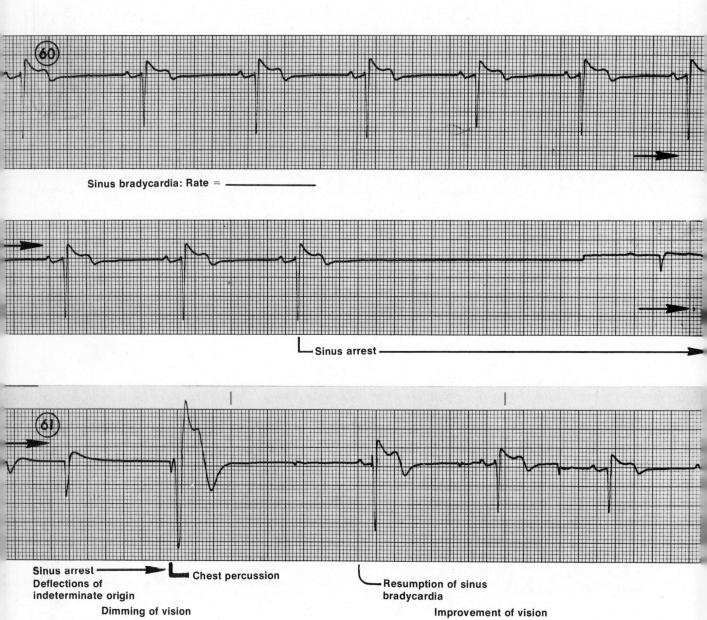

Sinus bradycardia: Rate = _____

Sinus arrest

Sinus arrest ⟶ Chest percussion
Deflections of
indeterminate origin   Resumption of sinus
                              bradycardia
Dimming of vision
                              Improvement of vision

Determine the entire duration of asystole (cessation of ventricular activity) (____ seconds). A sharp thump over the sternum with the fist induces a cardiac contraction. Note that the mechanically stimulated ventricular complex has a greater duration than the spontaneous complexes.

Sinus bradycardia may be treated with agents which increase sympathetic tone (e.g., isoproterenol) or which inhibit parasympathetic impulses (e.g., atropine).

These drugs may also be given to control vasovagal hyperactivity and for emergency treatment of severe sinus pauses or sinus arrest.

The following clinical sequence begins with a tracing showing severe sinus bradycardia in a 48-year-old man during induction of anesthesia for a surgical procedure. Treatment with a vagolytic agent was started.

8:10 AM:

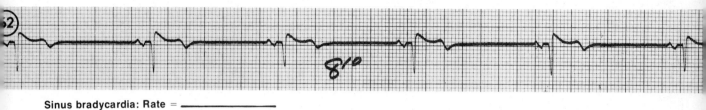

Sinus bradycardia: Rate = _____

8:11 AM: Atropine, 0.8 mg, was given intravenously.

8:13 AM:

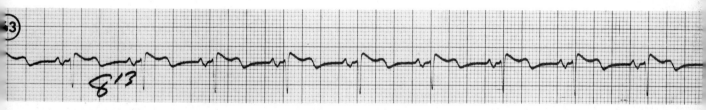

Normal sinus rhythm   Rate = _____

These reflex bradycardias are mediated through pressure-sensitive receptor nerves located in the carotid arteries and in the aortic arch. These are sensory fibers of the parasympathetic system which convey impulses in the vagus nerve to its nucleus in the brain stem. This stimulates responses of the nuclear centers, which in turn increase the activity of the effector vagal fibers directed to the heart, causing inhibition of sinus impulse formation. This response is commonly known as a **vasovagal reflex,** the term describing the reflex arc.

Some individuals are extremely sensitive to vagal reflexes which result in severe bradycardia. Diminution in blood pressure may occur, leading to lightheadedness and even syncope.

In hypersensitive patients, particularly those with recent myocardial infarctions, special care is necessary to avoid excessive cardiovascular reflexes during simple tasks such as shaving and washing, which may inadvertently produce carotid pressure-vagal stimulation.

Sinus Syndrome

A form of sinus irregularity can be seen with diseases (usually ischemic) which affect the sinus node, causing extreme variations in impulse-forming activity. Intermittent periods of excitation and depression of the sinus node may be present in which alternating sinus tachycardia and sinus bradycardia occur. This condition may be associated with episodes of cardiac syncope because of a tendency for developing sinus arrest. Severe sinus irregularity appearing in acute myocardial infarction is an ominous sign, usually requiring therapeutic intervention in the form of either pharmacologic agents or an electronic pacemaker. The **sinus syndrome** is also referred to as the sinoatrial syndrome or the sick sinus syndrome.

Marked sinus irregularity due to ischemic heart disease is evident in this tracing recorded from a 78-year-old man who has occasional dizzy spells.

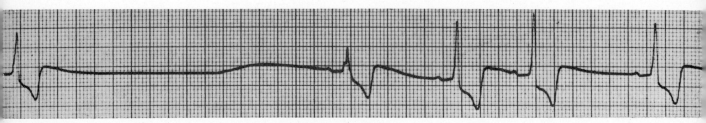

The Sinus Syndrome

Marked sinus irregularity is evident in this tracing from a 72-year-old woman. She had sustained two myocardial infarctions in previous years but had remained thereafter asymptomatic until recently, when brief episodes of lightheadedness began. These were most likely to occur during exertion or sudden standing.

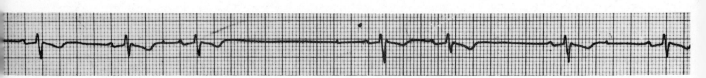

Sinus node activity is extremely erratic, presumably because of progressive ischemic disease. The symptoms were later established as related to periods of severe bradycardia. Short episodes of sinus tachycardia were also recorded but were not associated with symptoms or specific activities. These findings are typical of the sinus syndrome.

Dynamic Rhythm Profile

At this point, it would be interesting and helpful for the reader, working with a partner, to record and interpret his own electrocardiogram under a variety of conditions. The electrode placement may be according to that described for cardiac monitoring of the Coronary Care Unit patient, locating a single lead which has well-visualized components and is relatively free from movement artifact.

Procedure:

   I. Attach right arm and left arm electrodes.

     A. Select lead I on the machine.

     B. Record. Add the right leg electrode and record again; then compare.*

---

*Some electrocardiographic machines will not operate unless the right leg ground lead is attached.

II. Obtain a rhythm strip during the following conditions:
   A. Supine, normal breathing.
   B. Deep inspiration—hold for at least 30 seconds.
   C. Full, forced exhalation.
   D. Valsalva maneuver (strong expiratory force against a closed nose and mouth to make the ears "pop").
   E. Standing:
      1. Immediately.
      2. After one minute.
   F. Exercise:
      1. Immediately after exercise.
      2. After one minute of rest.
   G. Sitting—after rest and return of rate to baseline:
      1. During smoking.
   H. Carotid pressure (only under supervision of a physician).
III. Inspect each portion of the dynamic profile and correlate changes in rate with activity or maneuver. Also note any unusual beat forms or prominent irregularity of rhythm and set aside for later interpretation.
IV. Cut the electrocardiogram at convenient and uniform lengths and select representative sections. This series can be mounted in the same format as the example dynamic cardiac rhythm profile which follows. Use arrows or some other legend to indicate continuous, consecutive tracings.

The subject of this dynamic cardiac rhythm profile is a 24-year-old male physiologist in excellent health and moderately conditioned in athletics.

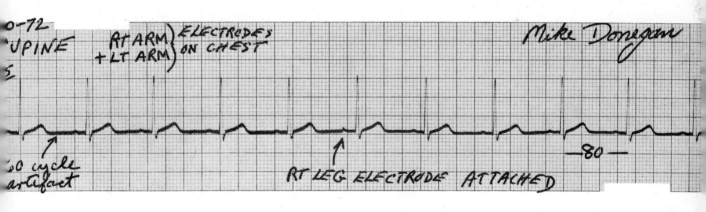

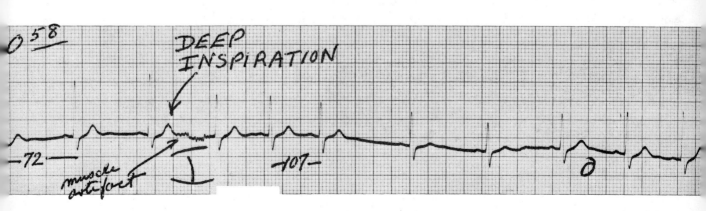

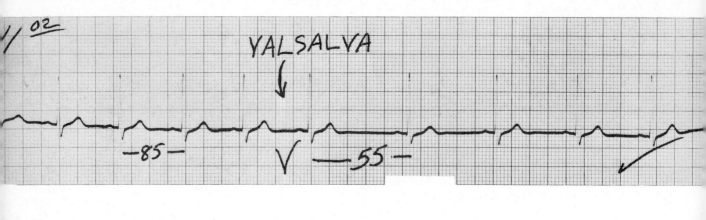

VALSALVA

—85—   —55—

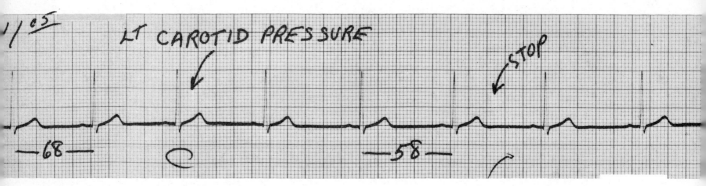

LT CAROTID PRESSURE   STOP

—68—   —58—

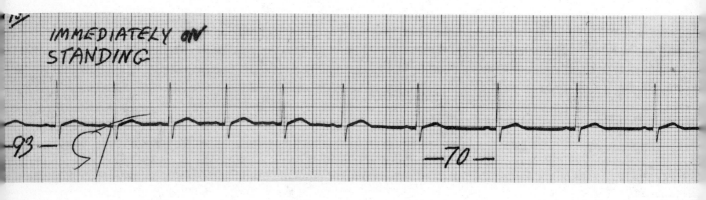

IMMEDIATELY ON
STANDING

—93—   —70—

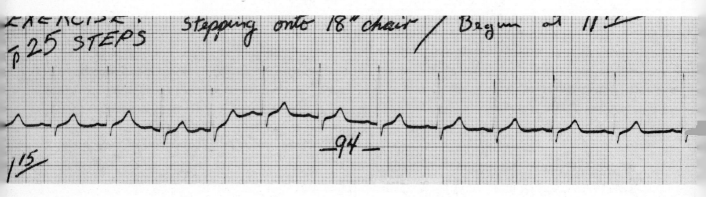

EXERCISE: stepping onto 18" chair / Begun at 11:13
T 25 STEPS

—94—

11:15

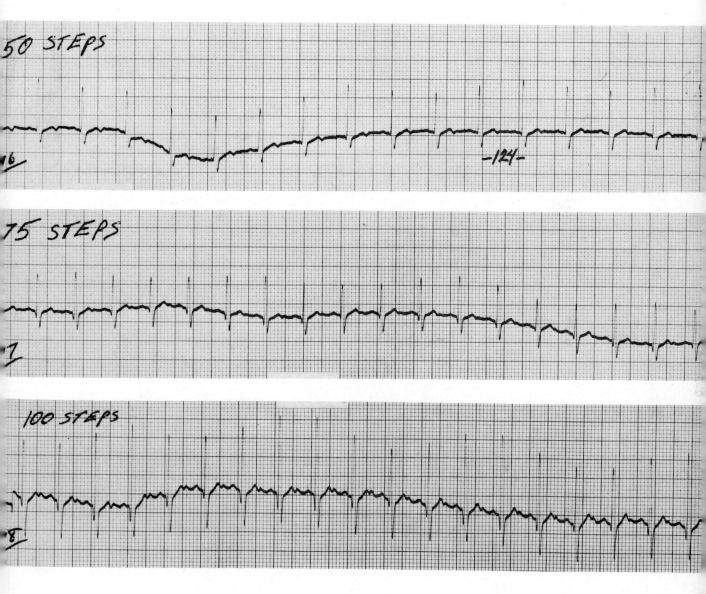

Preparation of a Cardiac Rhythm Notebook

A valuable collection of arrhythmias can be assembled from routine electro-cardiograms and monitoring tracings in hospitals of any size. These may be taken from clippings not selected for the permanent record. Almost all the examples used in this text are discarded portions of recordings from a community hospital of moderate size.

The search for and classification of cardiac rhythms can be an interesting and rewarding project for the member of a Cardiac Care Unit staff. A well-developed notebook may serve as a log of the Unit activities or as a ready bank of arrhythmias for review and teaching. The endeavor will increase rhythm scanning acuity and encourage careful interpretation, labeling, and display.

Examples in the notebook should be arranged by some orderly system. The format of this book or some other system may be followed. Each tracing should be clearly labeled with the name (or initials) of the patient and the date for reference.

Record pertinent drugs and activity. Interpretations may be written under each tracing or included on a separate answer sheet.

Tracings in this book have been cut at 20 cm (or 8 seconds) and mounted on regular-sized typing paper. Longer strips, if preferred, can be placed along the long axis of the paper, or a larger notebook size may be used. Changing rhythm patterns are highly desirable for teaching purposes. These can usually be cut and mounted as serial tracings, indicating continuity with bold arrows or some other symbol. A glue pencil is handy for mounting; rub the adhesive on the paper rather than directly on the electrocardiogram to avoid causing marks. Acetate folders are advantageous for protecting the tracing from slipping and from inadvertent marking such as with caliper points. Notebook tab dividers provide easy reference to rhythm categories.

Symbols can be placed on the electrocardiogram with any convenient marker, such as a ballpoint or fine-tipped felt pen. They are also available in dry transfer art-work sheets. For further information, see page 341.

SINUS NODE : IMPULSE CONDUCTION

Depression

S–AB = Sinoatrial block

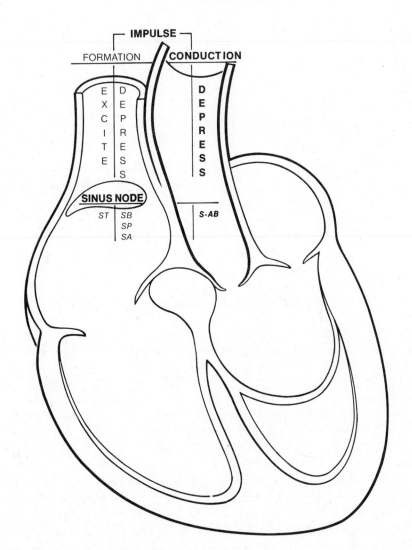

Sinoatrial Block

When the sinus node discharges but the impulse formed does not propagate into the atrial muscle because of conduction depression, **sinoatrial block** is present. The sinus node impulse is trapped and dissipated within the sinus node itself. The entire duration of the anticipated beat appears to be electrocardiographically silent. The subsequent beats pick up without any change in cadence.

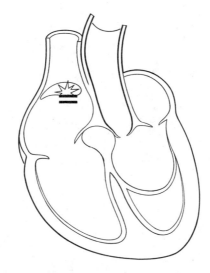

This phenomenon resembles a sinus pause or defect in impulse formation. However, actual on-time depolarization of the sinus node is presumed to have occurred, since there is no interruption of the sinus rhythm. It would seem unlikely that a pause in sinus impulse formation would occur for exactly one normal cycle length. The silent area then can be considered a defect in *impulse conduction* from the sinus node rather than a defect in impulse formation itself. Another name for this phenomenon is **sinus exit block.**

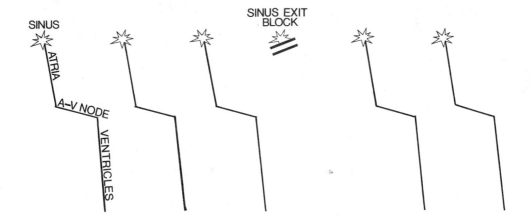

The stars represent sinus impulse formation and the lines the course and time of impulse conduction. Impulse blockage is depicted in the fourth cardiac cycle, in which the sinus impulse does not penetrate into the atria. Note that there is no change in the cadence of the sinus beat.

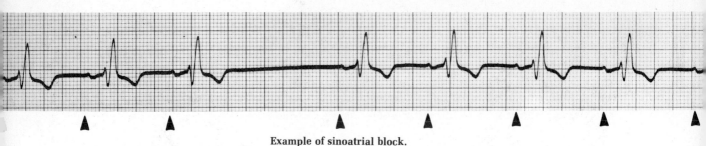

Example of sinoatrial block.

Normal sinus rhythm appears initially. After the third beat, a delay occurs. This appears to be a sinus pause (failure of sinus node impulse formation). However, when P waves are measured out with calipers, it can be demonstrated that subsequent P waves appear without any change of cadence. This is not likely to happen in sinus pause. More probably, the sinus node discharges an impulse on time during the apparent missed beat, but it does not exit from the sinus node to stimulate an atrial response. The basic rhythmicity of the sinus node is not disturbed.

The following sequence demonstrates sinoatrial block. This conduction defect was treated with a parasympathetic blocking agent.

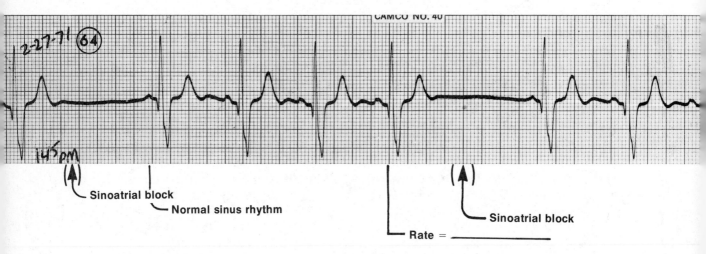

Sinoatrial block

Normal sinus rhythm

Rate = _____

Sinoatrial block

1:45 PM:

Sinoatrial block abolished by inhibiting vagal tone with a parasympathetic blocking agent.

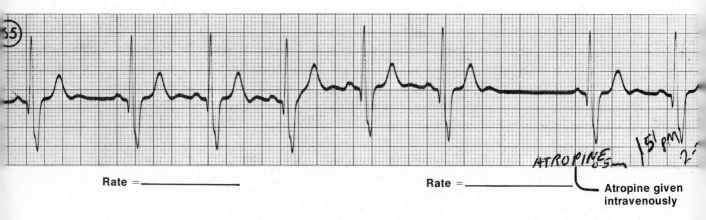

Rate = _____   Rate = _____   Atropine given intravenously

1:51 PM: Mark the site of the S-A block.

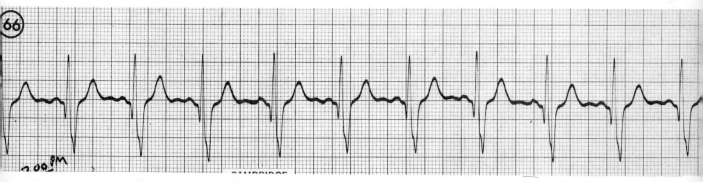

Rate = _____

2:00 PM: Nine minutes after the administration of atropine, the sinus rate has increased, and sinoatrial block is no longer present.

The pharmacologic suppression of parasympathetic activity resulted in acceleration of **impulse formation** (sinus rate increased) and **impulse conduction** (sinoatrial block abolished).

Chapter 4

THE ATRIA

IMPULSE FORMATION

Atrial tissue, like the sinus node, possesses the property of automaticity. Its natural rate of impulse formation is, however, not as fast as that of the sinus node. Consequently, the atria are periodically depolarized by impulses received from the sinus node before spontaneous atrial firing can occur. If sinus automaticity is sufficiently depressed, however, or if sinus impulses are blocked before reaching the atria, an impulse may be formed in an atrial focus.

Atrial Escape Beat

When an automatic focus within the atria escapes the controlling influence of the sinus node and initiates a cardiac contraction, the sequence is referred to as an **atrial escape beat.** The atrial impulse is propagated to other portions of the atria, to the sinus node and, by the ordinary conduction system, to the ventricles. Any such beat which originates outside of the sinus node is described as ectopic. These ectopic impulses can be considered normal responses of latent cardiac pacemakers which become expressed when the usual dominant pacemaker is inoperative.

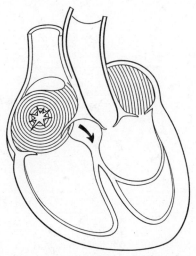

Schematic view of atrial impulse formation and conduction

Atrial depolarization from an ectopic atrial focus proceeds in a different direction than does that from the sinus node. This results in an electrocardiographic change, represented by a variation in P wave contour. The PR interval may also be altered. The impulse, after penetrating the A-V node, continues along normal conduction pathways so that the QRS complex and T wave of the beat are similar to those of sinus beats.

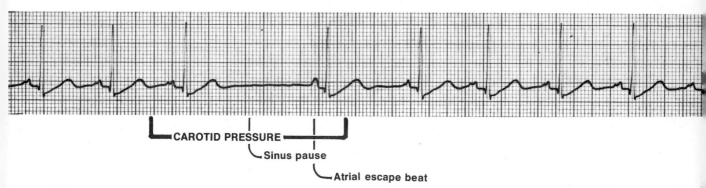

Note the delay in the rate of sinus beats (in this case induced by carotid pressure). During this slowing, a beat appears which has an altered P wave configuration. The associated QRS complex and T wave forms are identical to those of the sinus beats. This is an atrial escape beat.

A succession of atrial escape beats may occur with sustained suppression of the sinus node automaticity.

Atrial Escape Rhythm

Sustained atrial escape beats which result from sinus impulse formation slowing below a certain rate establish an **atrial escape rhythm.** Again, this is a normal physiological event which protects the heart from excessive depression of impulses from the sinus node.

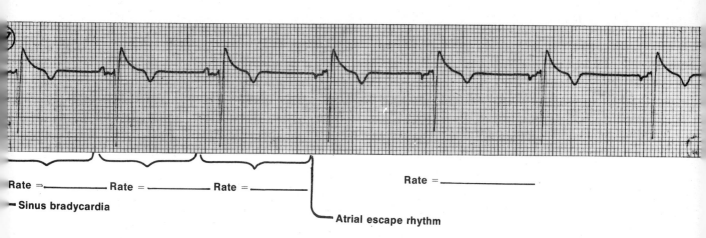

Progressive slowing of the sinus pacemaker leads to a sustained rhythm in which P waves have an altered configuration. QRS complexes and T waves remain unchanged. These are atrial escape beats which maintain a nearly constant rate.

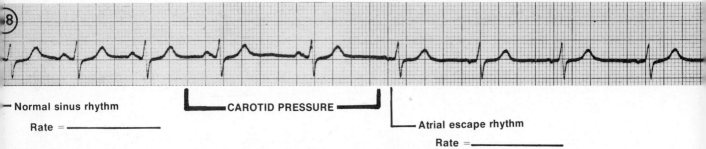

Normal sinus rhythm

Rate = _____

CAROTID PRESSURE

Atrial escape rhythm

Rate = _____

Atrial escape rhythm induced by vagotonic maneuver.

Following the slowing of the sinus rate with vagal stimulation, a rhythm super-cedes in which the P wave form and PR interval are altered. Presumably, a pace-maker is activated on suppression of the sinus node, and the atria are now de-polarized in a different sequence. This demonstrates a sustained escape rhythm from an atrial focus. Note that the escape rhythm rate is *slower* than that of the sinus rhythm.

A Wandering Pacemaker

Another variation of atrial rhythms is the shifting of impulse formation from focus to focus within the atrial tissue, virtually with every beat. Sinus beats may be interspersed throughout. P waves are of many forms, and the cadence tends to be somewhat irregular. Ventricular complexes are without alteration. This rhythm is termed a **wandering pacemaker.**

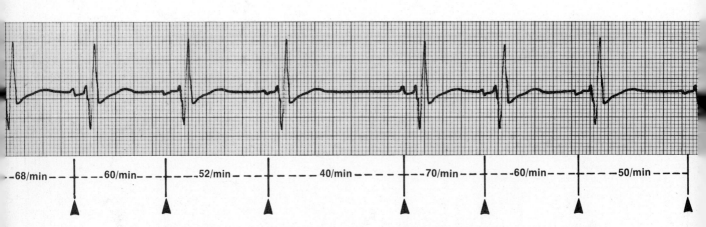

68/min — 60/min — 52/min — 40/min — 70/min — 60/min — 50/min

Note variable cycle rate and P wave configuration with similarity of QRS complexes and T waves.

A wandering pacemaker may be associated with ischemic disease involving the sinus node, or it may occur as a manifestation of an inflammatory state (e.g., acute rheumatic fever). Digitalis, probably by enhancing vagal tone, may cause the arrhyth-mia. Often, however, a wandering pacemaker is found without any other sign of cardiac disease.

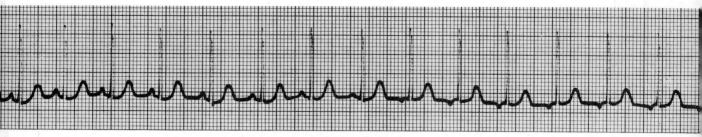

Wandering sinoatrial pacemaker.

Note the variation in the configuration of P waves.

ATRIUM : IMPULSE FORMATION

Excitation

APC = Atrial premature contraction
AT = Atrial tachycardia
AFl = Atrial flutter
AFib = Atrial fibrillation

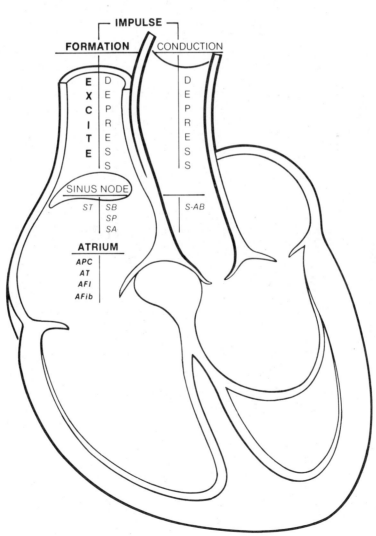

Atrial Premature Contractions

The atria may be excited to form impulses more rapidly than their usual rate of automaticity. Beats then result from atrial tissue at a faster rate than from the sinus node; this pre-empts sinus control of the cardiac rhythm. An isolated beat of this nature is known as an **atrial premature contraction.**

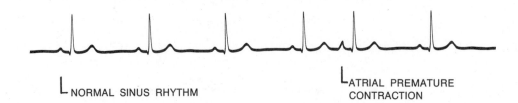

L NORMAL SINUS RHYTHM

L ATRIAL PREMATURE CONTRACTION

The pattern of normal sinus rhythm is interrupted by a beat with the following features:
1. It appears early in the cardiac cycle.
2. The P wave is altered in shape (as with atrial escape beats).
3. The QRS complex and T wave are similar to those of other beats (ventricular depolarization and repolarization proceed normally).

APC Pictorial

1. Normal sinus rhythm.
2. Atrial premature contraction originating from an impulse in the atria with
   a. conduction into atria in an aberrant direction.
   b. conduction into ventricles by normal pathways.

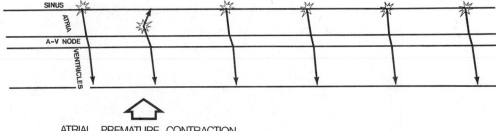

ATRIAL PREMATURE CONTRACTION

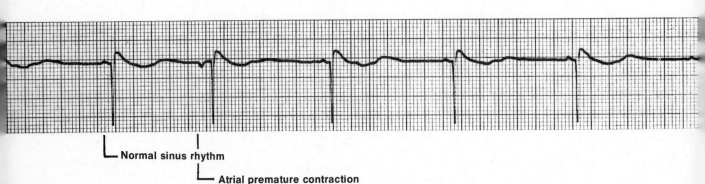

L Normal sinus rhythm

L Atrial premature contraction

Inspect the components of the atrial premature contraction. The P wave varies in form from that of the sinus-initiated beats; however, the QRS complex remains unchanged.

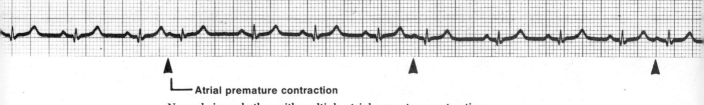

└─ **Atrial premature contraction**

Normal sinus rhythm with multiple atrial premature contractions.

Note the interruption of the sinus rhythm by early beats having altered P waves.

Examples of atrial premature contractions.

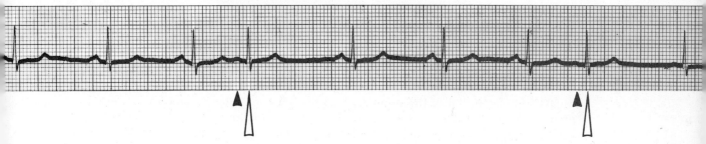

Basic rhythm: normal sinus rhythm. Rate = 71 per minute.
Ectopic beat(s) = two atrial premature contractions.

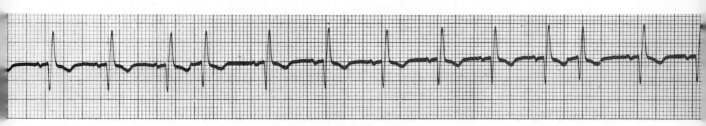

Basic rhythm: normal sinus rhythm. Rate = 92 per minute.
Ectopic beat(s) = two atrial premature contractions.

The frequency of atrial premature contractions is extremely variable. The examples below are arranged in order of increasing frequency. Identify and label each APC.

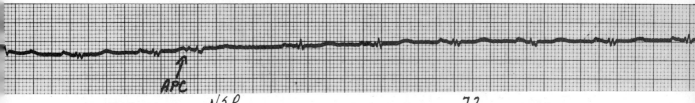

APC

Basic rhythm = _N S R_   Rate = _72_

Ectopic beats = _1 APC_

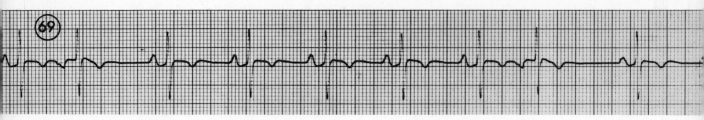

Basic rhythm = _NSR_   Rate = _____

Ectopic beats = _2 APC's_

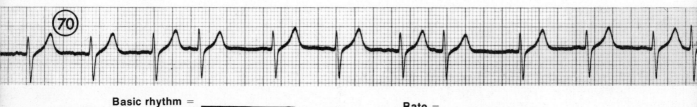

Basic rhythm = _____   Rate = _____

Ectopic beats = _____

Atrial premature contractions may appear so early that they occur before ventricular repolarization of the previous beat has been completed. The P wave of the premature beat is thereby superimposed on the T wave of the preceding beat. This combination of simultaneous events is usually not difficult to identify when other normal components are compared.

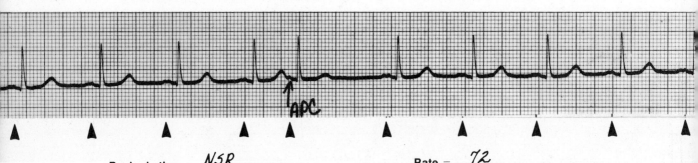

Basic rhythm = _NSR_   Rate = _72_

Ectopic beats = _1 APC_

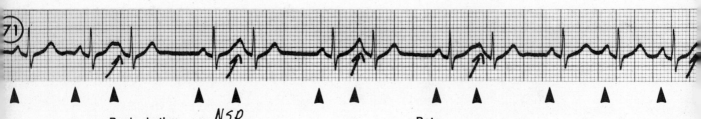

Basic rhythm = _NSR_   Rate = _____

Ectopic beats = _5 APC'S_

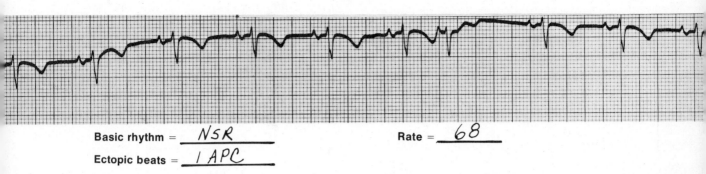

Basic rhythm = _NSR_   Rate = _68_

Ectopic beats = _1 APC_

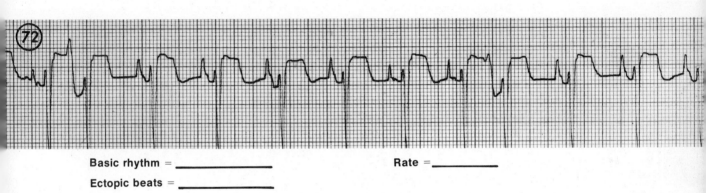

(72)

Basic rhythm = _____   Rate = _____

Ectopic beats = _____

An atrial premature contraction becomes less distinct when its P wave falls near the peak of the T wave. Sometimes the combined components can be recognized only by the increased amplitude of the T wave which precedes a premature QRS. For each of the following examples, determine basic rhythm and rate, locate the APC, and note:

1. the degree of prematurity by comparing the rates of normal and premature beats.
2. the contours of normal P, QRS, and T components as compared with those of premature beats.

Label the cardiac cycles; estimate rate per minute.

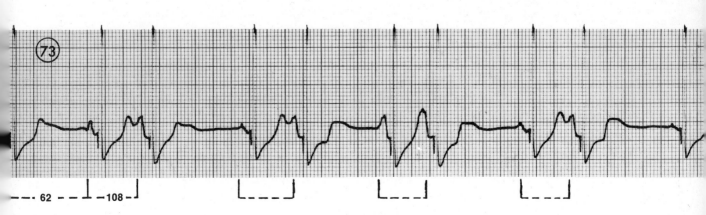

(73)

--- 62 --- --- 108 --

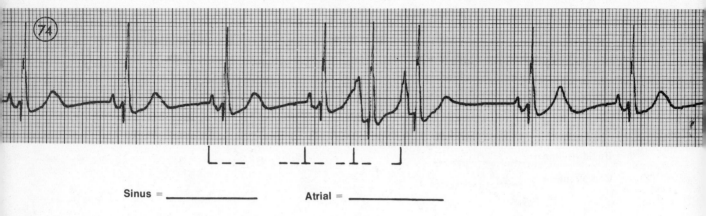

Sinus = _____   Atrial = _____

Locate all P waves of atrial premature contractions and mark.

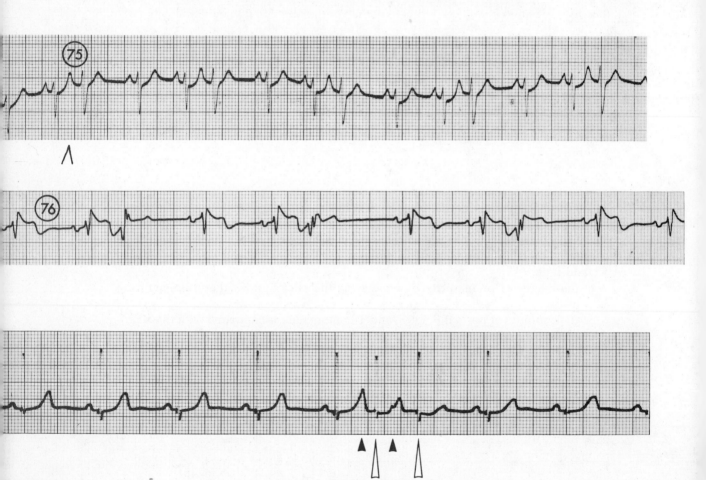

Atrial premature contractions occur in succession.

The P wave of the first of the paired APC's is superimposed on the T wave of the previous beat, causing the latter to appear taller and more peaked. The second atrial premature contraction occurs relatively earlier in the next cycle and can be identified before the T wave of the previous beat.

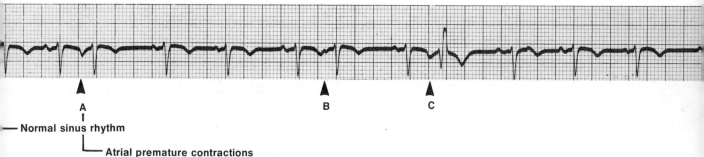

A

— Normal sinus rhythm

— Atrial premature contractions

Atrial premature contractions originating from multiple sites.

Compare atrial beats A, B, and C and note the dissimilarity of the P waves. The impulses which initiate each of these beats are presumed to originate in different areas or foci in the atria and, therefore, to depolarize the atria in different sequences. This phenomenon is termed **multifocal atrial premature contractions.** Alteration in conduction velocity in the ventricles associated with the QRS complex morphology at C will be described later.

Atrial premature contractions may assume a constant pattern in relation to normal beats. If every second beat is an APC, the term **atrial bigeminy** is applied.

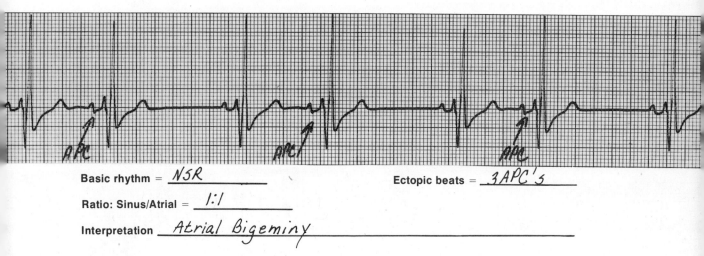

Basic rhythm = _NSR_   Ectopic beats = _3 APC's_

Ratio: Sinus/Atrial = _1:1_

Interpretation _Atrial Bigeminy_

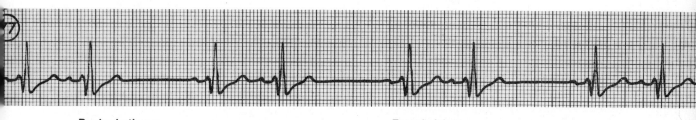

Basic rhythm = _____   Ectopic beats = _____

Ratio: Sinus/Atrial = _____

Interpretation _____

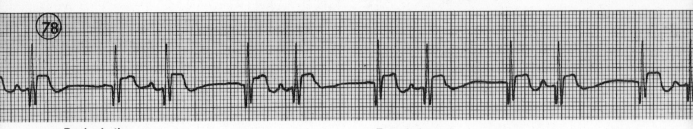

Basic rhythm = _____   **Ectopic beats** = _____

Ratio: Sinus/Atrial = _____

Interpretation _____

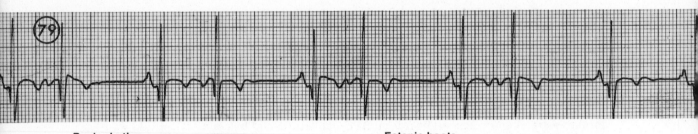

Basic rhythm = _____   **Ectopic beats** = _____

Ratio: Sinus/Atrial = _____

Interpretation _____

The following examples represent compound arrhythmias (i.e., they have more than one disturbance in rhythm). Note the sinus bradycardia (depression of impulse formation: sinus node) and atrial premature contractions (excitation of impulse formation: atria).

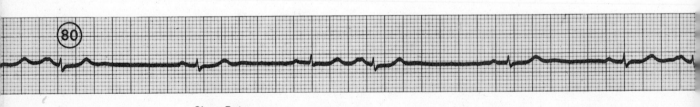

Sinus Rate = _____
Ectopic Rate = _____

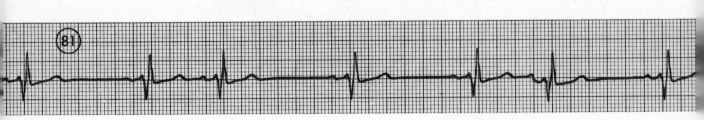

Sinus Rate = _____
Ectopic Rate = _____

Blocked Atrial Premature Contractions

An APC may take place so soon after the previous beat that ventricular recovery is not complete, and the ventricles cannot respond to the new stimulus. In other words, the premature impulse from the atria arrives at the ventricles at a time when they are refractory to depolarizing excitation. The impulse is dissipated within the conduction pathways, and ventricular contraction does not follow. Such an ectopic beat is described as *nonconducted, blocked,* or *dropped.* It can be identified by the appearance of an early P wave of abnormal configuration without a subsequent QRS complex.

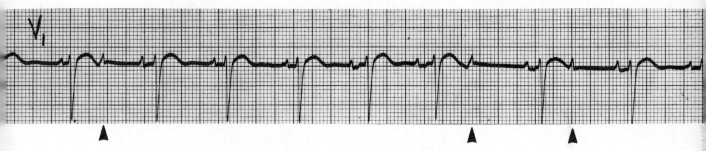

Examples of blocked atrial premature contractions.

The normal sinus rhythm, with a rate of 78 per minute, is interrupted by frequent atrial premature contractions, which are not conducted to stimulate the ventricles.

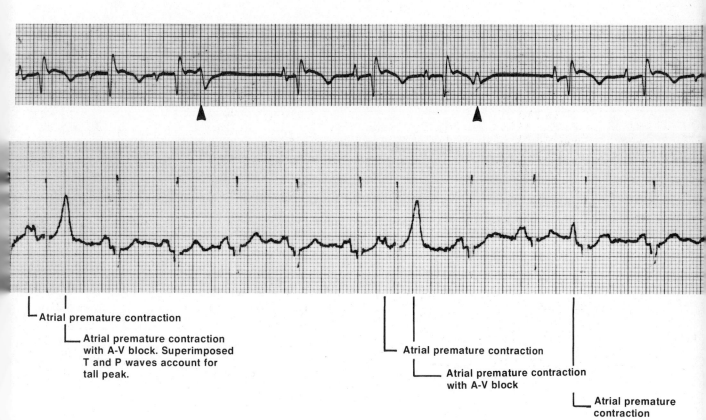

Atrial premature contraction

Atrial premature contraction with A-V block. Superimposed T and P waves account for tall peak.

Atrial premature contraction

Atrial premature contraction with A-V block

Atrial premature contraction

Conducted and nonconducted atrial premature contractions.

This sequence of atrial premature contractions, the first conducted and the second blocked, is repeated in this tracing. An isolated atrial premature contraction with A-V conduction appears toward the end of the strip.

Identify blocked APC's.

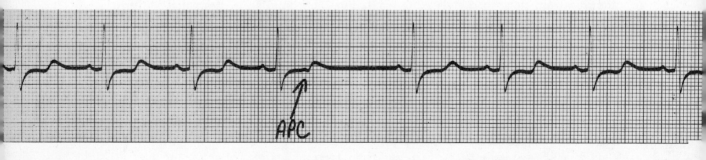

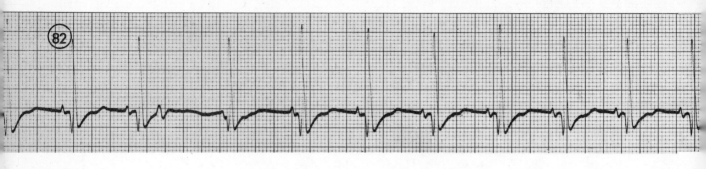

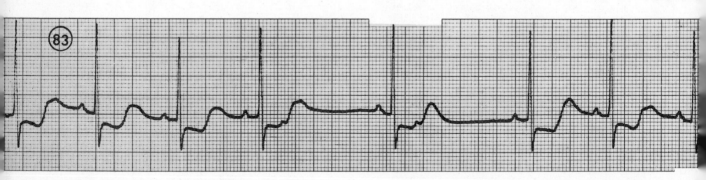

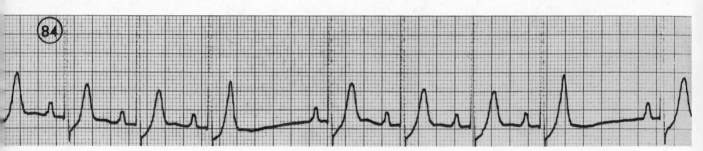

Normal sinus rhythm with pauses.

Note that the T wave preceding each pause is taller and more peaked than other T waves. Presumably an APC has occurred right at the time of the T wave's highest amplitude, causing it to be increased in amplitude and changing its contour somewhat. The APC happened so early in the normal cardiac cycle that the conduction mechanism had not recovered enough to carry this new impulse. The atrial and sinus nodes are depolarized, but further development of the beat is blocked (diagnosis: blocked atrial premature contractions).

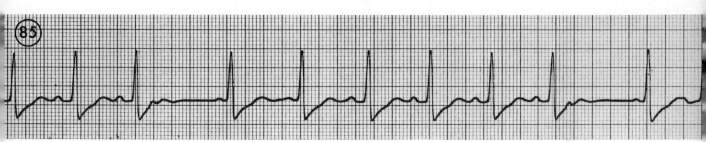

Identify the blocked APC's.

A dropped APC is an example of an electrical event within the cardiac cycle which is affected by the time relationship to the previous beat. This phenomenon involves repolarization and introduces an important concept in understanding arrhythmias—the **refractory period.**

The Refractory Period

Following depolarization, nerve and muscle cells restore their normal resting electrical potential over a period of time using metabolic energy. Immediately after discharge of stored energy, the cells cannot be driven to depolarize again, even with intense stimuli. However, as the processes of repolarization proceed, they gradually lose this refractoriness for stimulation and regain a state of excitability. The cells become responsive to progressively decreasing intensity of stimuli as physiological recovery continues. In the heart, this process occurs in impulse forming tissues, conduction pathways, and the myocardial fibers, but at different rates. The total refractory period begins at the moment of depolarization and ends when the cell has reestablished its normal sensitivity to stimuli.

The refractory period is made up of two phases, absolute and relative.

Immediately after depolarization, the tissue will not respond to a second stimulus, no matter how intense it is. This phase is known as the **absolute refractory period.**

As the tissue undergoes repolarization, it reaches a point at which it will respond to a stimulus, but only when this is of greater intensity than that required to initiate depolarization in the tissue during the resting stage. This later period of repolarization, in which there is decreased sensitivity to stimulation, is known as the **relative refractory period.**

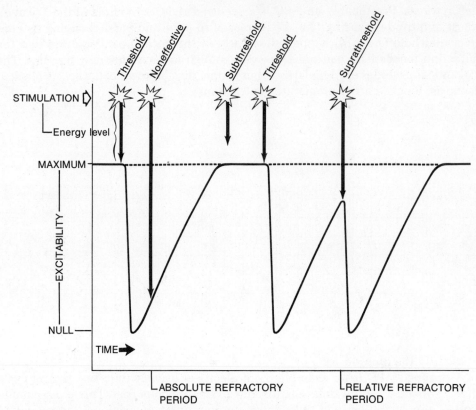

Graphic representation of the refractory period, in which the excitability of cells during varying phases of activity are related to magnitude of stimulation.

The resting cell is at the maximum point of excitability. In this state, the minimal intensity of stimulation which initiates depolarization is known as the **threshold stimulation.** Once activated, the cell changes rapidly from maximum to null excitability.

During the early phase of repolarization, the absolute refractory period, the cell cannot be stimulated again, no matter how great the intensity of energy applied.

When the cell has returned to its resting state (maximum excitability), a stimulus of less than threshold intensity will not induce depolarization. This is known as a **subthreshold stimulation.**

Following another threshold stimulation, the cell again undergoes depolarization, then repolarization. During the later phase of repolarization, the relative refractory period, the cell has attained a certain level of excitability at which energy which is greater than threshold stimulation can induce depolarization.

Atrial Tachycardia

Repetitive discharges from an excited atrial region result in a sustained ectopic rhythm with the following characteristics:
1. P waves have aberrant form.
2. The rate of atrial beats is rapid.

3. Atrial beats tend to occur at precise intervals (the term *regular* is aptly applied here).
4. Ventricular depolarization follows the usual pathways.

This arrhythmia is called **atrial tachycardia.** The rate of atrial beats in atrial tachycardia is usually greater than 120 and less than 200 per minute.

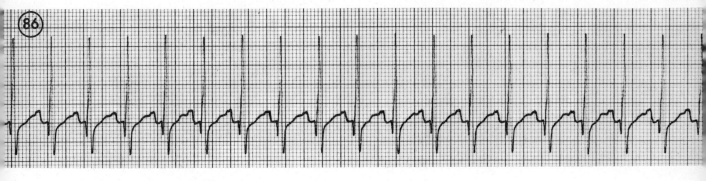

Rate =

Atrial tachycardia.

Note the regularity of beats and the similarity of P waves and of QRS complexes. T waves and P waves have become superimposed because of the rapid rate.

Atrial tachycardia usually appears suddenly and subsides just as abruptly, sometimes lasting for a few beats, a few minutes, hours, or days. These paroxysms may be precipitated by physiological or psychological stress. APC's may herald an episode of atrial tachycardia, but many times no triggering factor can be identified. Strong vagal stimulation tends to suppress the ectopic pacemaker. Sinus impulse formation can then regain its dominance, and atrial tachycardia is converted to NSR.

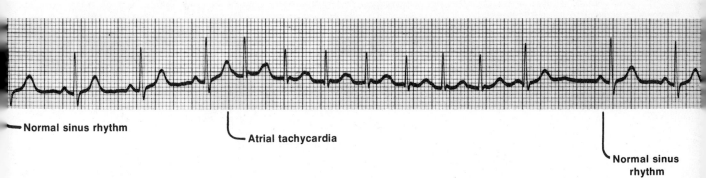

Normal sinus rhythm   Atrial tachycardia   Normal sinus rhythm

Paroxysmal atrial tachycardia is initiated by a typical APC. Note that the few beats of the tachycardia are *precisely* regular (measure R-R intervals with calipers). Near the end of the paroxysm, atrial beats become slightly irregular; then normal sinus rhythm is resumed. The sudden appearance and subsidence of the arrhythmia are characteristic of atrial tachycardia. Also note the change in the terminal portion of the QRS complex during the episode of tachycardia. This variation is due to altered ventricular conduction caused by the increased rate.

Compare these rhythms:

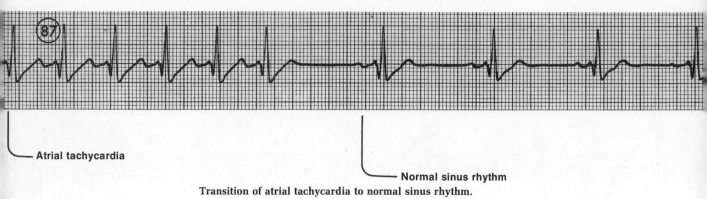

Atrial tachycardia

Normal sinus rhythm

Transition of atrial tachycardia to normal sinus rhythm.

A small P wave during the period of tachycardia can be identified on the down-slope of T waves.

	Atrial tachycardia	Normal sinus rhythm
Rate	_____	_____
Regular?	_____	_____

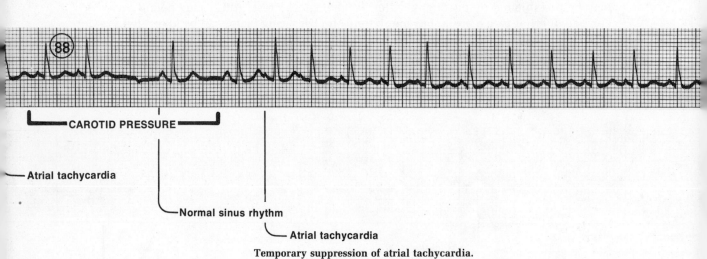

CAROTID PRESSURE

Atrial tachycardia

Normal sinus rhythm

Atrial tachycardia

Temporary suppression of atrial tachycardia.

Increased parasympathetic tone has converted atrial tachycardia to normal sinus rhythm, but the ectopic rhythm returned on removal of vagal stimulation.

	Atrial tachycardia	Normal sinus rhythm
Rate	_____	_____
Regular?	_____	_____

The abrupt onset and termination of atrial tachycardia help differentiate the arrhythmia from sinus tachycardia. Vagal stimulation in sinus tachycardia tends to cause gradual slowing followed by gradual resumption of rate when the stimulation is discontinued.

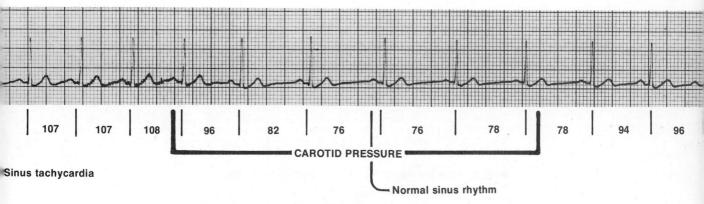

Sinus tachycardia

Normal sinus rhythm

Slowing of sinus tachycardia with vagal stimulation.

Note the gradual decrease in the sinus rate upon carotid pressure with gradual increase after release.

Patients with atrial tachycardia who are often in excellent health may be aware of palpitations or symptoms of diminished cardiac output due to the rapid rate. They frequently learn that yawning, gagging (Valsalva maneuver), breath holding, and rubbing the neck—all of which increase vagal tone—may suddenly abolish their symptoms.

Several classes of drugs are used to convert atrial tachycardia to normal sinus rhythm and to control recurrent attacks.

1. *Tranquilizers and sedatives:* reduce sympathetic stimulation from the central nervous system (e.g., Thorazine, phenobarbital).
2. *Adrenergic antagonists:* decrease sympathetic stimulation at cardiac nerve endings (e.g., reserpine, propranolol).
3. *Cholinergic stimulators:* suppress atrial ectopic impulse formation by increasing parasympathetic tone (e.g., digitalis, Tensilon).
4. *Direct cardiac suppressors:* inhibit automaticity of atrial tissue (e.g., quinidine, procainamide).

Atrial tachycardia can be converted with pharmacologic stimulation of the parasympathetic nervous system. This sequence is taken from a 38-year-old telephone operator who complained of a pounding sensation in her chest over 12 hours. Progressive weakness and a generalized soreness of the chest were also experienced. Librium and digitalis were given 2 hours before the tracing shown here was recorded. In addition, carotid pressure and the Valsalva maneuver were tried repeatedly to no avail.

6:20 PM: Atrial tachycardia:

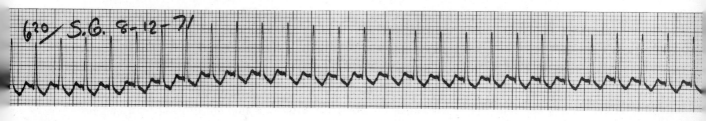

Rate = _____

6:21 PM: Tensilon (edrophonium chloride) was administered intravenously over one minute.

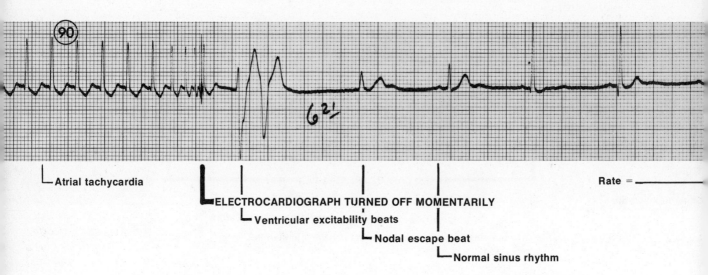

Atrial tachycardia

ELECTROCARDIOGRAPH TURNED OFF MOMENTARILY

Ventricular excitability beats

Nodal escape beat

Normal sinus rhythm

Rate =

6:21 PM: During the infusion of Tensilon, the rhythm converted to normal sinus rhythm. At the transitional period, ventricular excitability is demonstrated by abnormal beats. The patient's symptoms cleared rapidly.

Electrocardioversion

One of the most dramatic innovations in cardiology is the treatment of arrhythmias with electric shock. The electrical stimulation is applied directly to the chest and is used to convert rhythms of sustained, ectopic impulse formation excitation to a sinus rhythm.

This technique is performed with an electric power source (commonly called a **defibrillator**) and two broad electrodes placed on the chest wall. The most effective positions for the electrodes are directly anterior and posterior to the heart. The posterior electrode is designed in the shape of a table tennis paddle for placing under the back. If this type of flat electrode is not available, the left lateral chest position is usually satisfactory.

Many instruments are now available for electrocardioversion, each working according to the same principles but varying widely in design. The modern defibrillator discharges electric energy in the form of direct current within a small fraction of a second. The amount of electric energy is measured in terms of watts applied over one second (watts per second). This unit of energy is also referred to as a *joule*, after James Prescott Joule, an English physicist of the 19th century.

Because an electric shock delivered to the heart during a portion of ventricular repolarization is hazardous, the defibrillator is synchronized with the patient's electrocardiogram to fire automatically during ventricular depolarization. This is done by setting the control switch to **synchronize** (or its equivalent) and adjusting the instrument sensitivity level so that it detects one, and only one, spike in the QRS complex. The procedure outlined for selecting the monitoring lead can be followed. On activating the discharge button or switch, the instrument will fire immediately after the detected QRS spike. Except in conditions of great urgency, this synchronization of shock to ventricular depolarization should be tested.

A bulb indicator for testing is provided with the defibrillator and is installed in place of the electrode paddles, and a test shock is given using minimal electric energy. The discharge interferes with the electrocardiographic display, so that a brief period of electrical blackout occurs. When the proper synchronization has been demonstrated, the electrode paddles are then substituted for the indicator in preparation for the actual electrocardioversion.

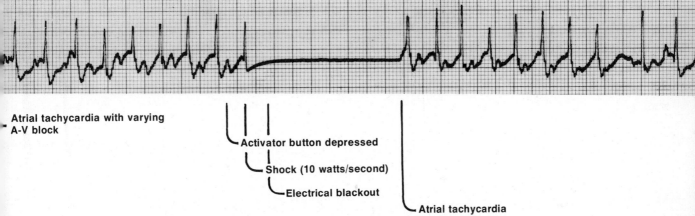

Atrial tachycardia with varying A-V block

Activator button depressed

Shock (10 watts/second)

Electrical blackout

Atrial tachycardia

The sequence of synchronized test shock in atrial tachycardia.

Following random activation of the discharge button, the actual firing occurs at the peak of the R wave. Therefore, the shock is synchronized with ventricular depolarization. The electrocardiogram is momentarily not visible immediately after the discharge. Of course, the arrhythmia is unaltered, since the discharge is not delivered to the patient during the test procedure.

The following example illustrates nonsynchronized test shock, an alternate method of activating the electric shock in which discharge occurs immediately upon pressing the discharge button. It is *not* timed with any event in the cardiac cycle and is used to treat arrhythmias with no definite QRS complexes. (It will be described in detail later.) The test is performed using the same electrocardiographic display as in the previous example. For this mode of delivery, the control switch is set on direct activation, which is usually designated **defibrillation.**

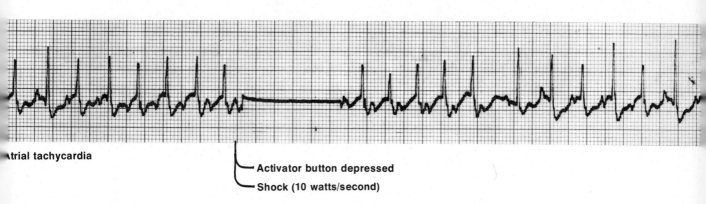

Atrial tachycardia

Activator button depressed

Shock (10 watts/second)

Note that the activator button depression and the electric shock occur simultaneously and have no relationship to the QRS complex or to any other electrical signal from the patient. The discharge is therefore not synchronous with ventricular depolarization. A transient period of electrical blackout again appears. The rhythm, as expected, is unchanged by this test shock.

After the testing procedure, the paddle electrodes are placed on the patient, and 50 watts per second are administered.

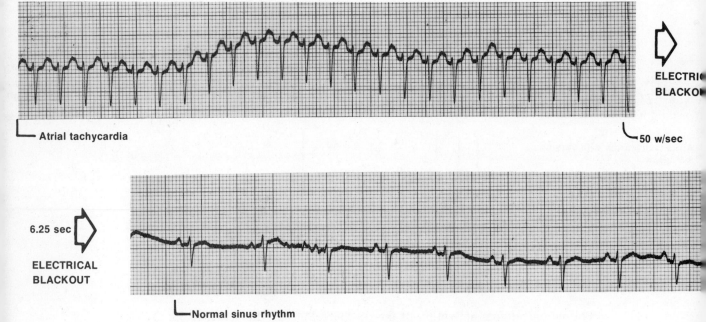

Atrial tachycardia

ELECTRIC BLACKO

50 w/sec

6.25 sec

ELECTRICAL BLACKOUT

Normal sinus rhythm

Example of electrocardioversion of atrial tachycardia.

Normal sinus rhythm appears following electric shock. During most of the electrical blackout period, the writer was completely off the graph paper.

While not completely understood, electric shock appears to work through two mechanisms:

1. Instant disruption of all responsive cardiac tissue.
2. Suppression of ectopic impulse formation activity.

At the moment of electric shock, all conductile and contractile cardiac tissue undergoes depolarization except that which is in its absolute refractory period. This tends to synchronize the processes of repolarization so that the heart responds in a coordinated manner to the next impulse. Whether or not the shock is successful in conversion of the arrhythmia depends on the integrity of the normal impulse formation and conduction system and the continued suppression of the excitable focus (or foci).

There is a high incidence of cardiac arrhythmias immediately after electric shock. They include severe sinus bradycardia and ectopic beats or tachycardia. These are usually very transient and are replaced by a more stable rhythm. Occasionally, however, these postshock arrhythmias need to be treated with appropriate, rapidly acting drugs.

Atrial Tachycardia with A-V Block

As the atrial rate becomes faster, the transmission capacity of the A-V node is exceeded. In other words, the interval at which atrial impulses assault the A-V node is shorter than the refractory period for that tissue. This critical limit is usually about 180 transmissions per minute in most adults. Beyond this, some atrial impulses are not transmitted, much as APC's may be blocked. This results in a physiological A-V node conduction defect.

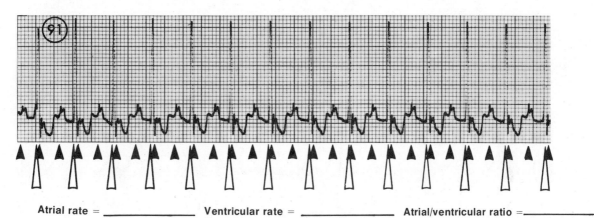

Atrial rate = _____   Ventricular rate = _____   Atrial/ventricular ratio =_____

Atrial tachycardia with 2:1 A-V block.

Note that every second atrial beat is not conducted.

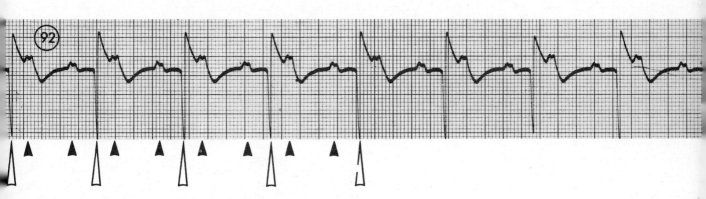

Atrial rate = _____   Ventricular rate = _____

Atrial/ventricular ratio = _____

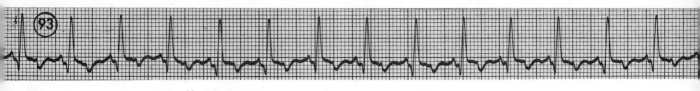

Atrial rate = _____   Ventricular rate = _____

Atrial/ventricular ratio =_____

Examples of atrial tachycardia with A-V block.

In the following examples of atrial tachycardia with A-V block, label atrial activity and determine atrial/ventricular ratio.

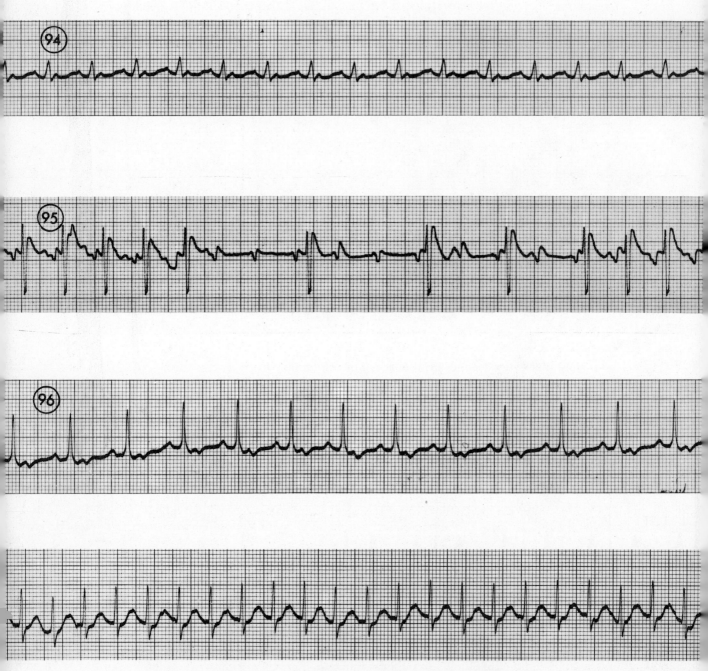

Atrial tachycardia verified with parasympathetic stimulation.

The tachycardia has a completely regular rate. Atrial activity cannot be clearly distinguished, but it becomes discernible in the following electrocardiogram.

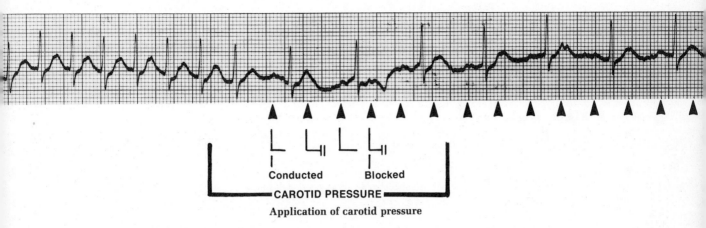

Application of carotid pressure

Vagal stimulation produces A-V block with consequent slowing of the ventricular rate and exposure of distinct, if complex, P waves. There is some variation of the atrial rate (check with calipers) under the influence of carotid pressure. A 2:1 A-V block now becomes evident. The rhythm prior to that can be interpreted as atrial tachycardia with 1:1 conduction.

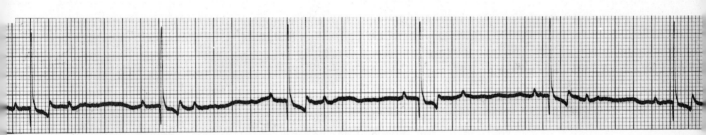

This arrhythmia appears to be a sinus rhythm with 2:1 A-V block, but it is not. Measure the atrial beats carefully with calipers or ruler and note that the blocked beat is premature. The interpretation, then, is sinus rhythm with blocked atrial premature contractions in bigeminal pattern. This distinction is important because 2:1 A-V conduction is serious, while blocked atrial premature contractions generally are not.

Digitalis has the special propensity for producing both excitation of impulse formation in the atrium and depression of impulse conduction in the A-V node. This dual effect frequently leads to atrial tachycardia with A-V block as an expression of digitalis toxicity. The following series presents an illustrative example.

A 58-year-old woman was admitted to the hospital after two days of rapid palpitations and dyspnea on mild exertion. Her maintenance dose of digitalis had been increased three weeks before because of nocturnal dyspnea due to rheumatic valvular disease (mitral regurgitation).

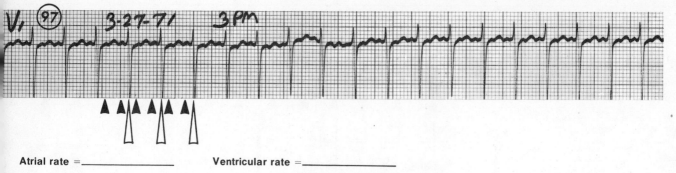

Atrial rate =_____   Ventricular rate =_____

Atrial tachycardia with 2:1 A-V block.

Atrial tachycardia with 2:1 A-V block is a common manifestation of toxicity from digitalis. There were no physical signs of congestive heart failure on admission, and serum electrolyte values were within normal limits. Digitalis was withheld.

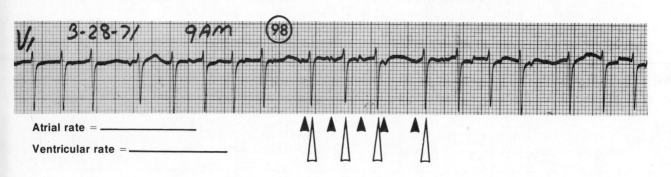

Atrial rate = _____

Ventricular rate = _____

On the following day, atrial tachycardia persisted. However, the atrial rate slowed somewhat and the severity of A-V block decreased. Observe that, after a pause in the ventricular rate, the PR intervals become progressively longer; then a blocked atrial beat occurs. The pattern then repeats itself. This is a complex form of A-V block which will be described later.

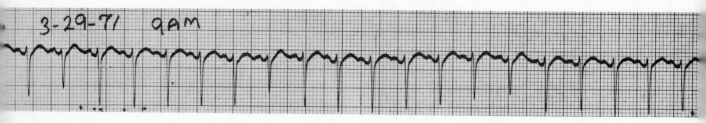

One day later, the atrial rate slowed further, and A-V block was no longer present. Atrial tachycardia with 1:1 A-V conduction was the diagnosis.

Several hours after the previous tracing, a sinus rhythm was found to have replaced atrial tachycardia. There is now no evidence of digitalis toxicity.

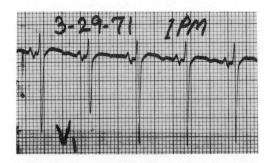

Atrial Flutter

When the atrial rate approaches 250 per minute, the forces of repolarization become more prominent, changing the shape of the recorded atrial wave itself. The wave tends to become bidirectional, and, at very rapid rates, it resembles the edge of a saw. These characteristic saw-toothed forms of atrial complexes are designated F waves and the arrhythmia **atrial flutter.**

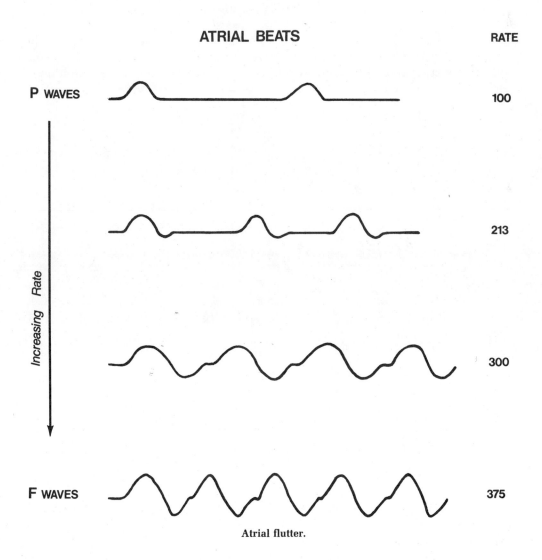

Atrial flutter.

Atrial beats at an extremely rapid rate are clearly seen in the middle portion of the following tracing, demonstrating the saw-toothed atrial configuration of atrial flutter. The pattern appears from a less obvious arrhythmia when briefly applied carotid pressure, during marked suppression of A-V conduction, is applied in a patient with an extremely sensitive vagal reflex.

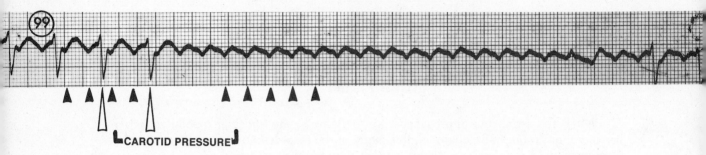

Atrial flutter with a rate of 237 per minute is apparent during a long period of ventricular inactivity induced by carotid pressure. Going back to the beginning of the tracing, similar but less obvious atrial beats can be found associated with ventricular beats in a ratio of 2:1. The same pattern reappears at the end of the tracing. The period of severely advanced A-V block represents the effect of parasympathetic stimulation on impulse conduction in the A-V node. The duration of ventricular inactivity is _____ seconds.

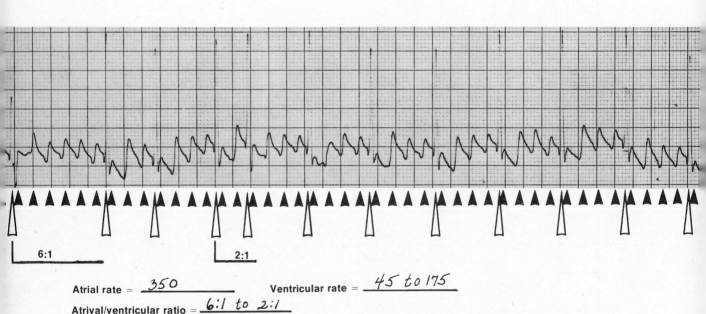

Atrial rate = *350* **Ventricular rate** = *45 to 175*
Atrival/ventricular ratio = *6:1 to 2:1*

Atrial flutter with variable atrioventricular ratio but constant F-R intervals.

Even though there is a large variation in the frequency of conducted atrial beats, the intervals between each QRS complex and the peak of the preceding F wave are virtually uniform.

These tracings are from the same standard electrocardiogram, but they represent different leads. Note the marked apparent dissimilarity in form. However, the interpretation of atrial flutter can be made after careful study of each lead.

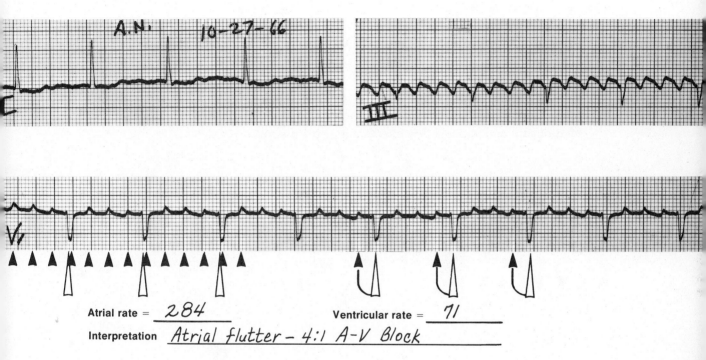

Atrial rate = _2 8 4_   Ventricular rate = _7 1_

Interpretation   _Atrial flutter – 4:1 A-V Block_

The above example of atrial flutter demonstrates a constant ratio of atrial and ventricular beats (e.g., 4:1). In addition, the conduction time between an F wave and the subsequent QRS complex (F-R interval) is also constant.

In the following tracings, examples of variability in the atrial/ventricular ratio or the F-R interval or both will be present.

Atrial flutter with varying degrees of A-V block, recorded from the same patient.

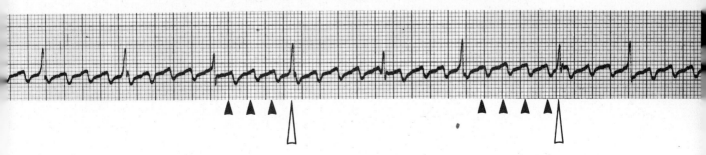

The atrial flutter with variable A-V conduction shows changes in both the number of atrial beats which precede each ventricular beat and the interval between the F wave and the QRS complex.

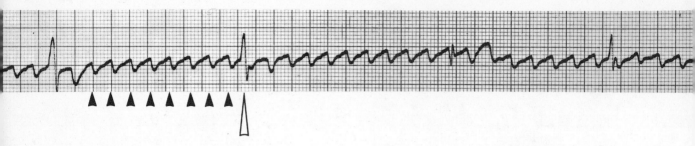

With deep-held inspiration and induced parasympathetic stimulation, physiological A-V block is markedly increased. A variable atrial/ventricular numerical
relationship and variable F-R intervals are still present.

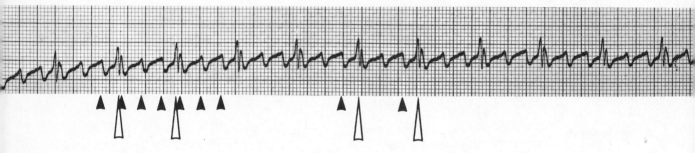

After light exercise, no change occurs in the atrial rate, but atrial conduction
is more frequent. The ventricular rate is, therefore, significantly increased. Now
there are a constant 3:1 atrial/ventricular ratio and constant F-R intervals.

Interpret the following tracings, giving complete rhythm diagnosis.

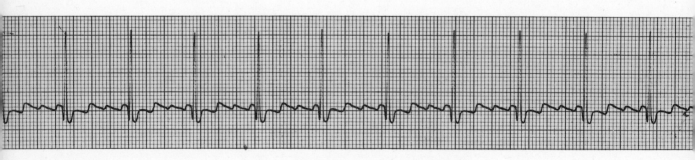

Atrial rate = _340_   Ventricular rate = _85_

A-V conduction: constant _✓_ or   variable _____

If constant, A-V ratio = _4:1_

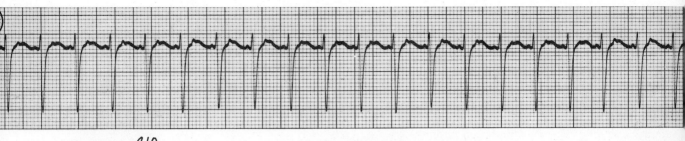

Atrial rate = _310_

Ventricular rate = _____

A-V conduction: constant_____ or variable _____

If constant, A-V ratio = _2:1_____

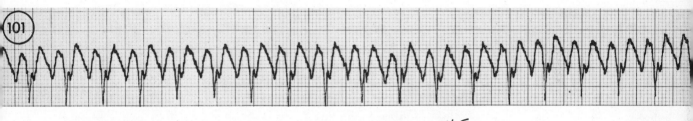

Atrial rate = _____

Ventricular rate = _145___

A-V conduction: constant _✓___ or variable _____

If constant, A-V ratio = _____

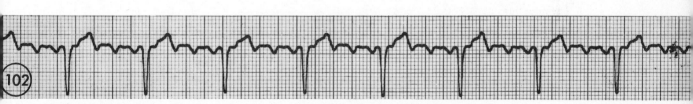

Atrial rate = _____

Ventricular rate = _____

A-V conduction: constant_____ or variable _____

If constant, A-V ratio = _____

Variable A-V conduction in atrial flutter occurs when incomplete recovery and variation in transmission occur in the A-V node because of the extremely rapid atrial firing rate. This results in changes in F-R intervals and contours.

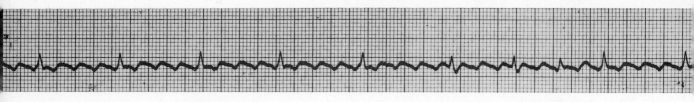

Atrial rate = *280*   Ventricular rate = *68-98*

A-V conduction: constant *✓* or variable *✓*

If constant, A-V ratio = *4:1 then variable then 4:1*

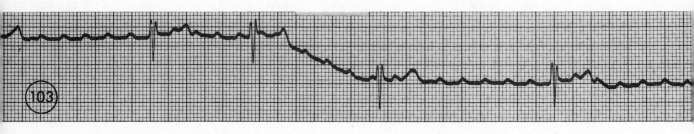

Atrial rate = _____   Ventricular rate = _____

A-V conduction: constant _____ or variable _____

If constant, A-V ratio = _____

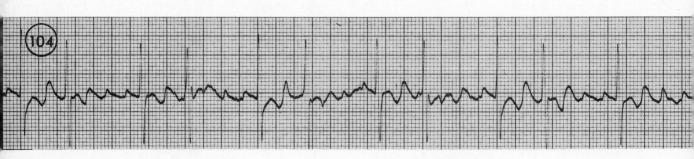

Atrial rate = _____   Ventricular rate = _____

A-V conduction: constant _____ or variable _____

If constant, A-V ratio = _____

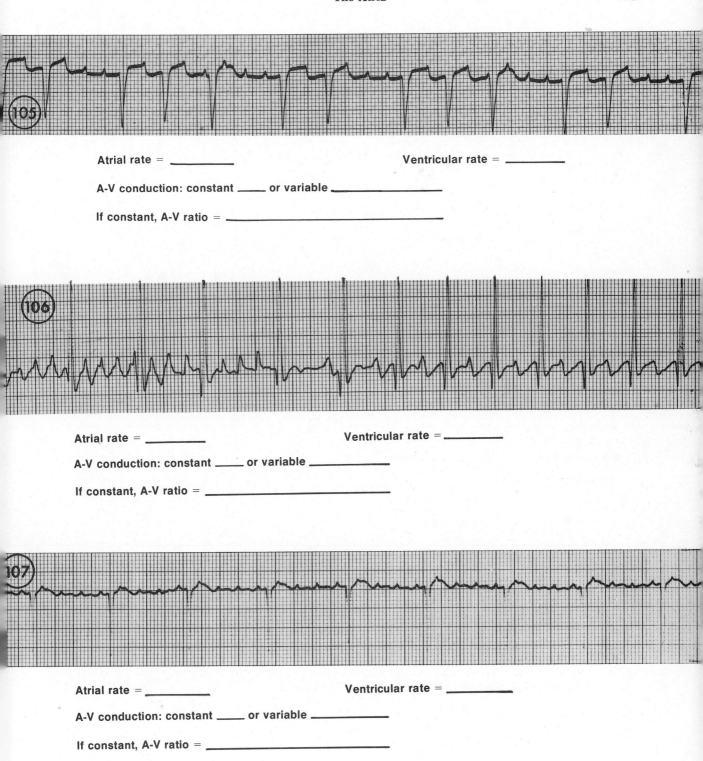

Atrial rate = _____   Ventricular rate = _____

A-V conduction: constant _____ or variable _____

If constant, A-V ratio = _____

Atrial rate = _____   Ventricular rate = _____

A-V conduction: constant _____ or variable _____

If constant, A-V ratio = _____

Atrial rate = _____   Ventricular rate = _____

A-V conduction: constant _____ or variable _____

If constant, A-V ratio = _____

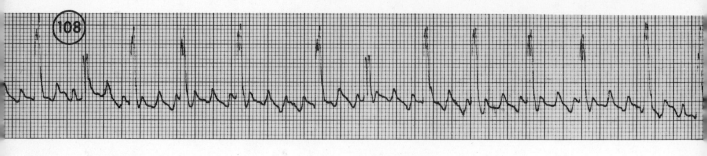

Atrial rate = _____   Ventricular rate = _____

A-V conduction: constant _____ or variable_____

If constant, A-V ratio = _____

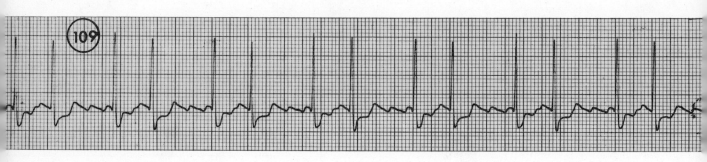

Atrial rate = _____   Ventricular rate = _____

A-V conduction: constant _____ or variable _____

If constant, A-V ratio =_____

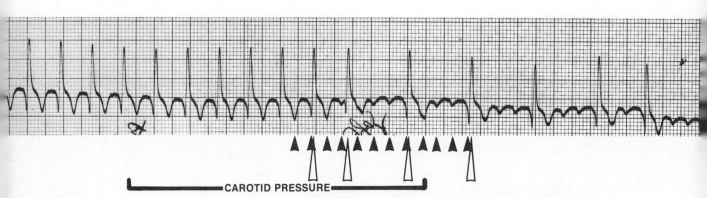

CAROTID PRESSURE

Atrial flutter demonstrated by suppression of ventricular responses with vagal stimulation.

As the ventricular rate slows with carotid pressure, the typical pattern of atrial flutter is revealed. The atrial rate is 346 per minute. Not all F waves can be morphologically identified, but they can be located by measuring out with calipers. F-R intervals are variable, and it is not certain which atrial beats are actually conducted to the ventricles. In the cycles having maximal A-V block, there is a 4:1 atrial/ventricular ratio.

A diagnosis of atrial flutter can now be given for the tachycardia present at the beginning of the tracing. There is a 2:1 A-V block in which the ventricular rate is

173 per minute (346 ÷ 2). In this example a difficult interpretation is clarified by increasing the degree of A-V block with vagal stimulation.

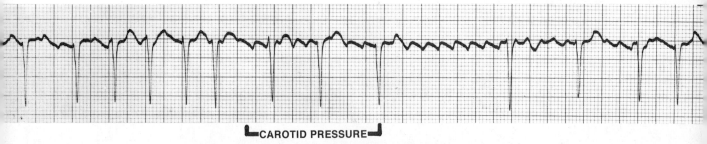

CAROTID PRESSURE

Diagnosis of supraventricular tachycardia using vagal stimulation.

From the earlier portion of the tracing, no precise interpretation can be made. Following carotid pressure and the resultant slowing of the ventricular rate, the pattern of atrial flutter emerges with an atrial rate of 360 per minute. Upon applying this information to the beginning of the tracing, the diagnosis of atrial flutter with variable A-V block can be assumed.

Atrial tachycardia and atrial flutter can be considered the same fundamental disorder of rhythm in which an excited atrial focus becomes the cardiac pacemaker. A distinction between the two tachyarrhythmias is made on the basis of *rate of atrial firing*, though no definite criteria have been generally accepted. The *saw-toothed F wave pattern* of typical atrial flutter and the degree of *physiological A-V block* are functions of tissue responsiveness in the atria and the A-V node, respectively; these vary among individuals for a given atrial pacemaker rate. When the rate is between 250 and 300 beats per minute, the designation of atrial tachycardia and atrial flutter becomes quite arbitrary. At these rates, unless typical undulations of atrial flutter are present in one lead, the term atrial tachycardia with a statement of the degrees of A-V block (if any) is more descriptive and, therefore, preferred.

Like atrial tachycardia, atrial flutter can sometimes be suppressed and the arrhythmia replaced by a sinus rhythm upon parasympathetic stimulation. In the following tracing, carotid pressure produces a slowing of the atrial rate of flutter, then cessation of atrial beats altogether. After this, sinus pacemaker activity emerges, at first at a slow rate, then speeding up to normal.

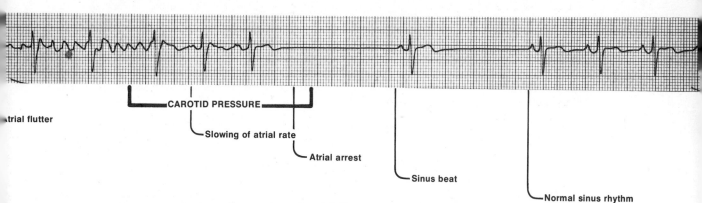

Atrial flutter

CAROTID PRESSURE

Slowing of atrial rate

Atrial arrest

Sinus beat

Normal sinus rhythm

Conversion of atrial flutter to normal sinus rhythm.

Note carefully the transitional activity of impulse formation. This recording has been photographically miniaturized to avoid a break in continuity.

The following series shows atrial impulse formation responses in a 46-year-old man following neurosurgical decompression of the cervical spine. The patient had no history of cardiac disease, and the preoperative electrocardiogram was within normal limits.

Sustained excitation of atrial impulse formation appeared during the recovery room period.

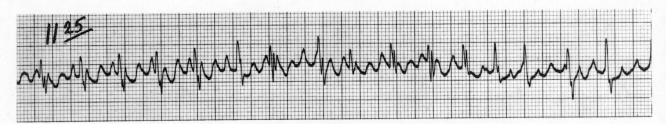

Atrial flutter with variable A-V block and rapid ventricular rate response.

An attempt was made to suppress the atrial arrhythmia by a vagotonic maneuver. Carotid pressure could not be performed because of the surgical procedure. Instead, pressure on an eyeball, which also exerts strong vagal stimulation, was applied.

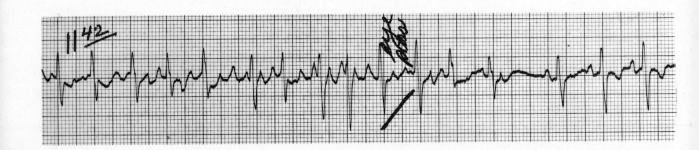

Atrial flutter is promptly converted to sinus tachycardia with reflex parasympathetic stimulation.

Continued excitation of atrial automaticity is expressed by frequent atrial premature contractions following conversion to a sinus rhythm.

Locate each atrial premature contraction _____, _____, _____.

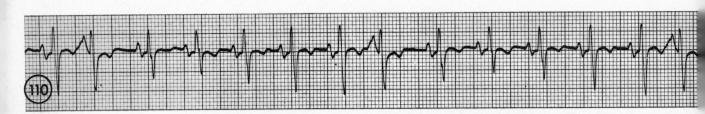

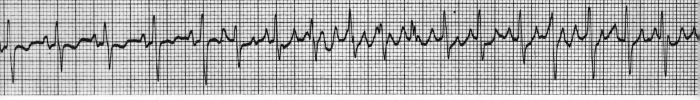

Recurrence of atrial flutter.

Note that atrial flutter begins with an atrial premature contraction. An important feature is that the APC is closer to the preceding normal beat than are those atrial premature contractions in the previous tracing. The sequence demonstrates a general principle: the greater the degree of prematurity of an ectopic beat, the more likely it is to induce a repetitive ectopic rhythm. This principle will be presented in subsequent examples.

Treatment of atrial flutter with electrical shock.

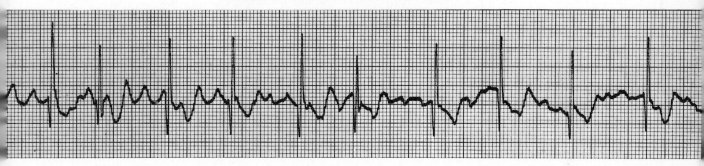

Atrial flutter with variable A-V conduction is evident. The flutter rate is also somewhat variable (check with calipers).

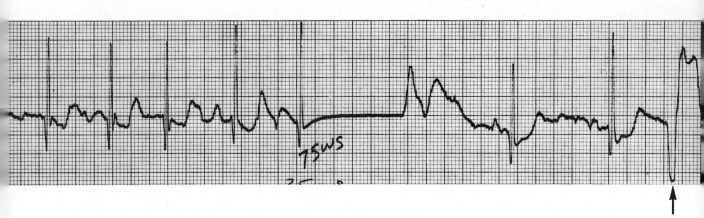

Precordial shock of 75 watts per second is applied. Normal sinus rhythm appears after the period of electrical blackout, but a beat from an excited ventricular focus (arrow) occurs.

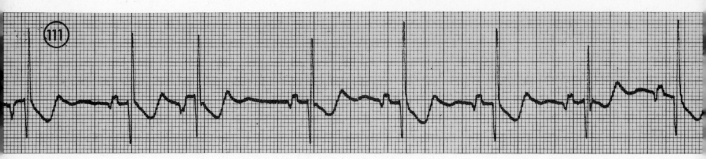

Following an atrial premature contraction (locate _____), stable normal sinus rhythm then supervenes.

Atrial Fibrillation

The atrial mass may react to more than 500 impulses per minute, completing each depolarization-repolarization cycle in time to respond to the ensuing impulse. However, an atrial ectopic focus may discharge impulses so rapidly that portions of the atria have not recovered from one depolarization wave when the next wave arrives. At extremely rapid atrial rates, minute areas of atrial tissue at any given moment are in various stages of depolarization and repolarization. The cardiodynamic result is complete disorder in which uncoordinated activity of the atria gives small contraction-relaxation events at innumerable sites, and effective muscular propulsion movement is abolished. This rhythm is **atrial fibrillation.**

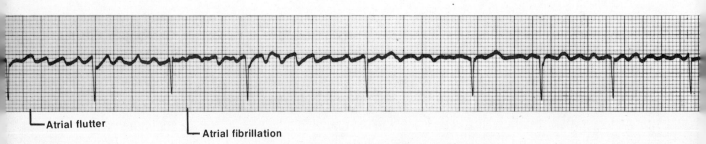

Atrial flutter

Atrial fibrillation

Transitional atrial flutter – atrial fibrillation pattern.

In places, typical atrial flutter appears to be present. In others, atrial activity is completely disorganized, as is characteristic in atrial fibrillation. Gradation between the two can be observed. This rhythm pattern is often referred to as **atrial flutter-fibrillation.**

Atrial fibrillation in the electrocardiogram is represented by continuous, irregular undulations of the baseline. Well-defined, small atrial complexes are termed f waves; these often cannot be clearly distinguished because of the electrical complexity throughout.

In the following examples of atrial fibrillation, determine the average rate using the three beat ruler and the three second interval markings; then compare.

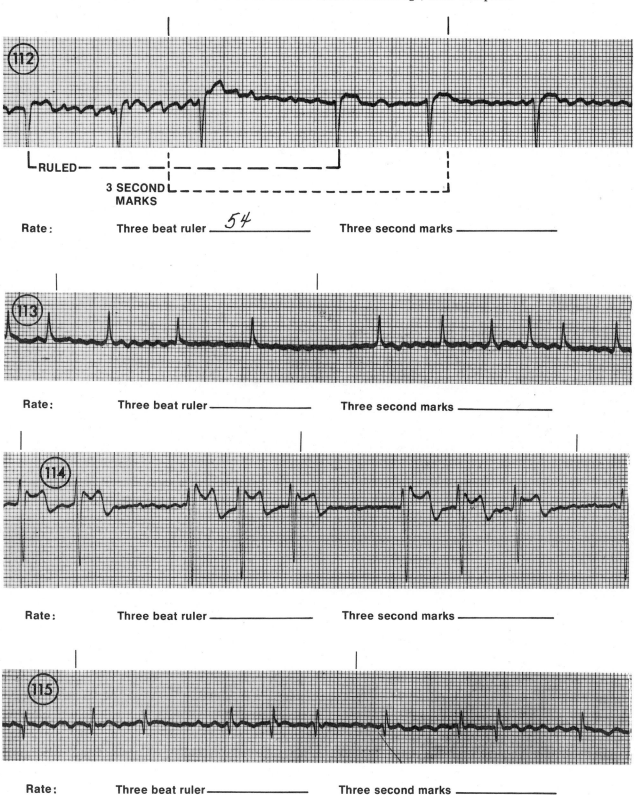

Rate: Three beat ruler ___54___ Three second marks _____

Rate: Three beat ruler _____ Three second marks _____

Rate: Three beat ruler _____ Three second marks _____

Rate: Three beat ruler _____ Three second marks _____

It is evident from the previous comparisons that rate determination in irregular rhythms is quite variable and depends upon the method used and the site selected for measurement.

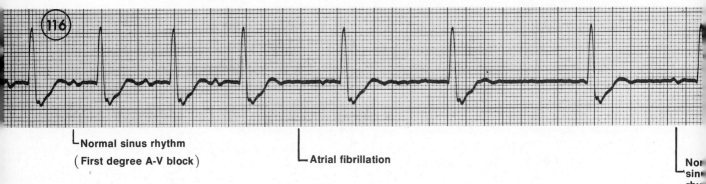

Normal sinus rhythm
(First degree A-V block)   Atrial fibrillation   Nor
                                                                                                      sin
                                                                                                      rhy

Example of a transitory period of atrial fibrillation.

Determine the rates: sinus _____
                     atrial fibrillation _____ (average)

Note the sudden change to an irregular rate and the similarity of the ventricular components of the two rhythm forms.

The mechanism for atrial fibrillation with its intricate electrical events is not fully understood. This arrhythmia appears to be related to atrial tachycardia and flutter, but having such extreme rapidity of atrial impulses that their orderly propagation disintegrates. The occasionally seen transition of atrial flutter to atrial fibrillation (or vice versa) suggests that these rhythms share a common mechanism.

TABLE 6.   Summary of Atrial Fibrillation

	Physiological Events	ECG Representation
Atria	1. Extremely rapid atrial excitation in uncoordinated sequences	Continuous uneven baseline activity
A-V Node	2. Overload of irregular atrial impulses; random transmission	Physiological A-V block
Ventricles	3. Irregular ventricular activation, though usual ventricular pathways	QRS complexes of usual configuration, appearing at irregular intervals.

The ventricles appear to respond randomly to the extremely rapid assault of f waves upon the A-V nodal system. In fact, irregularity of the ventricular rate is a hallmark of atrial fibrillation. The most common ventricular rate response in untreated atrial fibrillation is about 150 to 180 per minute, but this is quite variable. The intervals between beats allow differences in diastolic filling of the ventricles, especially at rapid rates. Cardiac output varies between beats, so that the force of the peripheral pulse is quite variable. Some of the weaker pulses may not be felt; this is especially true for rapid rates. The radial pulse deficit in atrial fibrillation is largely due to changes in pulsatile force, and a large discrepancy between apparent and real cardiac rate may be present. (For this reason the pulse rate of patients with atrial fibrillation should be taken by auscultation of the precordium or from the cardiac monitor, rather than by radial artery.)

The ventricular rate in atrial fibrillation should be expressed as an estimated average because of the marked irregularity usually present. The three beat ruler is preferable, and a portion of the electrocardiogram is selected which appears to have both slow and rapid ventricular beats. The ventricular rate may be given in general terms using the following criteria:

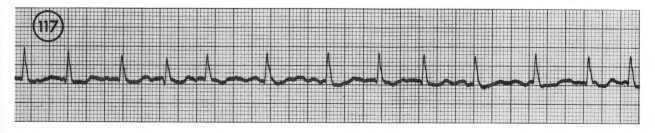

Rate = _____

Atrial fibrillation with rapid ventricular rate response (ventricular rate greater than 100).

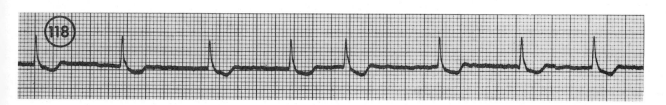

Rate = _____

Atrial fibrillation with moderate ventricular rate response (ventricular rate 60 to 100).

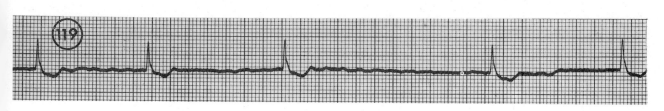

Rate = _____

Atrial fibrillation with slow ventricular rate response (ventricular rate less than 60).

The character of the f waves may be coarse or fine, but intermediary patterns are commonly present. It appears that coarse f waves are more common in atrial fibrillation of recent onset, but they become fine (and perhaps more rapid) as the arrhythmia is sustained over months and years.

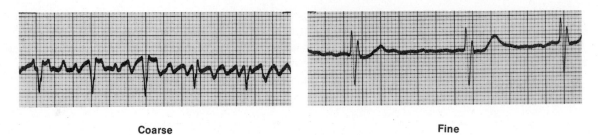

Coarse   Fine

Patterns of atrial fibrillation.

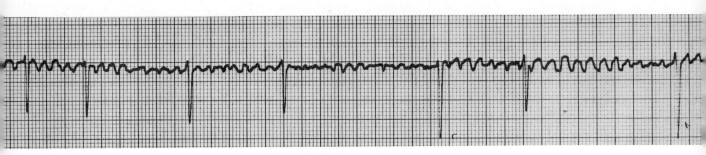

Atrial fibrillation with changing atrial pattern.

Note the transitions between coarse and fine atrial fibrillation.

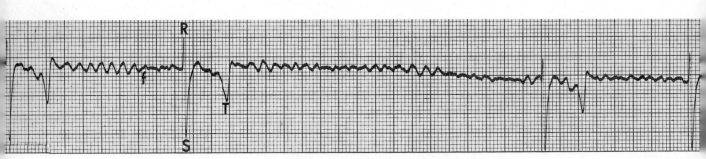

Example of coarse atrial fibrillation.

This electrocardiogram was taken from a three-year-old racehorse which was otherwise completely healthy. Atrial fibrillation is fairly common in the horse, in which the resting rate is relatively slow, but which usually speeds up markedly on exercise. Even in normal sinus rhythm, the resting heart rate is 28 to 30 beats per minute.

The ventricular rate in atrial fibrillation may be altered by changing the electrical resistance to impulse transmission in the A-V node. As in atrial tachycardia and atrial flutter, increasing parasympathetic tone will retard transmission frequency, thereby decelerating the ventricular rate. This is demonstrated in the following tracings using maneuvers which enhance vagal tone.

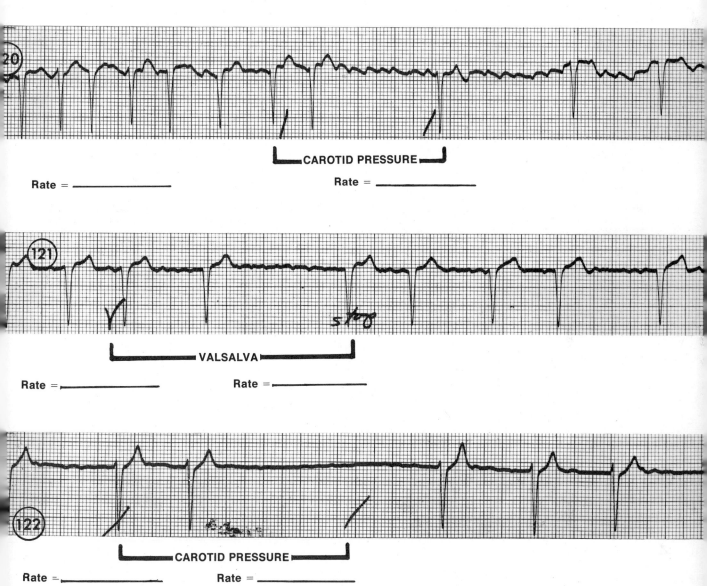

Rate = _____   Rate = _____
CAROTID PRESSURE

Rate =_____   Rate =_____
VALSALVA

Rate =_____   Rate = _____
CAROTID PRESSURE

The atria do not have an effective pumping action when fibrillating. Blood is not forcefully propelled into the ventricles from the atria but rather flows passively during the phase of ventricular relaxation. While synchronized atrial contractions are not an essential element of cardiac performance, they do augment overall cardiac output. Their contribution becomes more significant as the heart rate accelerates. The goal of therapy in atrial fibrillation is either to convert it to sinus rhythm or to maintain the ventricular response at a moderate rate.

Treatment of Atrial Fibrillation with Drugs

Drugs can be used to treat atrial fibrillation by:
1. *Conversion to normal sinus rhythm*: Drugs of depression, such as quinidine and procainamide, have been used extensively for this purpose. Relatively large doses are usually required for conversion, and toxic effects often appear.

2. *Slowing of ventricular rate:* This may be accomplished by increasing vagal tone, which in turn decreases the frequency with which atrial impulses are conducted through the A-V node. Digitalis is commonly given for this purpose. Propranolol, which has a direct suppressive action on conduction in the A-V node, also tends to slow the ventricular rate response.

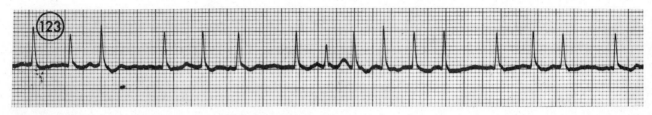

Rate = _____ (3 Beat Ruler)

Before digitalis.

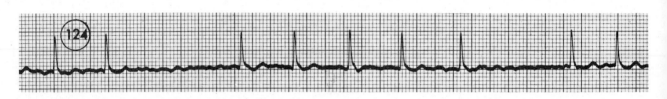

Rate = _____ (3 Beat Ruler)

After digitalis.

The accompanying clinical series is taken from an 82-year-old woman with congestive heart failure. Compare the rates and note progressive response to digitalis.

12/25 — 1:15 PM   Atrial fibrillation with rapid ventricular rate.

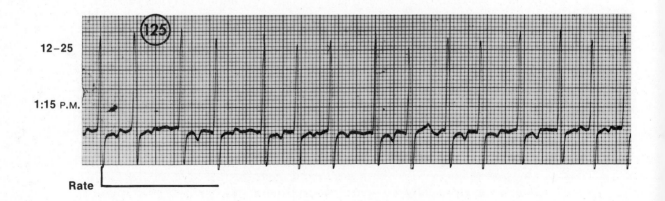

12-25

1:15 P.M.

Rate

4:00 PM   After digitalis, the ventricular rate has decreased somewhat.

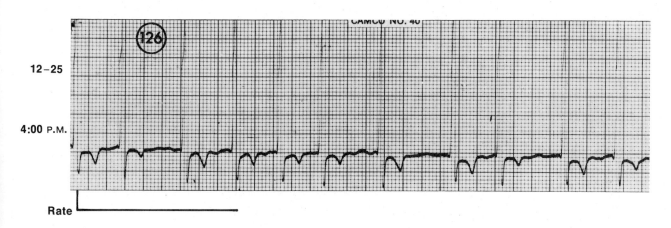

10:00 PM   With additive doses of digitalis, the ventricular rate has slowed further. Symptoms and signs of congestive heart failure have improved significantly (by the drug's effect on both myocardial contractility and rate slowing).

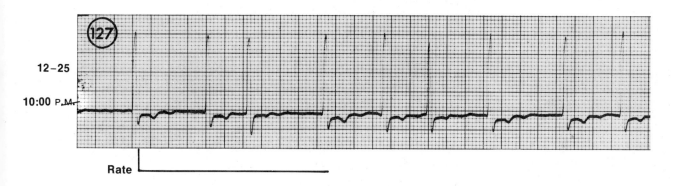

12/26— 2:30 AM   Digitalis effect is now very prominent as ventricular rate has become too slow. Note that some ventricular complexes are markedly widened and the terminal portion of the QRS disfigured; this represents a delay in forces of late depolarization. Excessive depression of impulse transmission in the A-V node and conduction velocity in the Purkinje system may be considered toxic effects of digitalis.

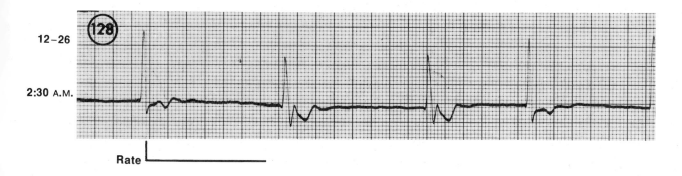

12/27 — 10:00 AM   After discontinuing digitalis for one day, the ventricular rate has again become rapid. Electrocardioversion is then performed after administration of quinidine to stabilize the atrial rhythm.

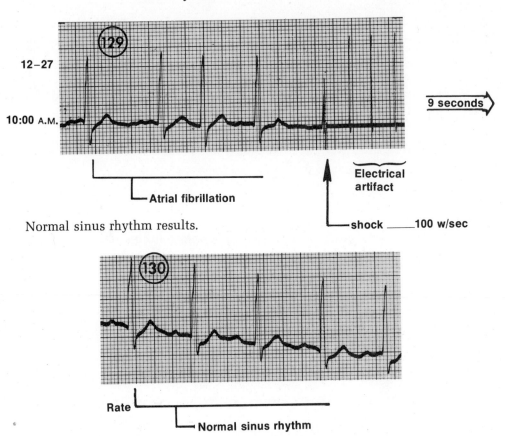

Normal sinus rhythm results.

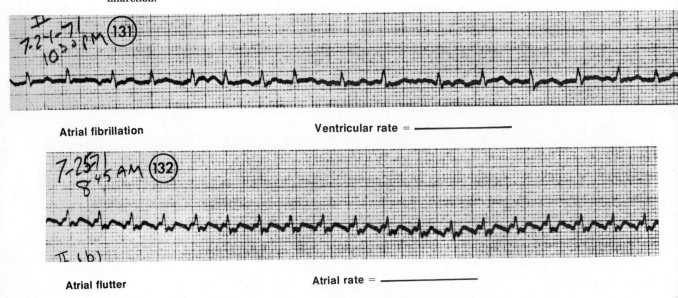

Rhythms of atrial excitation: sequential changes in an 83-year-old woman with an acute myocardial infarction.

Atrial fibrillation   Ventricular rate = _____

Atrial flutter   Atrial rate = _____

          Ventricular rate = _____

Note the 2:1 A-V block with a constant PR interval of conducted beats.
7/25/71—9:30 AM: digitalis started.

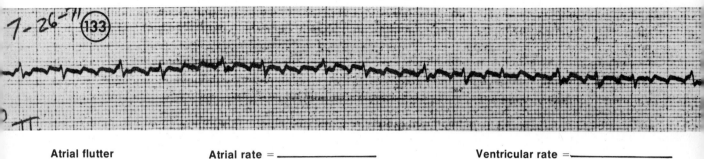

Atrial flutter   Atrial rate = _____   Ventricular rate =_____

The A-V ratio is now variable, and the F-R interval of conducted beats is inconstant. This change in A-V conduction may be due to the faster atrial rate and to the vagotonic effect of digitalis.

Response of atrial fibrillation to digitalis in a 54-year-old woman admitted with congestive heart failure.

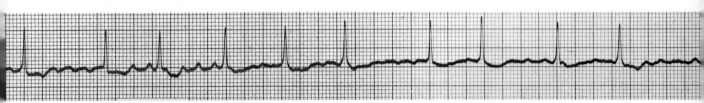

Atrial fibrillation with a moderate ventricular rate response is evident. The fibrillatory pattern is coarse at times and has an appearance of flutter.

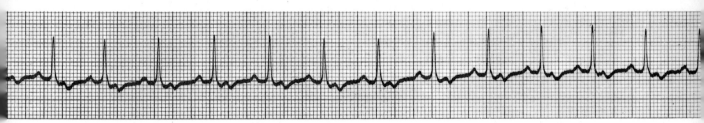

After administration of digitalis, atrial flutter with a 2:1 A-V block has supervened. The flutter rate has slowed considerably compared with the previous tracing. (This is an unpredictable response to digitalis.)

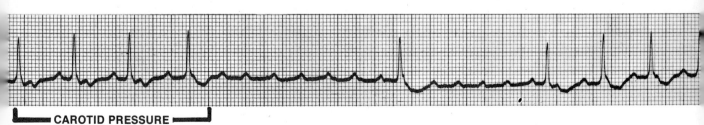

◄━ CAROTID PRESSURE ━►

Carotid pressure induces marked A-V block with a ratio of 8:1 in the initial period. The rhythm converted to normal sinus rhythm shortly after this tracing was made.

The ventricular rate increases with adrenergic stimulation. This sequence was recorded from a 79-year-old woman with atrial fibrillation. A rapid ventricular rate response was difficult to control on digitalis alone, so she was given propranolol in addition. Both agents suppress conduction in the A-V node. The day after starting this latter medication, the woman, on first arising, suddenly blacked out, losing consciousness momentarily. An electrocardiogram obtained within three minutes after onset revealed marked bradycardia.

11:45 AM: Atrial fibrillation with an extremely slow ventricular rate response is evident.

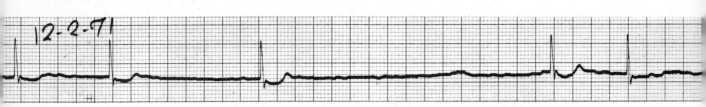

11:52 AM: Intravenous infusion of isoproterenol is started. This agent accelerates conduction velocity in the A-V node.

11:57 AM: Atrial fibrillation with moderate ventricular rate response is evident. By this time, the patient had returned to a fully alert state.

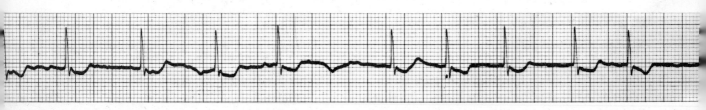

Increase of ventricular rate by parasympathetic block.

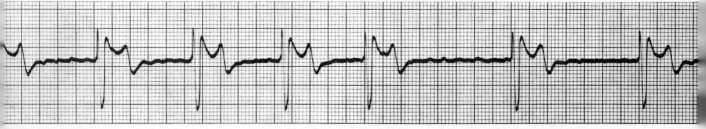

9:12 AM: Atrial fibrillation with excessively slow ventricular rate response (approximately 55 per minute) is evident.

9:15 AM: Atropine, 1 mg I.V., is administered. This agent blocks the inhibiting effect of the vagus nerve on A-V conduction velocity.

9:17 AM: Atrial fibrillation with more rapid ventricular rate response (approximately 78 per minute) is evident.

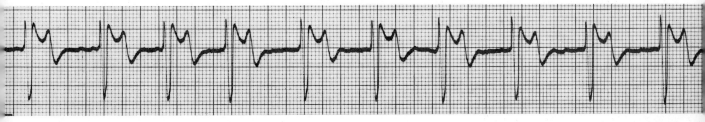

Electrocardioversion of Atrial Fibrillation

Application of this technique is identical to that used in atrial tachycardia and atrial flutter.

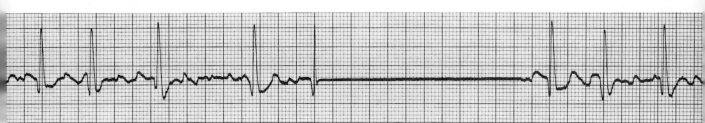

Atrial fibrillation: test electrical shock.

The basic rhythm is coarse atrial fibrillation and could even be designated atrial flutter with irregularity of flutter rate. The test shock of 8 watts per second (patient not connected to output system) demonstrates that the discharge is synchronous with the R spike of QRS. Having proved that the time of firing is satisfactory, the operator applies paddles to the chest.

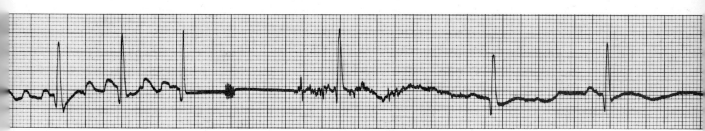

Atrial fibrillation: effective electrical shock.

After an electrical shock of 75 watts per second, sinus bradycardia emerges. Note that the actual shock occurs precisely in the QRS complex, as did that of the test shock.

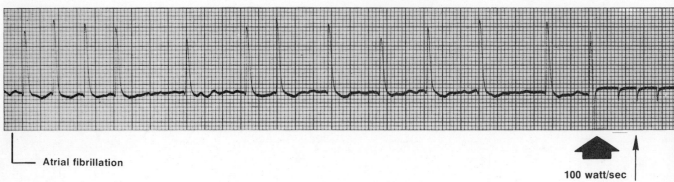

Atrial fibrillation

100 watt/sec

Machine artifact

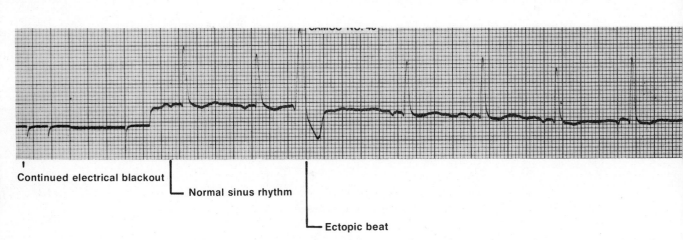

Continued electrical blackout

Normal sinus rhythm

Ectopic beat

Another example of atrial fibrillation treated with electrical shock.

By means of electrocardioversion, atrial fibrillation changes to NSR. An ectopic beat illustrates the transient rhythm instability which often follows the electric shock.

SELF-EVALUATION: STAGE 1

Label each tracing completely: components, rate, rhythm(s).

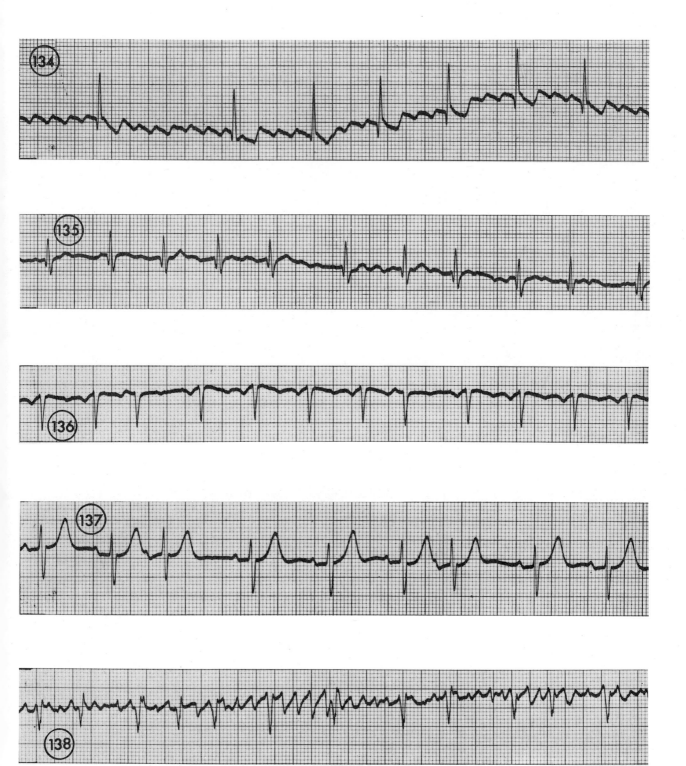

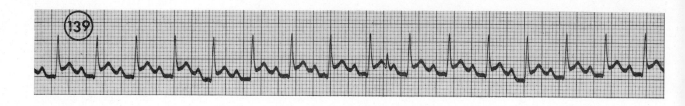

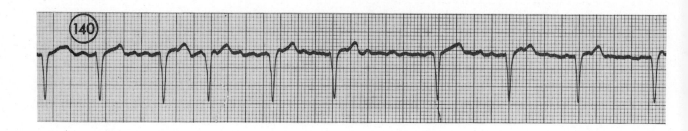

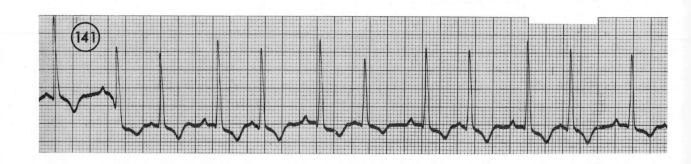

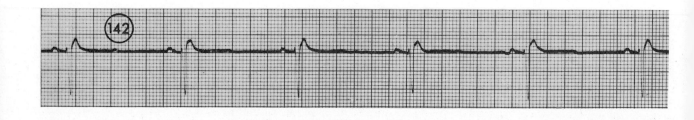

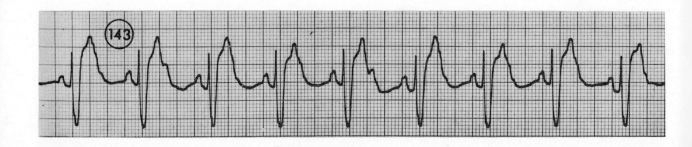

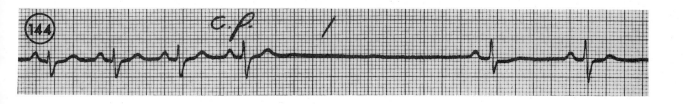

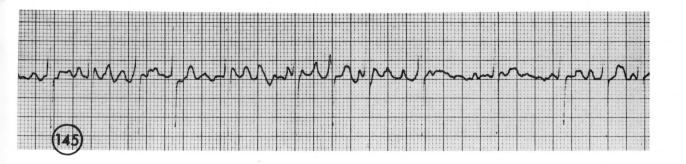

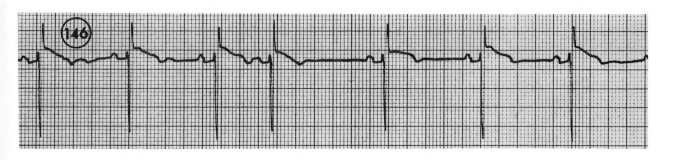

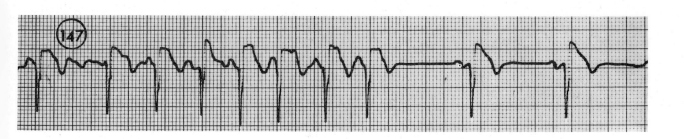

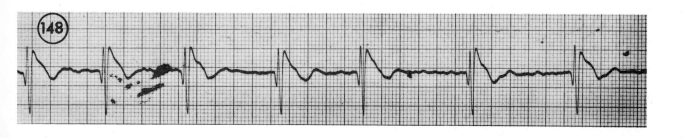

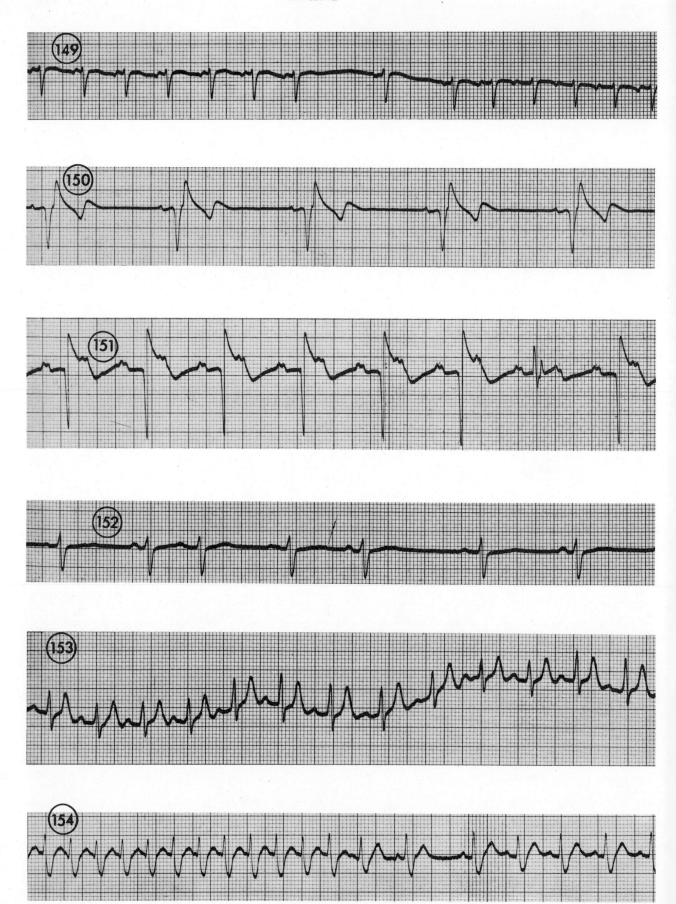

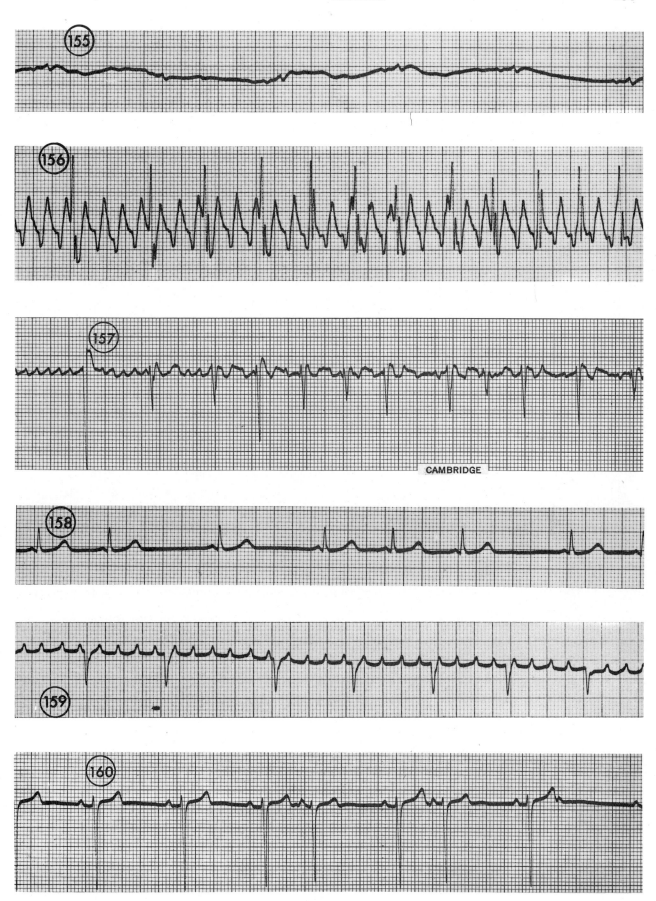

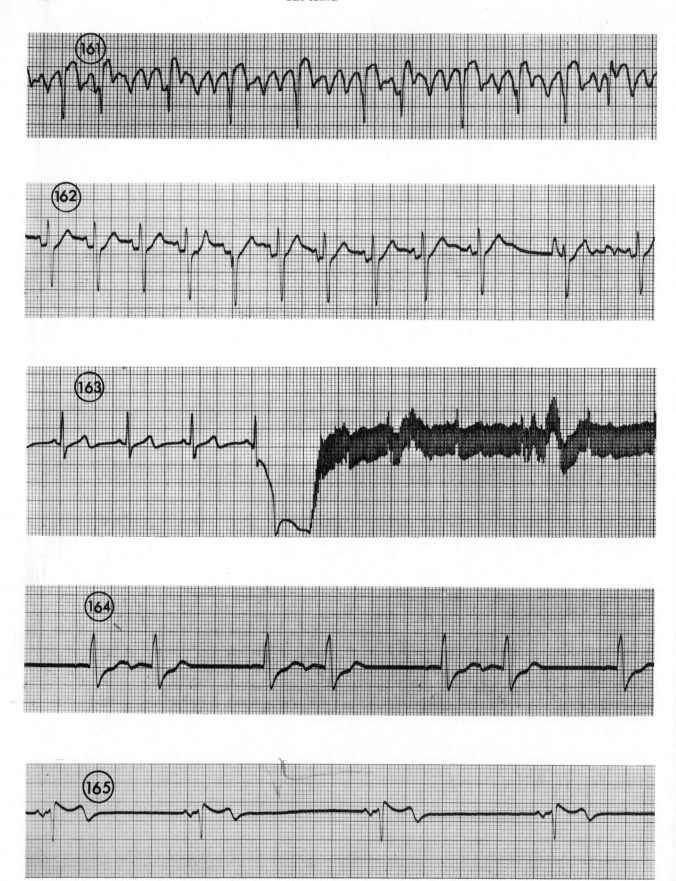

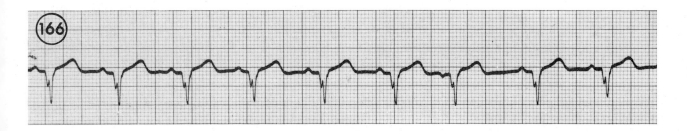

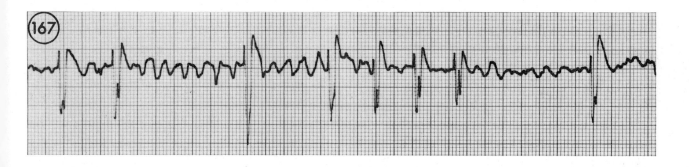

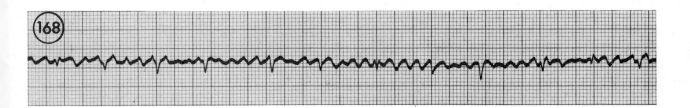

Chapter 5

THE ATRIOVENTRICULAR NODE

Impulses conveyed from the atria to the conduction system of the ventricles pass through the atrioventricular node. Impulse conduction velocity in this dense network of conduction fibers is relatively slow compared with other cardiac conduction fibers. This retardation of depolarizing forces has two distinct advantages in overall cardiac function:

1. Atrial contraction is completed before ventricular contraction begins. This allows more efficient emptying of atrial chambers and closure of the atrioventricular valves.
2. The ventricles are protected against the excessively rapid impulses generated in atrial tachycardia, flutter, and fibrillation.

The depolarization of the A-V node is electrically silent in the standard electrocardiogram because of the small amount of energy discharged. Recordings taken by intracardiac techniques reveal that conduction velocity in the A-V node is approximately one tenth that of the atria. This period is represented by an isoelectric line on the electrocardiogram which comprises the second portion of the PR interval. The PR interval begins with the onset of atrial depolarization and ends with the initial deflection of the QRS complex. (See figure at top of following page.)

The PR interval is normally from 0.12 to 0.20 second in duration. Some individuals without detectable heart disease exceed these limits. Nevertheless, for clinical work, it is important to memorize this range, and to consider intervals beyond it as deviations from normal. (See figure at bottom of following page.)

The natural resistance of conduction in the A-V node may be altered by physiological or pathological factors. Aberrant pathways cause accelerated conduction in the pre-excitation syndrome. Depression of A-V node conduction velocity leads to the various A-V nodal blocks. The autonomic nervous system exerts continuous extracardiac influences on conduction velocity at this relay center.

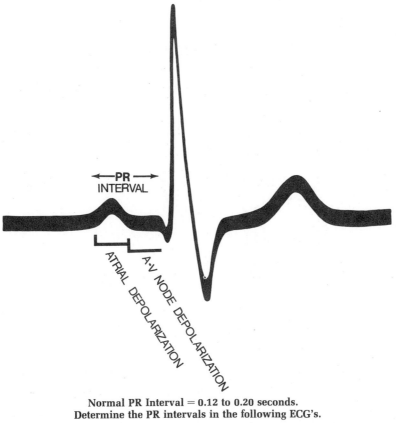

Normal PR Interval = 0.12 to 0.20 seconds.
Determine the PR intervals in the following ECG's.

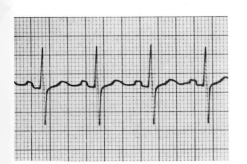

PR interval = _.14 sec._

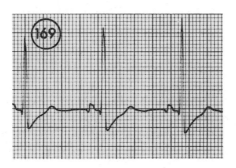

PR interval = _____

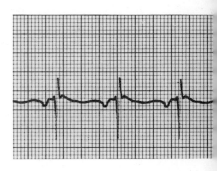

PR interval = _.12 sec._

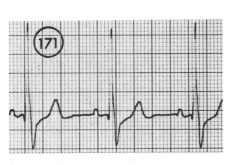

PR interval = _____

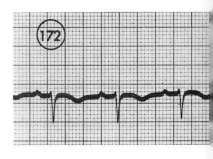

PR interval = _____

A-V NODE: IMPULSE CONDUCTION

Excitation

PES = Pre-excitation syndrome.

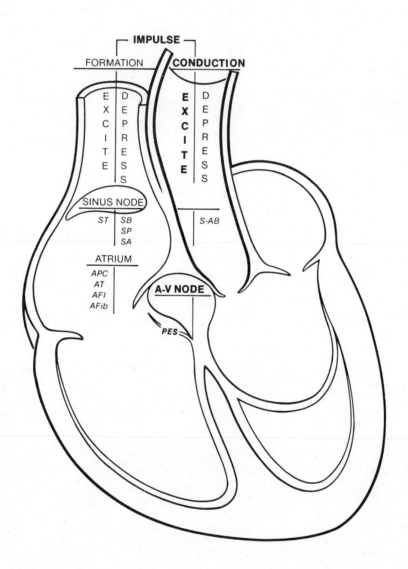

Pre-Excitation Syndrome

Pre-excitation syndrome (PES) refers to a rather uncommon congenital anomaly of conduction at the A-V node. Atrial impulses are transmitted to the ventricles at an accelerated rate, avoiding the normal conduction delay in the A-V node. It appears, from considerable experimental evidence, that conduction fibers near the A-V node operate as accessory pathways for impulse transmission, thereby short-circuiting the A-V node itself. This results in premature activation of the ventricles.

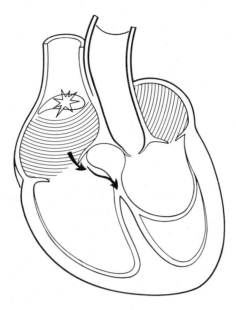

The electrocardiogram in the pre-excitation syndrome has the following characteristic features:

1. The PR interval is less than 0.10 second. This shortening of the PR interval represents early activation of the ventricles through aberrant conduction pathways which by-pass the A-V node.
2. The first portion of the QRS complex is distorted. Ventricular depolarization is initiated from an abnormal direction, producing a relatively slow moving, early QRS deflection, termed the **delta wave.**

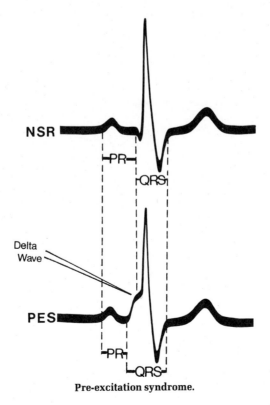

Pre-excitation syndrome.

The normal cardiac cycle is compared with that of pre-excitation. Note the delta wave produced by anomalous conduction around the A-V node and the resultant shortening of the PR interval and lengthening of the QRS complex. This alteration occurs at the junction of these two components. Also note that the P wave and central and terminal portions of the QRS complex remain normal.

K. F. is a 26-year-old man with typical electrocardiographic evidence of pre-excitation syndrome. Selected leads from the standard electrocardiogram are shown.

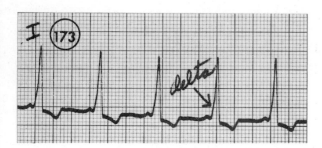

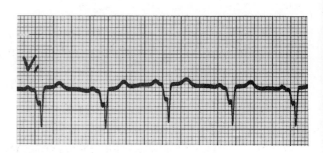

Rhythm = _____ Rate = _____ PR interval = _____

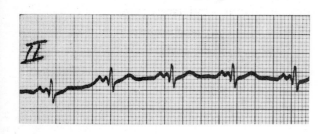

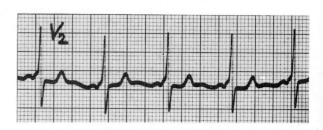

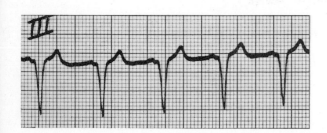

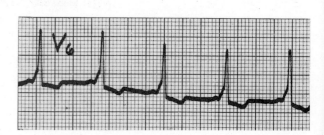

Determine: 1. Pacemaker = _____

2. Rate = _____

3. PR interval = _____

Mark the delta wave in each lead where discernible.

In 1930 Louis Wolff, John Parkinson, and Paul D. White published details on 11 cases of this anomaly in a communication entitled "Bundle-Branch Block with Short PR Interval in Healthy Young People Prone to Paroxysmal Tachycardia."* The pre-excitation phenomenon has since been commonly referred to by the eponym Wolff-Parkinson-White (or WPW) syndrome. Two illustrations from their original publication are presented.

A pre-excitation pattern is recorded following an episode of palpitations in a 21-year-old man.

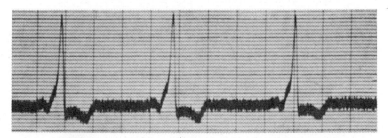

(Reproduced from Wolff, L., Parkinson, J., and White, P. D.: Bundle-branch block with short P-R interval in healthy young people prone to paroxysmal tachycardia. Amer. Heart J., 5:691, 1930, with permission.)

The transition from pre-excitation pattern to normal A-V conduction and ventricular activation was recorded in a 16-year-old boy with a history of attacks of tachycardia while playing football.

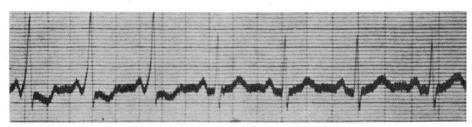

(Reproduced from Wolff, L., Parkinson, J., and White, P. D.: Bundle-branch block with short P-R interval in healthy young people prone to paroxysmal tachycardia. Amer. Heart J., 5: 693, 1930, with permission.)

*Amer. Heart J., Vol. V, No. 6, August, 1930, p. 691.

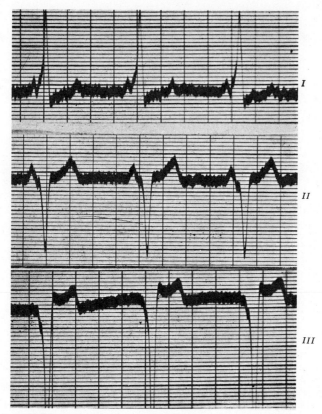

I

II

III

(Reproduced from Wolff, L., Parkinson, J., and White, P. D.: Bundle-branch block with short P-R interval in healthy young people prone to paroxysmal tachycardia. Amer. Heart J., 5:700, 1930, with permission.)

This electrocardiogram appeared in the original publication by Wolff, Parkinson, and White on the pre-excitation syndrome, then referred to as an intraventricular conduction defect with a short PR interval. This example was taken from a 44-year-old widow, first examined in 1927. She had experienced attacks of palpitations since age 7. These episodes "lasted from a few minutes to several hours (intermittently) and were easily terminated by taking a deep breath and holding it, or by lying down." An electrocardiogram taken later, during an attack, revealed "auricular paroxysmal tachycardia at a rate of 230."

The pre-excitation pattern may be continuous or intermittent. Rarely, it appears in brief succession and even in isolated beats. Increasing vagal tone may shift normal A-V node transmission to anomalous pathways in susceptible persons.

The following tracing from a 37-year-old man was recorded with a magnetic tape recording of the cardiac rhythm over ten hours. The electrocardiogram was then reproduced from the tape.

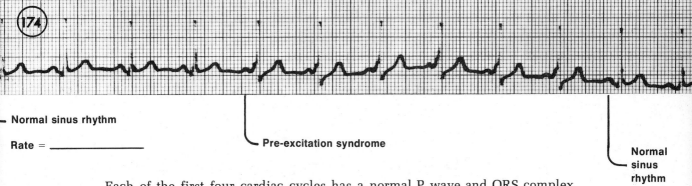

— **Normal sinus rhythm**

Rate = _____

Pre-excitation syndrome

Normal sinus rhythm

Each of the first four cardiac cycles has a normal P wave and QRS complex configuration and a normal PR interval. PR interval = _____ seconds

In the fifth cardiac cycle, the PR interval is drastically shorter. PR interval = _____ seconds

Particularly note the slurring of the initial portion of the QRS complex, the delta wave. This abnormal sequence repeats itself up to the tenth cardiac cycle; then the original ECG pattern is resumed.

The most important clinical feature of pre-excitation syndrome is the associated high frequency of cardiac arrhythmias. Impulses transmitted from the atria to the ventricles through this anomalous route tend to turn back, returning to the atria through the A-V node or along the accessory fibers themselves. Thus the atria may be stimulated a second time by the same impulse.

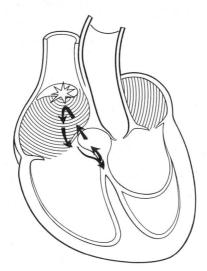

Re-entry phenomenon.

This atrial **re-entry phenomenon** appears to be responsible for the increased incidence of atrial premature contractions and sustained rhythms of atrial excitation in persons with pre-excitation syndrome. While some individuals remain entirely asymptomatic, others are severely incapacitated by recurring atrial tachycardia, flutter, or fibrillation.

Drug therapy for the prevention and control of recurring paroxysmal tachycardia in pre-excitation syndrome is directed at selective blocking of impulse conduction through the accessory pathways or at least inhibiting the retrograde conduction, while causing minimal interference with normally directed A-V conduction. Digitalis, quinidine, procainamide, and most recently propranolol have been used with varying degrees of success, but their effects on the pre-excitation phenomenon are unpredictable. In some intractable cases, a surgical approach in which the region of accessory pathways was severed has been beneficial.

Label the following examples.

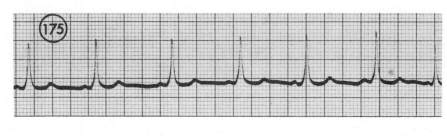

Rate = _____   PR interval = _____

Indicate the delta wave.

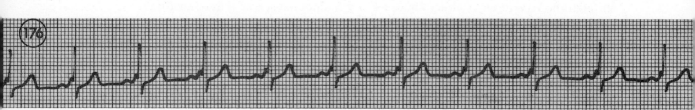

Rate = _____   PR interval = _____

Indicate the delta wave.

TABLE 7.   Summary of Pre-Excitation Syndrome

Cardiac Sequence	Mechanism	ECG
1. Sinus impulse	Normal	—
2. Atrial depolarization	Normal	Normal P wave
3. A-V node accessory pathways	Relatively rapid conduction, skirting the A-V nodal system	Short PR interval (less than 0.10 sec)
4. Ventricular depolarization	One ventricle activated early	Initial QRS slurred (delta wave) (∴ widened QRS)
5. Retrograde conduction from ventricles to atria	Atria re-entry impulse	Tendency to supraventricular paroxysmal arrhythmias

A-V NODE: IMPULSE CONDUCTION

Depression

1° = First degree A-V block
2° = Second degree A-V block
3° = Third degree A-V block

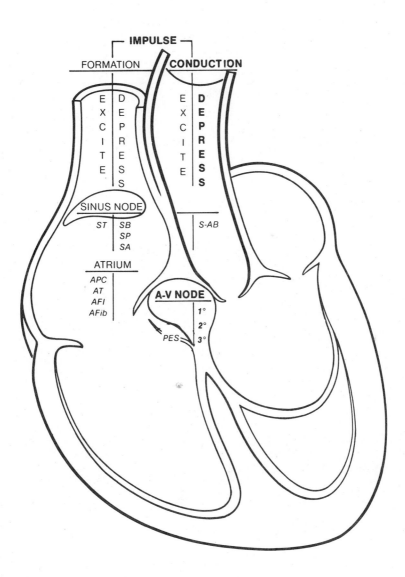

First Degree A-V Block

First degree A-V block (1°) refers to simple prolongation of the PR interval, representing *delayed* conduction velocity through the A-V node.

First degree A-V block = PR interval greater than 0.20 second.

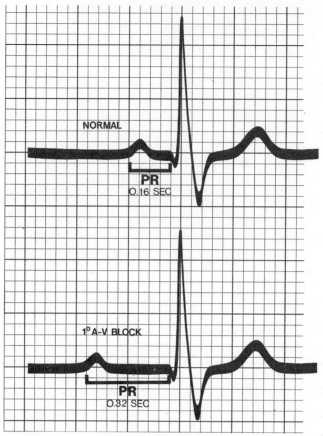

NORMAL

PR
0.16 SEC

1° A-V BLOCK

PR
0.32 SEC

First degree A-V block.

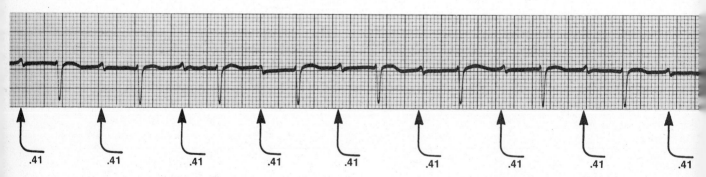

.41   .41   .41   .41   .41   .41   .41   .41   .41

First degree A-V block may result from disease within the A-V node (ischemia, infarction) or from infections (rheumatic fever, myocarditis). Patients in the CCU who develop delayed A-V conduction velocity should be observed with particular attention for progressive rhythms of depression. Increased parasympathetic tone will slow conduction velocity in the area. Activities and drugs which intensify vagal stimulation may exaggerate the A-V conduction defect.

In the following examples of first degree A-V block, identify the components, determine the cardiac rate, and measure the PR intervals.

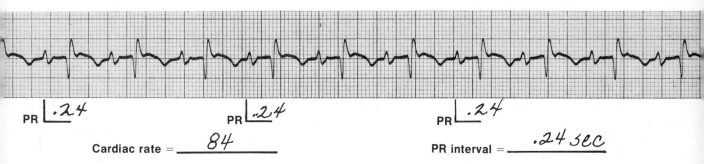

PR └.24   PR └.24   PR └.24

Cardiac rate = _____84_____   PR interval = ___.24 sec___

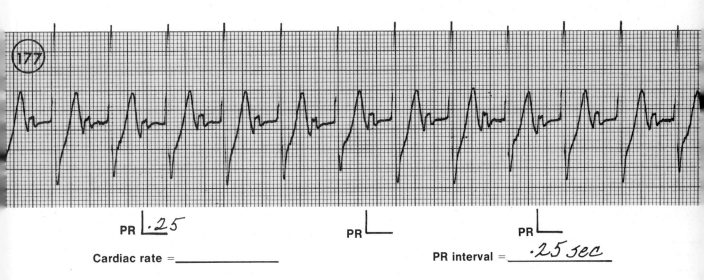

(177)

PR └.25   PR └_   PR └_

Cardiac rate = _____   PR interval = __.25 sec__

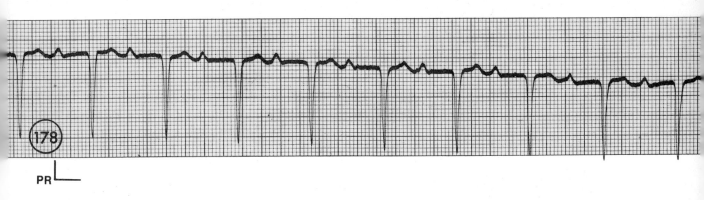

(178)

PR └_

Cardiac rate = _____   PR interval = _____

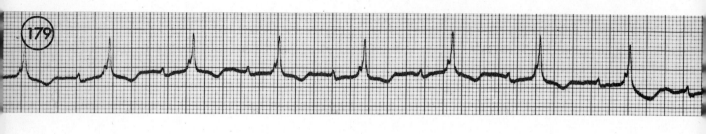

Cardiac rate = _____   **PR interval =** _____

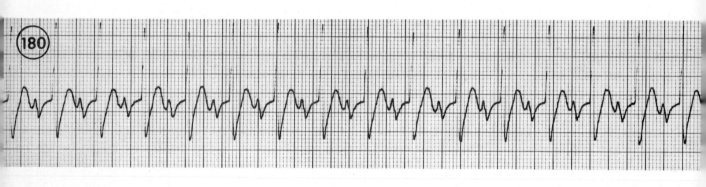

Cardiac rate = _____   **PR interval =** _____

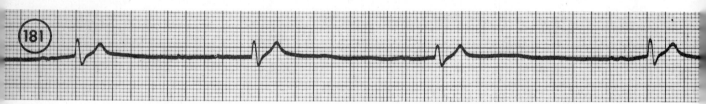

Cardiac rate = _____   **PR interval =** _____

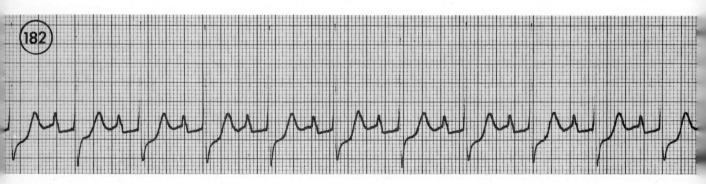

Cardiac rate = _____   **PR interval =** _____

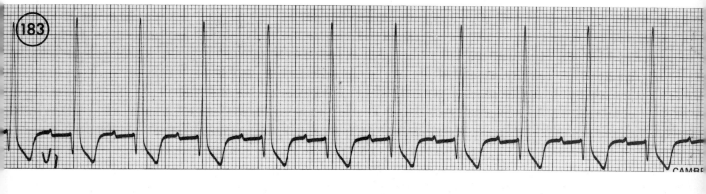

Cardiac rate = _____   PR interval = _____

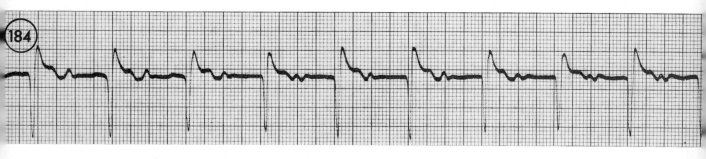

Cardiac rate = _____   PR interval = _____

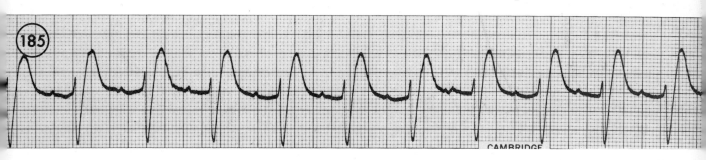

Cardiac rate = _____   PR interval = _____

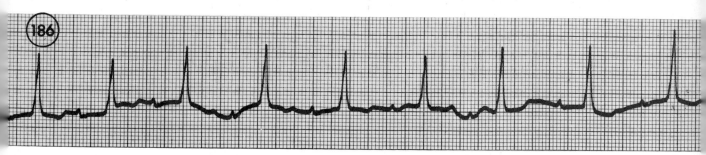

Cardiac rate = _____   PR interval = _____

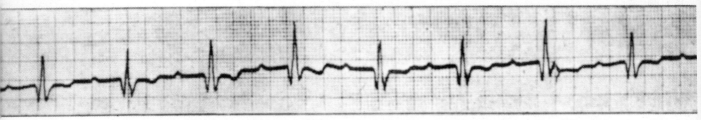

First degree A-V block in a 54-year-old man in Cape Town, South Africa. (Reproduced from New York Daily News, January 22, 1968, with permission of The Associated Press.)

This is an historic electrocardiogram which appeared in the headlines of the *New York Daily News* on January 22, 1968, following the first human heart homo-transplantation.

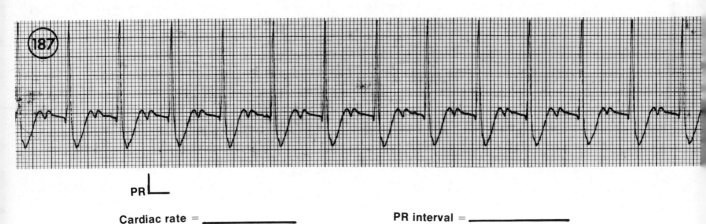

PR └─

Cardiac rate = _____   PR interval = _____

P waves occur so close to the T wave of a preceding beat that they may appear as a complex T wave form. The more angular appearance and the absence of a P wave elsewhere help to identify them.

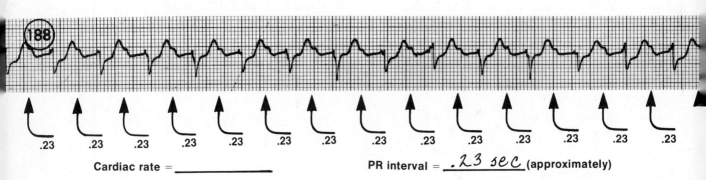

.23   .23   .23   .23   .23   .23   .23   .23   .23   .23   .23   .23   .23   .23

Cardiac rate = _____   PR interval = *.23 sec* (approximately)

In this example of T-P combined waves, the PR interval cannot be accurately measured because the initial portion of the P wave is obscured.

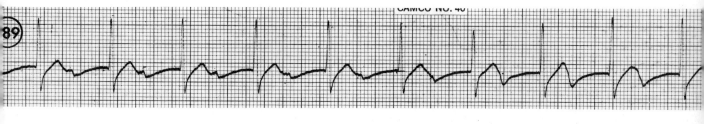

Cardiac rate = _____   **PR interval** = _____

P waves are more positively identified in this tracing. Slight changes in rate alter the timing relationship between T and P waves. As rate increases, the P waves appear further "into" the previous T wave, causing changes in the terminal T wave form and in the shape of the T wave peak. Thus, at the faster rate, P wave and T wave peaks are more closely superimposed. As rate slows again, the P waves occur relatively later and emerge from the previous T wave.

Depression of conduction velocity in the A-V node may be treated with drugs with excitatory effects on impulse conduction:

1. Sympathetic stimulators (catecholamine agents, e.g., isoproterenol)
2. Parasympathetic inhibitors (vagal blocking agents, e.g., atropine)

These drugs of excitation will tend to shorten the PR interval and may correct first degree A-V block, or at least decrease it. In the CCU, control of the conduction delay may prevent development of higher degrees of block in an unstable conducting system. Isoproterenol is often satisfactory since the effective dose can be carefully controlled with intravenous infusions.

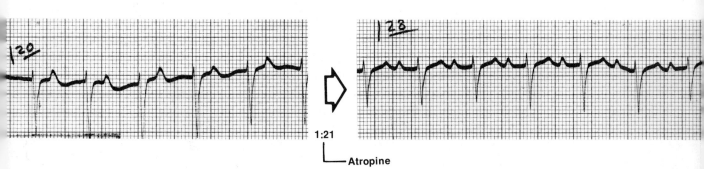

1:21

└─ Atropine

First degree A-V block revealed with parasympathetic block.

1:20 PM: The rhythm appears to be of nodal origin. However, on comparing each T wave, a slight change in form can be seen, suggesting that P and T waves may be superimposed.

1:21 PM: Atropine was given at this time to test this possibility.

1:28 PM: First degree A-V block is now obvious with a PR interval of 0.22 second (estimated initially as 0.36 second). The P wave has "moved out" of the T wave (note decreased T amplitude) as conduction velocity is increased in the A-V node. Interestingly, there has been *no* change in *rate* of sinus impulse formation.

By definition, each sinus impulse in first degree A-V block eventually leads to ventricular depolarization, regardless of the severity of delay in A-V conduction time. This *complete* penetration of all sinus beats through the A-V node differentiates first degree A-V block from the more severe degrees of conduction disturbances.

In first degree A-V block, the magnitude of the conduction delay has much clinical significance. Therefore, an informative description of the arrhythmia should include either the actual length of the PR interval or an expression of the severity of the slowing of A-V conduction. The table below provides arbitrary limits for grading first degree A-V block.

TABLE 8

	PR Interval	Grade
Normal	0.12 — 0.20 second	
First Degree A-V Block	0.21 — 0.24 second	Slight
	0.25 — 0.29 second	Moderate
	0.30 second or over	Severe

Conduction velocity may be so severely depressed in the A-V node that some of the sinus impulses fail to penetrate the A-V node. This results in intermittent absence of ventricular depolarization from a sinus beat, a condition termed **second degree A-V block.**

Second Degree A-V Block

Depression of impulse conduction in the A-V node and the major pathways may result in the failure of some of the sinus beats to penetrate the ventricles. This is known as **second degree** or **intermittent A-V block.**

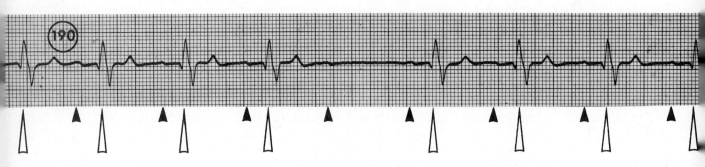

Basic rhythm: normal sinus rhythm (rate = _____) with prolongation of A-V conduction (PR interval = _____ sec).

Sinus beat No. 5 occurs at the expected time, but no QRS complex or T wave follows. The sinus impulse is blocked, and the ventricular beat is dropped.

Sinus beat No. 6 is conducted, and the basic sinus rhythm is resumed without interruption of cadence.

Diagnosis = second degree or intermittent A-V block.

The pre-existing prolonged PR interval suggests an adverse factor operating in the A-V node relay system. It can be appreciated that a further delay in conduction velocity beyond a critical level may result in dissipation of the impulse somewhere in the conduction pathways, and no effective ventricular stimulation will follow.

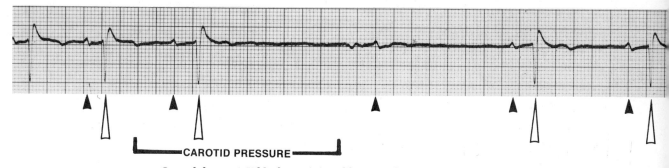

Second degree A-V block precipitated by carotid pressure.

Basic NSR with PR interval = 0.20 second (beats No. 1 and No. 2).

Vagal stimulation effected by carotid pressure causes

    a. severe slowing of sinus impulse formation.

    b. retardation of A-V node conduction velocity leading to prolongation of PR interval (0.26 second in beat No. 3) and blocked sinus impulse (beat No. 4).

Sinus beats resume, with sinus bradycardia and slightly prolonged PR interval as residual effects of vagal stimulation (beats No. 5 and No. 6).

The following ECG was taken during an episode of vomiting in a 52-year-old man with an acute myocardial infarction. Normal sinus rhythm had been present during his previous two days in the Cardiac Care Unit. Intermittent failure of sinus impulse conduction is evoked by the strong parasympathetic stimulation of vomiting. Thus a defect of A-V nodal conduction is revealed.

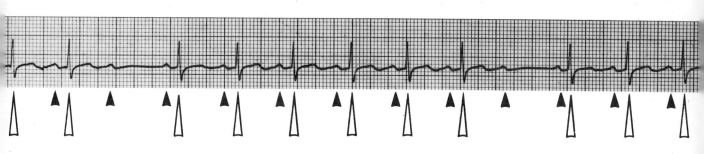

The vagotonic effect of vomiting or other forms of straining commonly results in a significant delay in nodal conduction velocity, particularly in the heart already affected by acute ischemic disease. Certain cardiac drugs used in the treatment of myocardial infarction also enhance vagal tone. Thus the vagotonic effects of vomiting and digitalis superimposed on acute ischemic injury in the A-V nodal area may induce serious problems of impulse conduction. The PR interval should be studied in detail in the CCU for signs of impending A-V node conduction malfunction during these provocative acts.

Label each P wave. Mark the blocked sinus beat and the place where the QRS should appear.

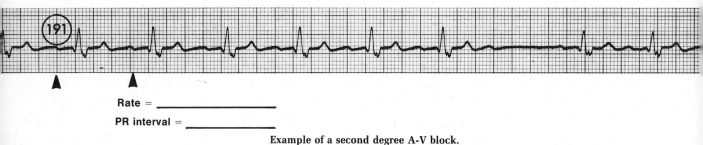

Rate = _____

PR interval = _____

Example of a second degree A-V block.

Serial rhythm strips from a 50-year-old woman with an acute myocardial infarction.

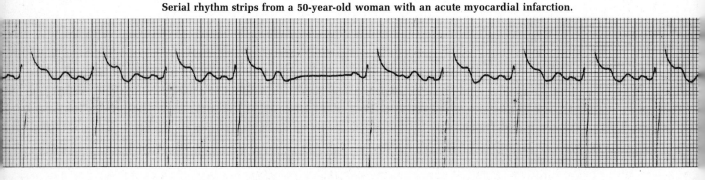

Sinus rhythm with instance of failure of A-V node conduction. Note that the blocked sinus or atrial beat occurs sooner after the previous beat than conducted sinus beats.

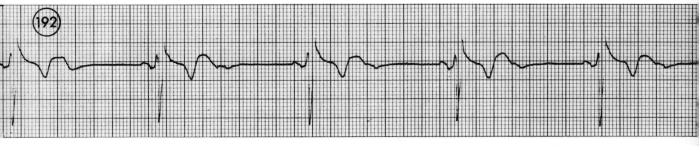

Atrial rate = _____

Ventricular rate = _____

The A-V conduction block has increased so that one hour later every other sinus beat is blocked. This produces two atrial contractions for every ventricular contraction, a condition designated as second degree A-V block with 2:1 A-V ratio. The atrial rate, then, is exactly twice the ventricular rate.

Because of slight changes in the sinus rate from beat to beat, nonconducted P waves appear in a variable time relationship to the previous T waves.

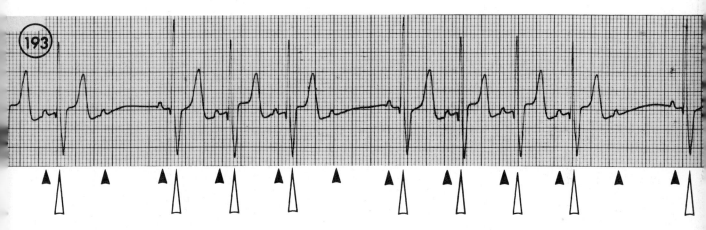

All P waves and QRS complexes are marked. Which sinus beats are blocked?

_____

Note that each conducted sinus beat has identical PR intervals of _____ second.

In the first group of beats the ratio of atrial to ventricular contractions is 3:2. In the second, the ratio is 4:3. In the third, the ratio is _____ : _____.

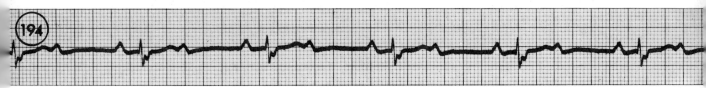

Sinus rhythm with A-V block.

Mark all sinus and ventricular components. What is the atrioventricular ratio? _____

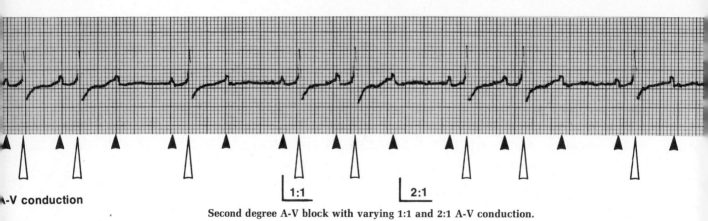

A-V conduction

| 1:1 | 2:1 |

Second degree A-V block with varying 1:1 and 2:1 A-V conduction.

The following electrocardiograms are examples of second degree A-V block for interpretation.

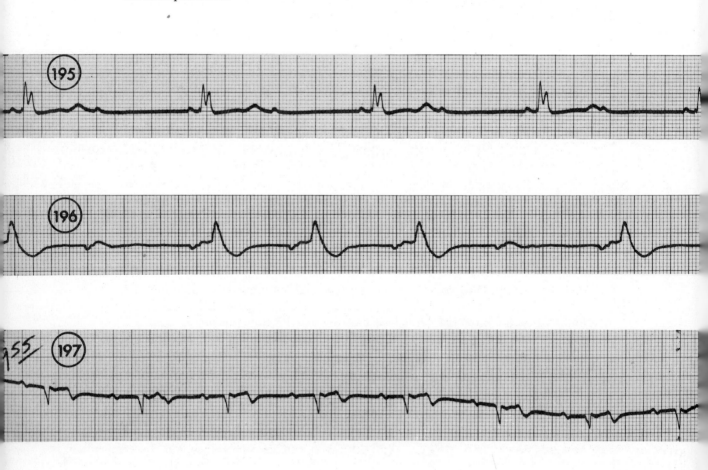

(195)

(196)

(197)

Advanced A-V Block

The following examples illustrate second degree A-V block in which relatively few of the sinus-initiated impulses penetrate the A-V node to stimulate the ventricles. **Advanced A-V block,** as in these strips, results in severe slowing of the ventricular rate and often in symptomatic bradycardia (lightheadedness, weakness, fainting). In these arrhythmias, any maneuver or drug action which stimulates the vagus nerve may further increase the A-V nodal block (by increasing conduction delay) and intensify the bradycardia.

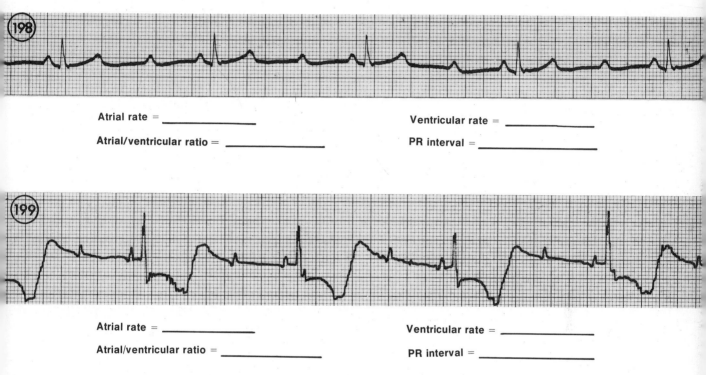

Atrial rate = _____   Ventricular rate = _____

Atrial/ventricular ratio = _____   PR interval = _____

Atrial rate = _____   Ventricular rate = _____

Atrial/ventricular ratio = _____   PR interval = _____

These sequential tracings are from an 81-year-old man with recurring episodes of dizziness and syncope. A cardiac arrhythmia was suspected as the cause, and the patient was admitted to the Cardiac Care Unit for observation.

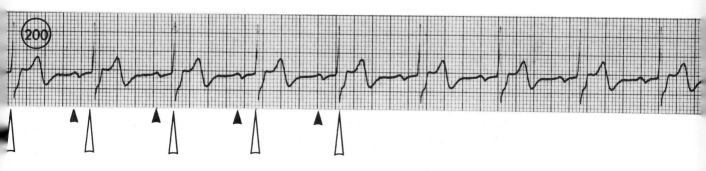

3:50 PM: The patient is alert and without symptoms. The cardiac monitor reveals (_____), with a rate of _____ per minute and a PR interval at the upper limit of normal (_____ second).

4:06 PM: The pulse detector loses the R component signal which activates the alarm system and automatic pen recorder. The next two strips are continuous tracings subsequently obtained.

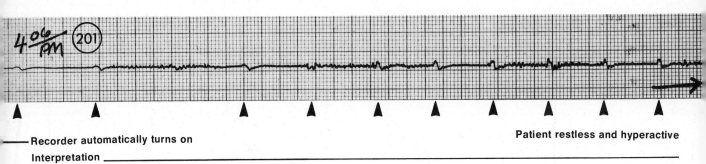

Recorder automatically turns on   **Patient restless and hyperactive**

Interpretation _____

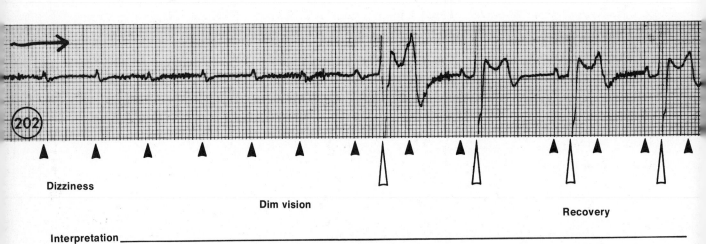

Dizziness

   Dim vision

                          Recovery

Interpretation _____

   This sequence reveals a series of atrial waves without ventricular complexes for several seconds, during which time the patient developed the symptoms and behavior of acute cerebral circulatory arrest. With spontaneous recovery of A-V conduction, symptoms quickly disappear, and the cause of his original complaints is clarified. Note, however, that the recovery rhythm appears to be 2:1 A-V block. Also note the increase in sinus rate during the period of ventricular inactivity, presumably caused by cardiovascular reflexes. The duration of documented ventricular inactivity is _____ seconds.

   By 4:08 PM, an intravenous infusion of isoproterenol is started.

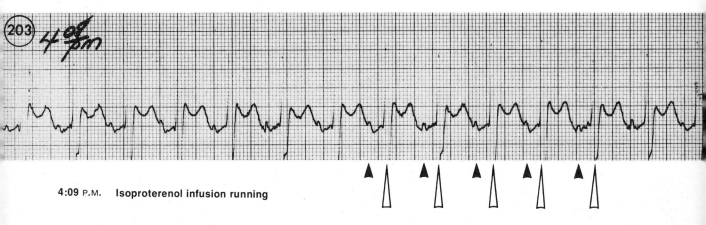

4:09 P.M.   Isoproterenol infusion running

Within a minute, all sinus beats are conducted. The accelerating effect of isoproterenol on sinus impulse formation is reflected in the sinus tachycardia now present (rate = _____).

Wenckebach Phenomenon

A special form of second degree A-V block exhibits progressively increasing PR intervals interrupted by periodic blocked sinus beats and is known as the **Wenckebach phenomenon.** This arrhythmia is often perplexing for the beginner, but with developed awareness and experience, it is usually not difficult to interpret. It is, in fact, one of the most interesting of all arrhythmias. Furthermore, it is one which generally can be effectively treated when recognized. This form of second degree A-V block occurs with relative frequency in acute myocardial infarction.

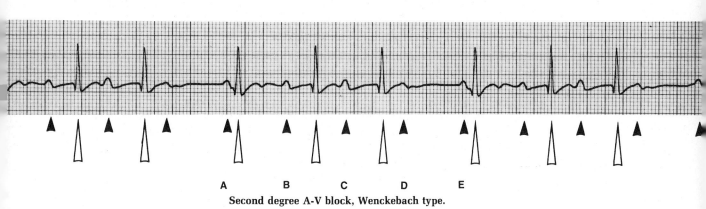

A   B   C   D   E

Second degree A-V block, Wenckebach type.

Beginning with the normal cardiac cycle at A, the PR interval is 0.12 second. In the following cycle at B, the configuration of components is unchanged. However, the PR interval has increased to 0.32 second. In the next beat, C, the PR interval is now 0.41 second. There has been a progressive increase in the duration of the A-V conduction time. Obviously, this progression cannot continue indefinitely, and the following events illustrate resolution of the process.

A P wave appears in the expected time, D, but no QRS complex follows. This blocked beat establishes the rhythm as a form of second degree A-V block. The next beat is of particular interest. Note that the sinus cadence remains constant (D-E). Then note that the PR interval at E is short, similar to that at A. In subsequent beats, the PR interval gets longer and longer. Then a blocked beat occurs. The cycle has repeated itself in four beats.

Complete the diagrams and determine the PR intervals.

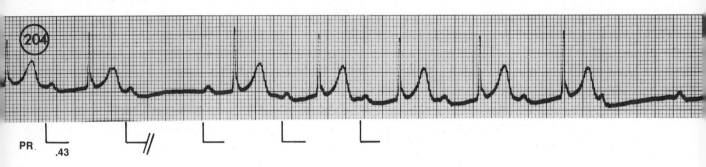

PR   .43

Upon scanning this electrocardiogram, the pause in the ventricular rate is obvious. A blocked sinus beat seems to occur in this area. In complex rhythms, it is often helpful to begin interpretation immediately after such a pause, if it is present. In this example, the first cycle after the earliest pause in the ventricular rate has a prolonged PR interval. Using a ruler or calipers, observe that this interval becomes gradually longer in subsequent beats. Then a blocked sinus beat occurs. A cycle can be made out at the end of the strip in which the PR interval is shortened to the same length as that following the first blocked sinus beat and pause in ventricular contraction.

In diagrammatic form, complete the labeling of all PR intervals and blocked beats.

The A-V node appears to fatigue with each beat as the conduction time becomes successively longer until one impulse fails to be transmitted. However, after a period of rest (during the blocked sinus beat), the A-V node recovers more fully. A-V conduction is improved, and the PR interval after the pause is relatively short, only to increase in subsequent beats.

In each of the following examples of intermittent A-V block with Wenckebach phenomenon, mark all PR intervals and determine lengths. Mark all blocked atrial beats. Give atrial/ventricular ratios.

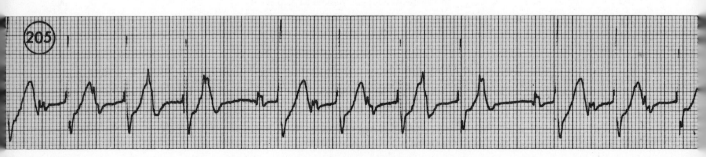

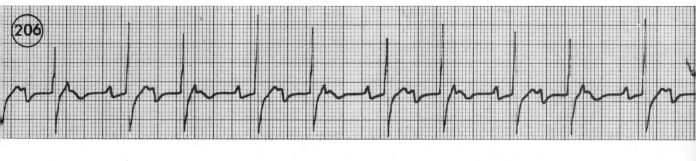

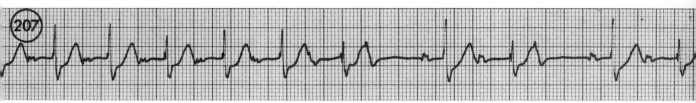

The following ECG's demonstrate Wenckebach arrhythmia with a high degree of A-V block, in which the dropped beat occurs after only two or three completed cardiac cycles.

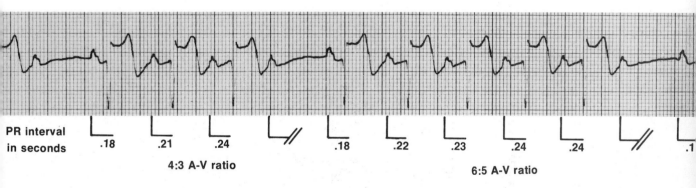

Complete the labelling.

Locate the Wenckebach phenomenon in the following tracings.

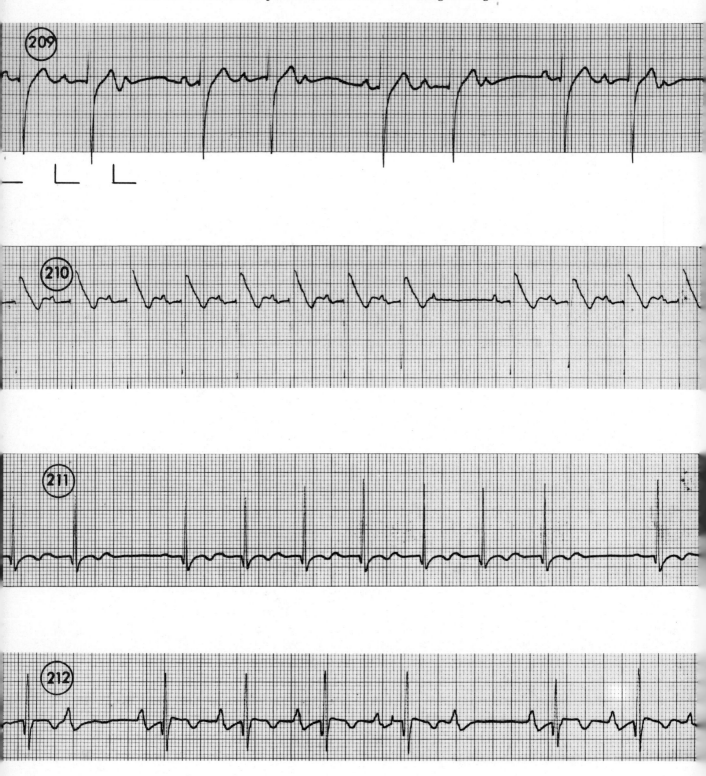

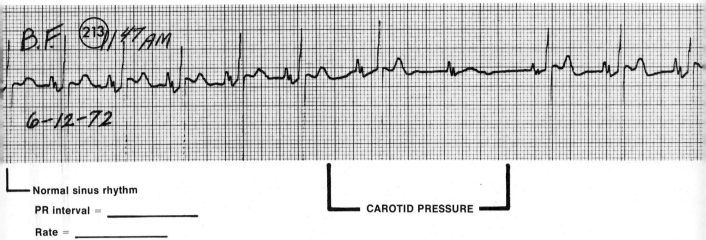

Normal sinus rhythm

PR interval = _____

Rate = _____

CAROTID PRESSURE

Demonstration of an A-V nodal conduction dysfunction with a provocative vagotonic maneuver.

Application of carotid pressure induces:
1. Slowing of the sinus rate.
2. Prolongation of the PR interval.
3. Complete block of A-V conduction.

Full recovery of the cardiac rhythm occurs following the release of carotid pressure. The above sequence is that of the Wenckebach phenomenon as an isolated event. This is an abnormal response to carotid pressure which took place in a 52-year-old man who was recovering from an acute myocardial infarction, complicated by prolonged second degree A-V block of the Wenckebach type with spontaneous remission.

On the following day, carotid pressure induced similar slowing of the sinus rate and some prolongation of the PR interval, but there were no blocked beats. Further recovery was demonstrated the day after when carotid pressure again resulted in sinus slowing but no change in A-V conduction.

Types of Second Degree A-V Block

Two forms of second degree A-V block have been presented. Both are characterized by intermittent failure of impulses originating in the sinus node to pass through the atrioventricular conduction system. In the first form presented, conducted beats have a constant A-V transmission time. In the second, sequential lengthening of A-V conduction time occurs until a beat is blocked.

These forms of intermittent A-V block have important clinical distinctions. The form with *constant PR intervals* is usually associated with organic disease of the major conduction tracts leading into the ventricles. The arrhythmia usually indicates a permanent conduction defect which frequently leads to a complete block of all A-V node impulses. The form with *lengthening PR intervals* is more often transient, appearing as a complication of acute cardiac disease, such as myocardial infarction. It usually involves the A-V node itself and is not often a forerunner of progressive A-V node conduction failure.

Development of terminology for the forms of second degree A-V block has had a complicated history which has tended to complicate the subject matter itself. Karl Wenckebach, professor of medicine at the University of Groningen in Holland, described both forms in 1906 in the early days of electrocardiography. However, his name has become firmly affixed to the form with progressively increasing PR intervals. The eponym is so widely accepted that it serves as a convenient and easily communicated term for this complex phenomenon. The arrhythmia is properly designated as intermittent (or second degree) A-V block of the Wenckebach type.

In 1924, Walter Mobitz, a German physician, classified both of these forms of intermittent A-V block as Type I and Type II. His name has become associated with the form characterized by constant PR intervals, but the eponym is not uniformly used, and it has no historical priority. We prefer to designate this form as intermittent (or second degree) A-V block with constant PR intervals.

The proposed nomenclature of Type I and Type II appears to confuse the beginner rather than help him. This system has not been used in this text. In fact, the types were presented in reverse order because the constant PR interval form is easier to understand.

A description of intermittent A-V block should include some indication of the severity of the conduction defect. As a guide for expressing this, the following table is provided and may be applied to either form of intermittent A-V block.

TABLE 9

Grade of A-V Block	Frequency Ratio: Blocked Beat per Conducted Beats	
Occasional	1 (or fewer)	10
Moderate	1	5–9
Advanced	1 (or greater)	4

While the previous description of the intermittent A-V block pertains to sinus rhythms, these phenomena may occur in rhythms of atrial excitation. The following examples of atrial tachycardia present intermittent A-V block in various patterns.

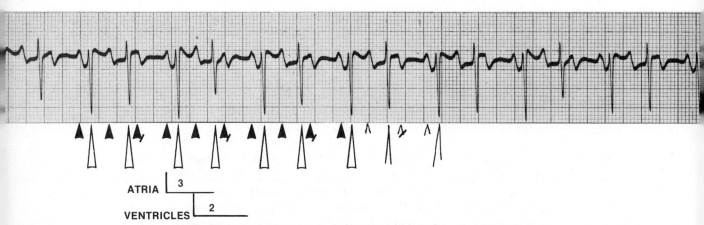

ATRIA $\quad$ 3

VENTRICLES $\quad$ 2

Wenckebach phenomenon in the presence of a rhythm of atrial excitation.

Complete the labeling and indicate blocked atrial beats.

PR intervals are variable, and a delay in ventricular activity occurs after every two ventricular beats. Starting after a pause in the ventricular rate, the PR interval is 0.12 second. In the next cardiac cycle, the PR interval is 0.22 second. The atrial beat following this is blocked. The sequence then repeats itself, demonstrating

Wenckebach phenomenon in atrial tachycardia with a consistent atrial/ventricular ratio of 3:2. Atrial rate = 190. Ventricular rate = 127.

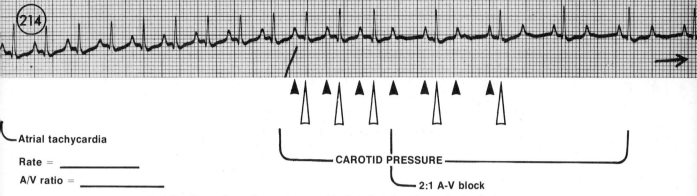

Atrial tachycardia

Rate = _____

A/V ratio = _____

Atrial tachycardia with varying A-V block induced with vagal stimulation.

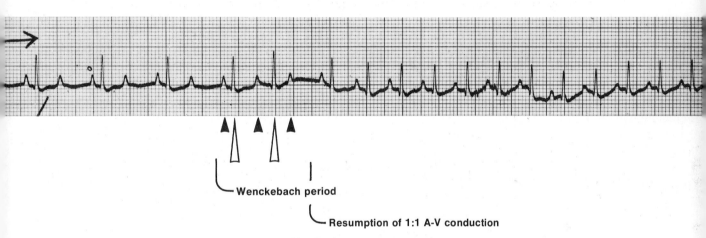

The single sequence of the Wenckebach phenomenon represents a transitional rhythm between 2:1 A-V block and 1:1 A-V conduction.

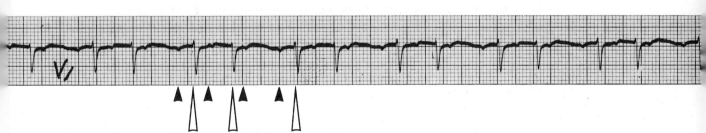

Example of atrial tachycardia with a recurring pattern of A-V block.

Atrial tachycardia in which every third atrial beat is blocked is evident. The PR interval following a blocked beat is short. In the subsequent cycle, the PR interval is longer. Then a blocked atrial beat occurs again. This is the Wenckebach phenomenon appearing in atrial tachycardia, in which there is a recurring 3:2 atrial/ventricular ratio.

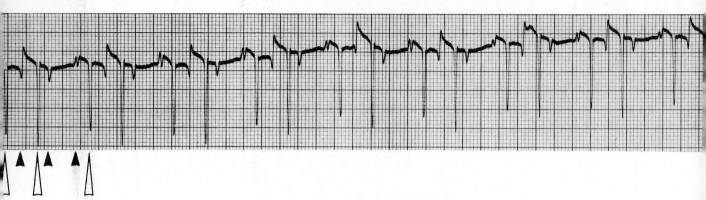

Digitalis-induced atrial tachycardia with A-V block.

Atrial tachycardia is present with second degree A-V block of the Wenckebach type. The subject is a 16-year-old mongrel dog which had been given digitalis for shortness of breath. Each Wenckebach period is made up of three atrial and two ventricular beats. Use diagrammatic notations to label the entire tracing.

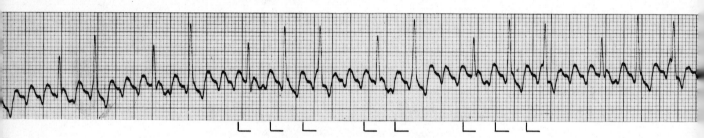

Atrial flutter with Wenckebach phenomenon.

Ventricular response to atrial flutter occurs in groups of two and three beats. After each pause in the ventricular rate, the F-R interval increases progressively in consecutive cardiac cycles. This follows the pattern of intermittent A-V block of the Wenckebach type. The A-V block is due not to an abnormality of the conduction system but rather to a physiological response to impulse overload from the atrial excitation.

Third Degree A-V Block

Impulse propagation in the A-V node and major conduction pathways may be so severely depressed that *no* impulses are transmitted between the atria and the ventricles. This condition is known as **complete** or **third degree A-V block.** Since the ventricles cannot receive stimuli from sinus or atrial pacemakers, the ventricles may fail to beat.

A 56-year-old man who incurred a massive intracerebral hemorrhage developed complete A-V block. Progressively severe A-V block appears in these serial tracings which leads to interruption of all impulse conduction from the sinus node and absence of all ventricular activity. The entire sequence shown here occurred in less than one minute.

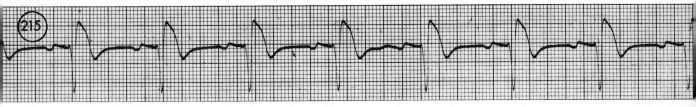

PR interval = _____

First degree A-V block.

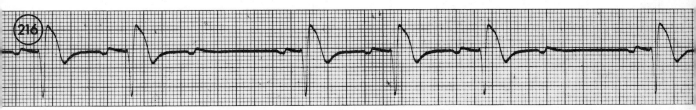

Second degree A-V block (intermittent failure of A-V node conduction).

Locate blocked sinus beats.

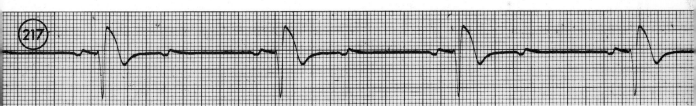

Second degree A-V block of increased severity is evident with an atrial/ventricular ratio of _____.

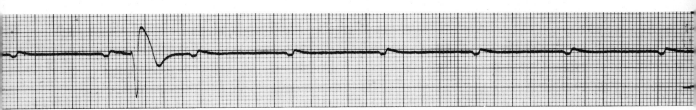

After a ventricular contraction, evidently from an impulse conducted through the A-V node, there is cessation of further ventricular activity. Rhythmic sinus impulse formation with atrial contractions continues, but impulse transmission between atria and ventricles has become totally blocked. The patient at this point manifested signs of cardiac and respiratory arrest and could not be resuscitated.

On cessation of ventricular contractions, evidence of circulatory arrest appears within a few seconds. When disease affects the A-V node and major conduction pathways between the atria and ventricles so that impulses can no longer pass, the ventricles are no longer stimulated from above. Survival then depends upon the development of sustained pacemaker activity beyond the conduction disturbance. Tissue adjacent to the A-V node and in the ventricles normally has the capability for automaticity. These subsidiary pacemakers will be discussed in subsequent chapters according to their sites of origin.

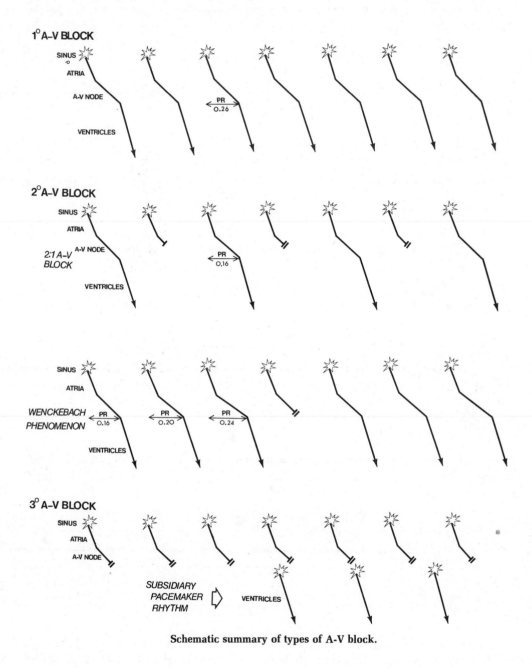

Schematic summary of types of A-V block.

Chapter 6

THE ATRIOVENTRICULAR JUNCTION

A-V JUNCTION: IMPULSE FORMATION

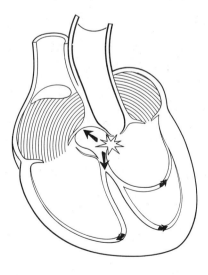

Spontaneous impulses may be generated in the region of the A-V node which, under certain conditions, assumes the role of cardiac pacemaker. Recordings from microelectrodes placed directly into the region indicate that the A-V node itself does not possess the capacity for impulse formation. Rather, short fibers adjacent to the node which have continuity with atrial fibers possess latent properties of automaticity. Pacemaker activity at this site is referred to as an A-V *junctional* rhythm. However, common usage of the term A-V *nodal* rhythm is so well established in the arrhythmia vocabulary that this convention, although imprecise, will be followed.

Nodal Escape Beats

Nodal beats may be activated through an escape mechanism, comparable to that of the atria. Like atrial automaticity, self-excitation in the A-V junctional tissue is normally precluded by impulses received from the higher, more rapid pacemaker sources. With depression of impulse formation or conduction from primary pacemaker sites, a latent automatic focus in the A-V junctional tissue escapes their inhibitory influence and initiates an impulse. This is a normal physiological response to a defect in usually dominant impulse formation and conduction activity. It represents another intrinsic mechanism which protects against excessive cardiac slowing.

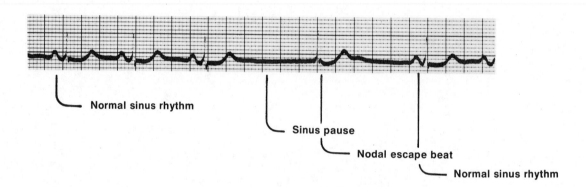

Normal sinus rhythm

Sinus pause

Nodal escape beat

Normal sinus rhythm

Following the sinus pause, a cardiac cycle occurs. This beat has a normal-appearing QRS complex and T wave, representing ventricular depolarization and repolarization. However, a P wave which would normally precede the QRS complex is not recognizable. The complex is presumed to have been initiated by an impulse originating in an intermediary location in the electrical pathway, since this impulse activates the ventricles, but *not* the atria, in a normal way.

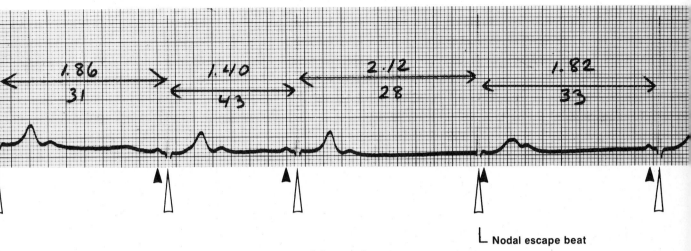

A-V nodal escape beat.

Severe sinus bradycardia is present. Note that the fourth ventricular complex is not preceded by a P wave. The complex resembles that of normal beats, however. It appears that an impulse was fired spontaneously from A-V junctional tissue when a sinus impulse failed to reach it by 2 seconds. A P wave, presumably formed from a sinus impulse, is found at the terminal portion of the nodal QRS complex. It can then be determined that the sinus pacemaker has slowed to 28 per minute, allowing the nodal pacemaker to escape. Following this, the sinus pacemaker speeds up, and sinus bradycardia is resumed.

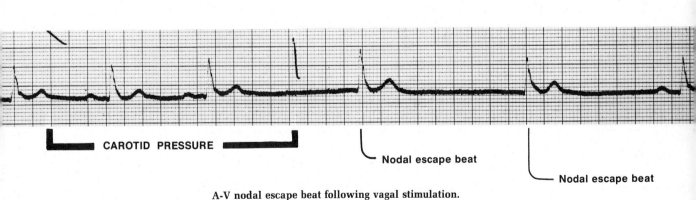

A-V nodal escape beat following vagal stimulation.

Nodal escape beats appear during slowing of the sinus node pacemaker induced by carotid pressure. The presence of sinus bradycardia with first degree A-V block before carotid stimulation suggests that vagal tone is already high, and an exaggerated parasympathetic response can be expected.

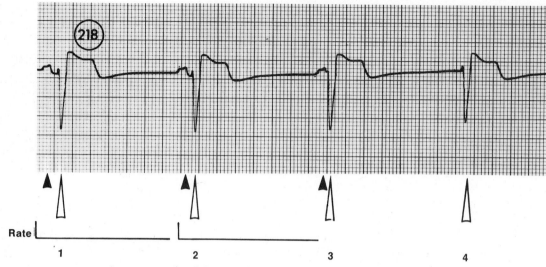

Appearance of nodal escape beats on slowing of the sinus pacemaker.

Sinus bradycardia with a nodal escape beat at No. 4 is evident. Note, however, that the P waves of the preceding beats appear to be moving closer to the QRS complexes. In beat No. 3, in fact, the isoelectric line produced by normal A-V nodal delay is almost nonexistent. Also note the slight slowing of the sinus rate.

It is presumed that this slowing in sinus impulse formation, even though very slight, allowed the release of automatic firing from an A-V junctional site. This escape pacemaker rate is close to that of the sinus rate. The result, in beats No. 2 and No. 3, is a nodal escape beat which begins *after* the atria have been depolarized and before this wave front can penetrate the A-V node, accounting for the changing relationship of P to QRS. In beat No. 4, the escape impulse begins before atrial excitation.

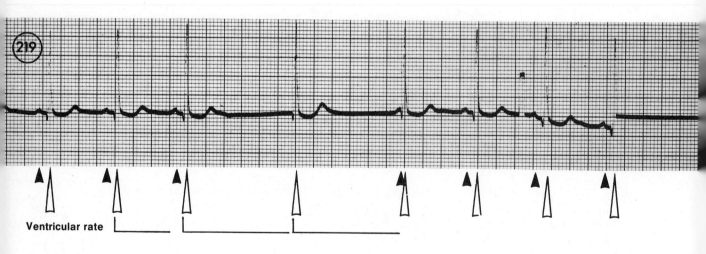

A delay in the sinus rate allows a nodal beat to escape. There is no sign of a P wave which may actually have occurred during the QRS formation but been completely concealed. In the following beat, a normal P wave appears to be developing, but before it can be completed, another nodal escape beat occurs. This P wave is assumed to originate in the sinus node because of its similarity in form to normal P waves. Subsequently, the sinus rate increases and takes over the cardiac rhythm.

Locate the standardization marker _____.

Impulses from the A-V junctional tissues have the following characteristics of propagation:

1. Forward or **antegrade** conduction into the ventricles along the normal conduction system. A-V nodal beats ordinarily have normal QRS complexes.
2. Backward or **retrograde** conduction into the atria, effecting depolarization of the atria and sinus node. This reversal in the usual direction of electrical flow through the atria produces P waves which:
   a. have opposite polarity, hence altered configuration.
   b. may vary in time relationship to QRS, depending upon the chronological activation of atria and ventricles. The P waves may appear *before, during,* or *after* their associated QRS complexes.

It is important to identify retrograde P waves in any of these three possible positions in order to interpret rhythms of A-V junctional origin.

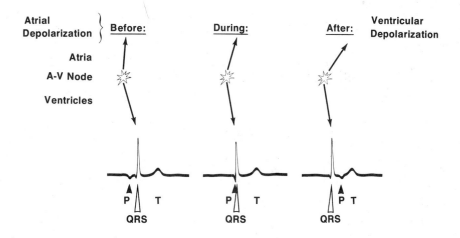

Sometimes retrograde conduction does not occur at all because of A-V nodal block and the subsequent absence of atrial depolarization. Of course, a P wave associated with the QRS would be absent.

Nodal escape beats may occur in succession if sinus node slowing is sustained or if sinus arrest occurs. This establishes a secondary escape rhythm with an A-V node junctional pacemaker, commonly termed an **idionodal rhythm** or, simply, **nodal rhythm.** The natural rate of impulse formation in this tissue is usually 40 to 60 per minute. Sustained nodal rhythms may occur when sinus node impulse formation has been suppressed by excessive vagal tone or disrupted through disease (ischemia, rheumatoid or sarcoid plaques, amyloid deposits).

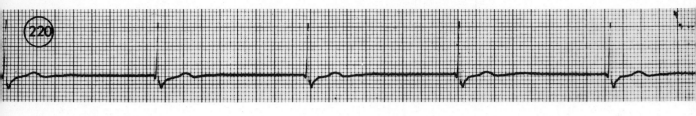

——————— **Sustained nodal rhythm**

Rate = ———————————   **Examples of nodal rhythms.**

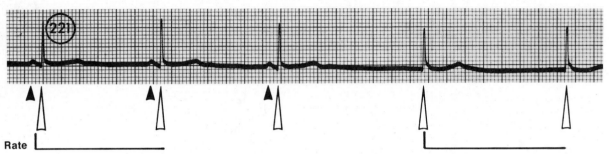

Rate

Slowing of sinus rhythm with replacement by nodal rhythm.

A nodal escape rhythm developed in a 77-year-old woman with a history of lightheadedness on first standing and on walking. Treatment with an adrenergic agent is demonstrated.

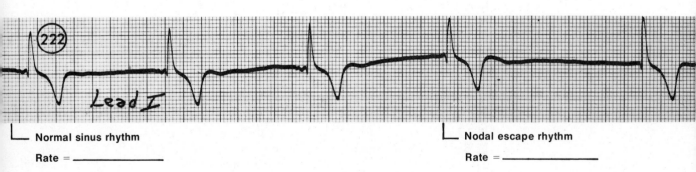

Normal sinus rhythm   **Nodal escape rhythm**

Rate = ———————————   Rate = ———————————

The following tracing was taken 30 minutes after administration of Proternol, a sustained-action oral preparation of isoproterenol.

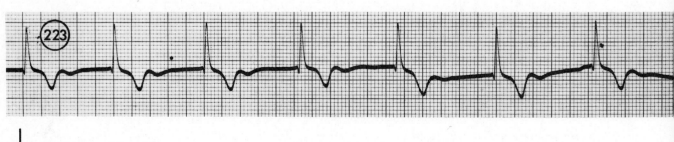

Sustained nodal rhythm

Rate = ———————————

A sinus rhythm could not be restored by adrenergic stimulation. However, the pacemaker in the A-V junctional tissues was driven at a faster rate, and symptoms were no longer produced during exertion.

Complete A-V Block

The preceding electrocardiograms demonstrate potential pacemakers located in the A-V junction which become activated on slowing or absence of impulse formation in the sinus node and atria. Examples will now be given of similar activation of these subsidiary pacemakers when higher impulses occur which are *not transmitted* to the ventricles. By this mechanism, ventricular contractions are sustained despite severe degrees of A-V block.

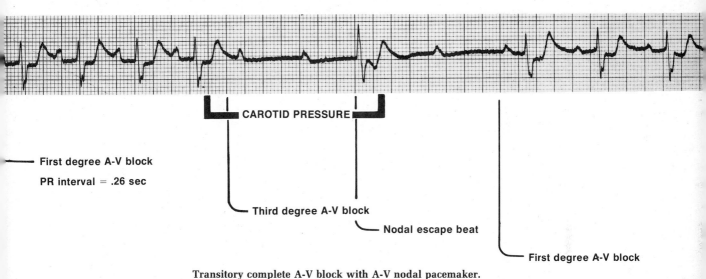

Transitory complete A-V block with A-V nodal pacemaker.

Conversion of delayed A-V node conduction to complete A-V block is induced by vagal stimulation. Prolonged ventricular standstill is prevented by an impulse originating in the A-V junctional tissues.

The following electrocardiogram exhibits cessation of all impulse conduction in the atrioventricular pathway, in which separate rhythms coexist in the atria and the ventricles independently.

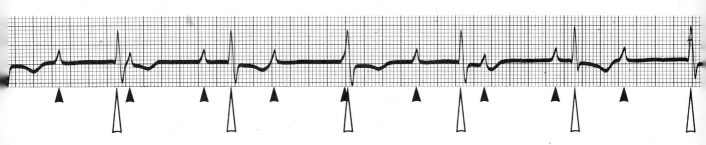

The first P wave–QRS complex combination appears to be a normal cardiac cycle having a normal PR interval. The next cycle has an extremely long PR interval. Then a blocked P wave follows. Up to this point, the Wenckebach type of intermittent, or second degree, A-V block appears to be present. Note that in subsequent beats, however, this pattern does not recur. The P waves fall with great variability in time relationship to QRS complexes. There are no dropped ventricular beats. In fact, the ventricular rhythm is entirely regular with a rate differing from that of the atria. The ventricles, then, beat with no relationship to the atria. This is characteristic of complete A-V block, in which no impulses pass between the atria and ventricles. A supraventricular pacemaker is maintained, while an escape pacemaker is activated distal to the impulse blockade. There are many variations of this basic pattern.

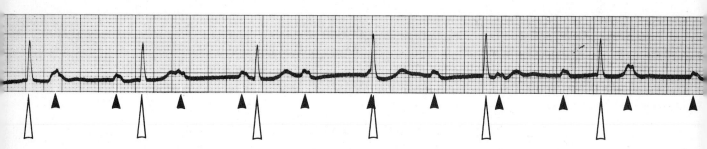

Sinus rhythm: Rate = 86 per minute. A-V nodal rhythm: Rate = 48 per minute. Identify all P waves and QRS complexes, using calipers.

Apparent PR intervals are not constant, and there is no pattern to their variability. No relationship between atrial and ventricular activity can be determined. QRS complexes are of normal duration and form. Note how the fourth QRS complex is distorted by a P wave which has its onset just before the ventricular depolarization sequence begins. This is complete A-V block with independently operating sinus and A-V nodal pacemakers.

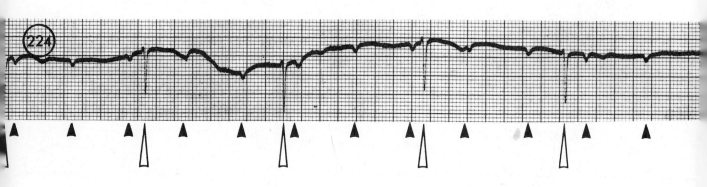

Sinus rate = _____   A-V nodal rate = _____

Is there any relationship between sinus and A-V nodal beats? *No*
Interpretation *complete A-V block with A-V nodal pacemaker*

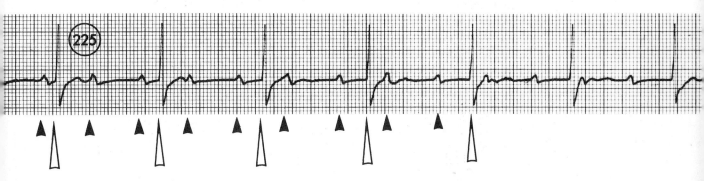

Sinus rate = _____ A-V nodal rate = _____
Is there any relationship between sinus and A-V nodal beats? _____
Interpretation *complete A-V block with A-V nodal pacemaker*

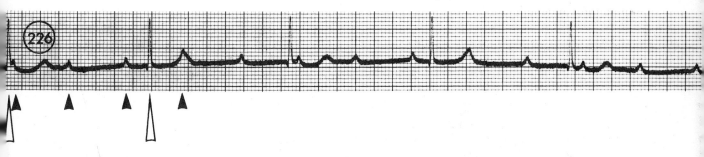

Label all P waves and QRS complexes.
Sinus rate = _____ A-V nodal rate = _____
Is there any relationship between sinus and A-V nodal beats? _____
Interpretation _____

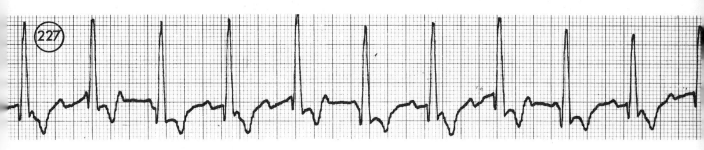

Label completely.
Atrial rate = _____ Ventricular rate = _____
Atrioventricular activity: Related _____ Unrelated _____
Interpretation _____

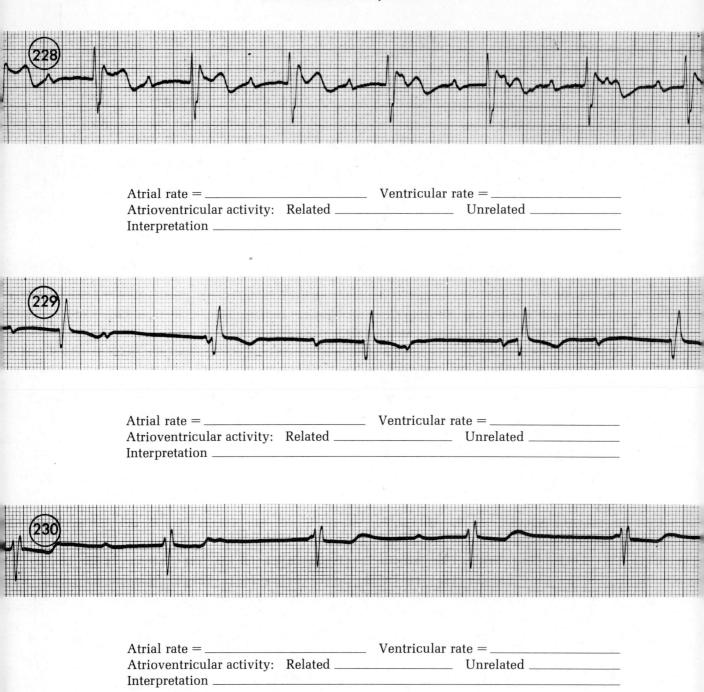

Atrial rate = _____   Ventricular rate = _____

Atrioventricular activity: Related _____   Unrelated _____

Interpretation _____

Atrial rate = _____   Ventricular rate = _____

Atrioventricular activity: Related _____   Unrelated _____

Interpretation _____

Atrial rate = _____   Ventricular rate = _____

Atrioventricular activity: Related _____   Unrelated _____

Interpretation _____

Complete A-V block may occur with a variety of supraventricular rhythms. Examples have been presented demonstrating sinus tachycardia, sinus bradycardia, and atrial tachycardia. In the following tracing, complete A-V block appears with atrial fibrillation.

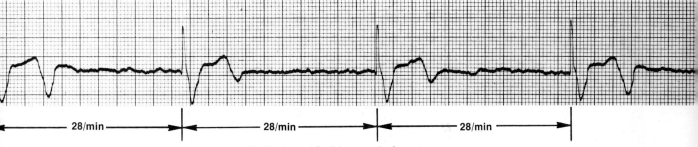

Atrial fibrillation with slow ventricular rate.

Note that the initial components of QRS are of normal appearance but that the terminal part is markedly delayed. This represents a slowing of conduction velocity in the ventricular pathways due to block.

More importantly, examine the ventricular rhythm using calipers and note that it is extremely regular. Since the supraventricular rhythm is totally irregular, the ventricular rhythm could only be regular if complete A-V block existed with an operating pacemaker below the block. In this illustration, third degree A-V block was induced by digitalis and represents a toxic effect of the drug. An A-V junctional pacemaker with a conduction defect drives the ventricles.

The patient with atrial fibrillation who develops a regular rhythm on digitalis may have a serious form of drug toxicity. It is extremely important to recognize this complication of drug therapy.

The following series demonstrates progression and regression of various forms of A-V block in acute myocardial infarction and the responses of impulse formation and conduction to a sympathetic stimulating agent.

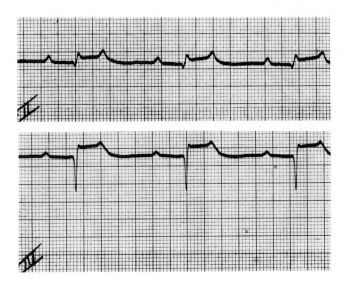

6/9/71 — 12:45 PM: Portions of the standard electrocardiogram taken on admission of a 54-year-old man with chest pain and the electrocardiographic pattern of acute myocardial infarction reveal intermittent A-V conduction with 2:1 A-V block. The ventricular rate was _____*47*_____ per minute.

1:15 PM: On transfer of the patient to the Cardiac Care Unit, the cardiac monitor disclosed complete A-V block with a nodal pacemaker having a rate of 46 per minute.

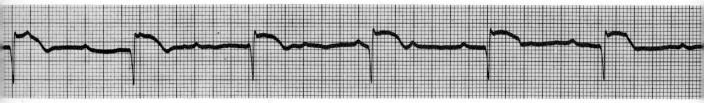

1:20 PM: Isoproterenol was given by intravenous infusion, 1 mg/1000 cc 5 per cent D/W at 50 drops per minute.

1:27 PM: Second degree A-V block has been reestablished, but the rhythm is now of the Wenckebach type with an atrioventricular ratio of 3:2. The ventricular rate is 76 per minute.

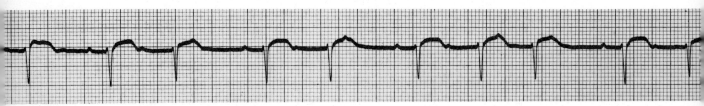

2:12 PM: Complete A-V block has reappeared, even though the concentration of isoproterenol has been increased to 2 mg/1000 cc 5 per cent D/W, and the infusion rate sped up to 100 drops per minute. The idionodal rate has increased from 46 to 64 per minute.

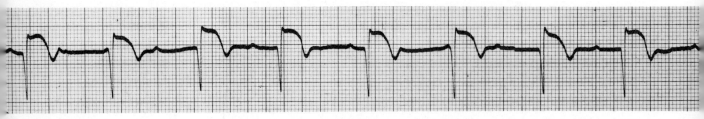

Complete A-V block persisted through the subsequent two days, while the infusion of isoproterenol was continued at 50 drops per minute at the same concentration. An interesting development during this time was the transient appearance of atrial fibrillation, demonstrated in the next electrocardiogram.

6/11/71—8:45 AM: Complete A-V block is evident. Following the sixth ventricular beat, atrial fibrillation is present. Note that there is no change in the ventricular rate or regularity because of the conduction abnormality.

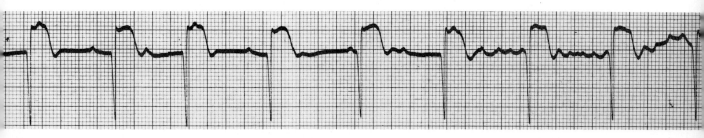

12:45 PM: Second degree A-V block has reappeared and is again of the Wenckebach type with an atrial/ventricular ratio of 3:2. The isoproterenol is still being infused at 2 mg/1000 cc 5 per cent D/W at 50 drops per minute.

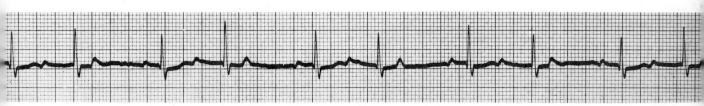

12:52 PM: The rate of the infusion is increased from 50 to 100 drops per minute. Continuous tracings reveal improvement in A-V conduction.

The severity of second degree A-V block decreases from a 3:2 to an 8:7 atrial/ventricular ratio because of the increased adrenergic stimulation.

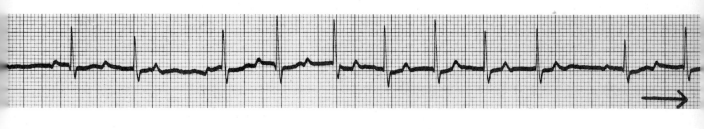

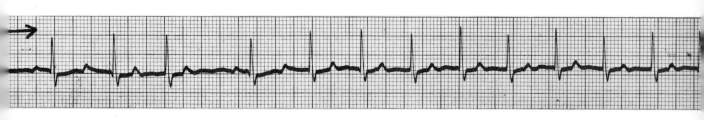

Then a 4:3 ratio appears, followed by complete sinus capture, in which the PR interval is prolonged. The sinus rate is 117 per minute, and the PR interval 0.33 second. This first degree A-V block persists, even as the isoproterenol concentration and infusion rate are gradually reduced.

By 6/12/71, the isoproterenol concentration has been reduced to 1 mg/1000 cc 5 per cent D/W and the infusion rate slowed to 25 drops per minute.

10:30 AM: The PR interval has been decreased to within normal limits (0.19 second). An atrial premature contraction occurs which is blocked. The PR interval immediately following the resultant ventricular pause is even shorter (0.13 second).

Isoproterenol was discontinued at 2:00 PM after gradually decreasing its infusion rate.

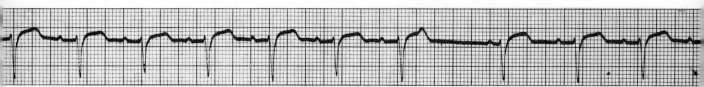

3:00 PM: Stable normal sinus rhythm is maintained without pharmacological agents.

The subsequent course of recovery from acute myocardial infarction remained entirely uneventful.

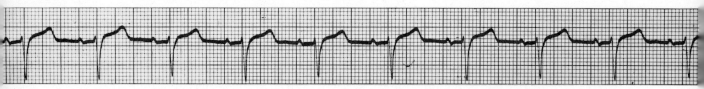

The A-V nodal escape beat was described as a normal response from a latent pacemaker in the A-V junctional tissue which is activated by depression of a pacemaker of a higher order (e.g., sinus or atrial) or by the failure of impulses from these pacemakers to reach the A-V node. The A-V junctional tissue may also be excited so that it produces impulses at a rate faster than the normally dominating pacemakers. This is abnormal acceleration of automaticity and, like that in the atria, it produces impulses singly or in succession. These may appear as **nodal premature contractions** or as **nodal tachycardia.**

A-V JUNCTION: IMPULSE FORMATION

Excitation

NPC = Nodal premature contraction
NT = Nodal tachycardia

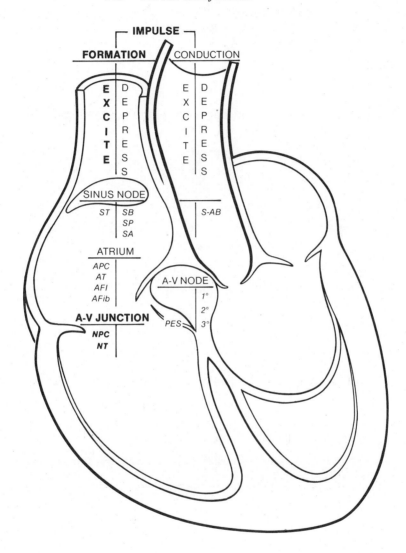

Nodal Premature Contractions

Nodal premature contractions typically have the following characteristics:
1. They occur early in the cardiac cycle.
2. Atrial and ventricular contractions are controlled from an impulse formed in the A-V junction through retrograde and antegrade conduction, as with nodal escape beats.
3. The sinus node pacemaker changes cadence after being reset by the retrograde impulse.
4. Ventricular depolarization follows the normal sequences.

Nodal premature contraction with retrograde conduction.

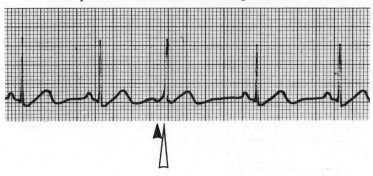

An NPC with a retrograde P wave appears before the QRS complex.

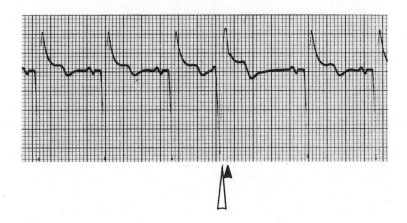

An NPC with a retrograde P wave occurs during ventricular depolarization.

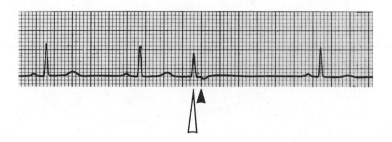

An NPC with a retrograde P wave appears after the QRS complex.

Nodal Tachycardia

Nodal tachycardia is produced by sustained excitation of a pacemaker in the A-V junctional tissue. The individual beats have the same characteristics as nodal premature contractions, having retrograde atrial conduction and normal ventricular depolarization. As the intrinsic rate of automaticity in the A-V junction is about 40 to 60 a minute, an accelerated nodal rhythm (as opposed to an nodal escape rhythm) is considered any rate faster than 60. While there is no agreement on exact criteria, the term nodal tachycardia is applied when the rate of a functioning A-V junctional pacemaker is greater than 100 per minute.

Nodal tachycardia and atrial tachycardia have several common features:

1. Accelerated local impulse formation.
2. Precisely regular cadence (in contrast to NSR).
3. Tendency for paroxysms with abrupt onset and termination.
4. Conversion to normal sinus rhythm by
   a. suppressor drugs.
   b. strong vagal stimulation.
   c. electrical countershock.

Nodal tachycardia　　　　　　　　　　**Normal sinus rhythm**

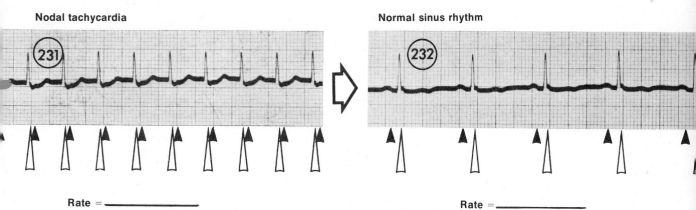

Rate = _____　　　　　　　Rate = _____

Conversion of nodal tachycardia to normal sinus rhythm.

Compare the area immediately following the QRS complexes. Note that there is a slight but definite change after conversion. This indicates that a retrograde P wave was present during the nodal tachycardia.

Tracings which demonstrate rhythms originating from an A-V junctional site follow. Check the regularity of the rate with calipers. Note the relationship of retrograde P waves to QRS complexes where possible.

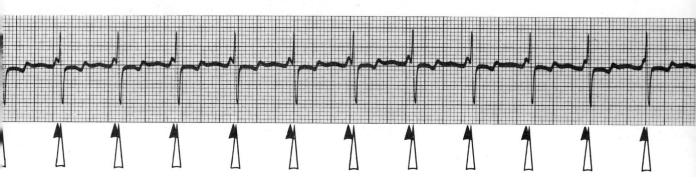

Accelerated nodal rhythm. Rate = 94. Retrograde P wave precedes the QRS complex.

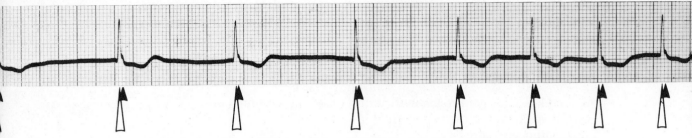

Nodal rhythm with variable rate. Rate = 45-90. Retrograde P wave follows the QRS complex.

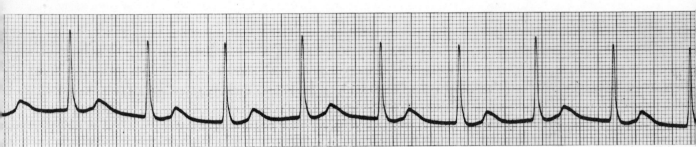

Accelerated nodal rhythm. Rate = 71. P waves not identifiable.

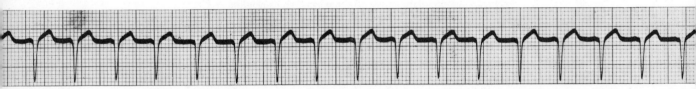

Nodal tachycardia. Rate = 135. P waves appear to be present before the QRS complexes.

Compare the rhythms before and after treatment with precordial direct-current shock. The patient was a 38-year-old woman, who was having a fluttering sensation in her chest with generalized weakness and restlessness for 3½ hours prior to treatment.

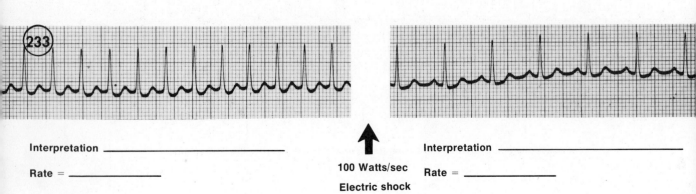

Interpretation _____

Rate = _____

100 Watts/sec
Electric shock

Interpretation _____

Rate = _____

A-V nodal tachycardia occurs as a paroxysmal arrhythmia in otherwise normal individuals. It is also seen as a relatively unusual complication of myocardial infarction or inflammatory diseases of the heart. Digitalis may cause excitation of impulse formation in the A-V junctional tissue, much as in the atria. In fact, A-V nodal tachycardia most commonly occurs as a toxic manifestation of digitalis effect.

Electrocardiographic evidence of digitalis toxicity is present in a 56-year-old man with congestive heart failure due to ischemic heart disease and hypokalemia after vigorous treatment with a thiazide diuretic.

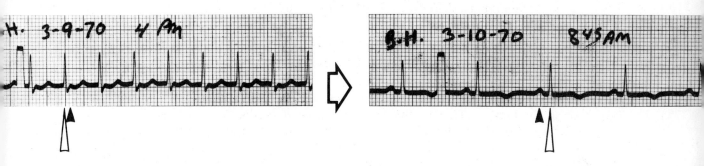

On 3/9/70, tachycardia with a regular rate of 162 per minute was present. P waves and T waves could not be differentiated. QRS complexes were of normal duration. Nodal tachycardia was suspected.

Potassium chloride was then administered orally, and both digitalis and the diuretic were withheld.

By 3/10/70, normal sinus rhythm had replaced the tachycardia. P waves were then obvious, and the terminal portions of QRS complexes had changed so that the S wave was no longer present. It is now clear in retrospect that the terminal QRS complex in the earlier tracing was, in reality, a retrograde P wave from an A-V nodal impulse. This establishes the original arrhythmia as nodal tachycardia.

Unidirectional Block

Impulses from an A-V junctional pacemaker may be blocked in one direction or another. This is more likely in impulses directed toward the atria than those directed toward the ventricles, since conduction tends to be slower in retrograde than in the usual antegrade direction.

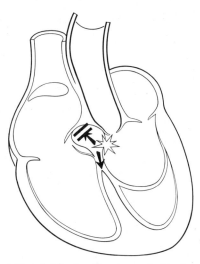

A-V nodal beat with retrograde block.

The tendency for unidirectional block becomes more prominent as the ectopic pacemaker rate increases. A-V nodal tachycardia is commonly associated with retrograde conduction block, resulting in A-V dissociation. The sustained, accelerated A-V junctional pacemaker controls the ventricular rhythm, but not the atrial. However, nonpenetrating retrograde impulses keep the fibers of the A-V node in a state of refractoriness. This creates a block of depolarizing waves originating in the atria. The result is independent atrial and ventricular rhythms from two distinct pacemakers. The conduction defect in the A-V node represents a physiologic block due to excessively rapid stimulation and is *not* due to abnormal depression of conduction velocity.

A-V Dissociation

The A-V nodal rhythms thus far presented have manifested bidirectional impulse conduction. That is, the impulse initiated in the A-V junctional tissue is propagated both in the usual direction (antegrade to the ventricles) and in the reverse direction (retrograde to the atria). This single ectopic impulse, emanating from midway in the normal electrical pathway, controls the sequences of both atrial and ventricular contractions.

On analyzing a single A-V nodal contraction in which no retrograde P wave can be identified, it cannot be determined if retrograde conduction is blocked or whether an A-V nodal–stimulated P wave occurs simultaneously with QRS but is obscured. This differentiation is made by examining the atrial rhythm. If the A-V nodal impulse produces a change in the periodicity of atrial beats, it is assumed that the ectopic impulse is conducted through the atria. If there is no interruption of the atrial rhythmicity, the retrograde impulse must have been blocked. In this case, the ventricles respond to one pacemaker (A-V nodal) and the atria to another (sinus or atrial), and the resultant rhythmic contractions are dissociated from each other. This complex rhythm, involving two pacemakers and a unidirectional block, is a form of A-V dissociation taking place during a single cardiac cycle.

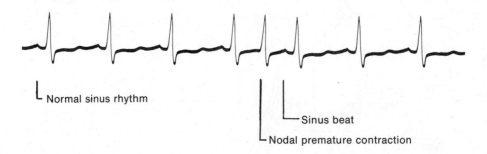

Normal sinus rhythm

Sinus beat

Nodal premature contraction

The nodal premature contraction does not interrupt the regularity or shape of the established atrial response. It is therefore assumed that the premature impulse was not transmitted through the atria to the sinus node. A unidirectional (retrograde) block was present.

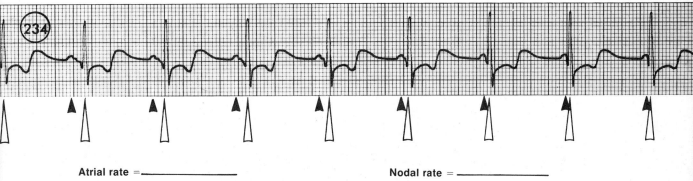

Atrial rate =_____   Nodal rate = _____

Isorhythmic A-V dissociation.

Both the atrial and the ventricular beats recur at regular intervals, but the PR intervals become progressively *shorter*. Finally, P waves merge with QRS complexes, and, presumably, conduction cannot take place through the A-V conduction system. Therefore, the atria and ventricles must be controlled by separate pacemakers (e.g., sinus and A-V nodal, respectively), which operate at nearly the same rate. This close rate proximity of independent chamber beating is referred to as **isorhythmic A-V dissociation.**

Supraventricular Tachycardia

At very rapid rates, sinus tachycardia, atrial tachycardia, and A-V nodal tachycardia may be difficult or impossible to distinguish, since electrical activity just before the QRS is blended with the T wave of the previous beat. Thus P waves cannot be satisfactorily discerned. When a positive interpretation cannot be reached because of this, the term **supraventricular tachycardia** is used. This implies that one cannot be sure of the pacemaker origin but that it is at one of three sites — sinus, atrium, or A-V junction.

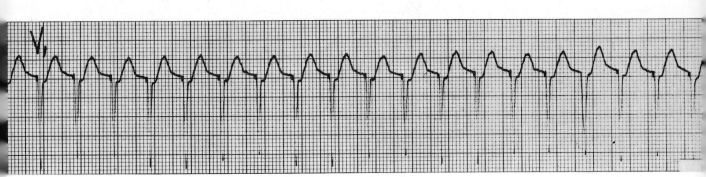

Supraventricular tachycardia.

A P wave cannot be identified with any degree of certainty. QRS complexes are of normal configuration and duration for lead V_1.

Interpretation of a supraventricular tachycardia can often be made by maneuvers which induce a change in the rate of impulse formation. In the following tracing, P waves cannot be identified in the initial portion. The diagnosis could be sinus, atrial, or nodal tachycardia.

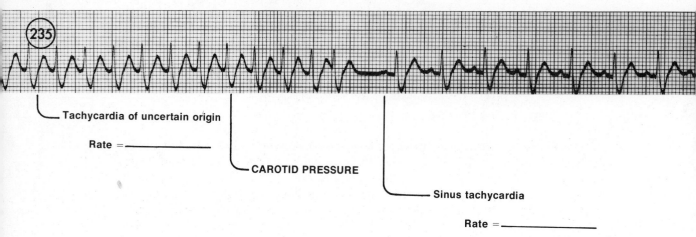

Tachycardia of uncertain origin

Rate =_____

CAROTID PRESSURE

Sinus tachycardia

Rate =_____

Vagal stimulation induces abrupt slowing of the heart rate, and a well-defined sinus rhythm emerges. This sudden slowing is characteristic of the response of atrial and nodal tachycardia to carotid pressure or other vagotonic action and is distinguished from the gradual slowing response usually seen with sinus tachycardia.

A few minutes after the previous ECG was taken, a tracing was obtained demonstrating premature contractions, then recurrence of the original tachycardia. This record contains the clue to a precise diagnosis.

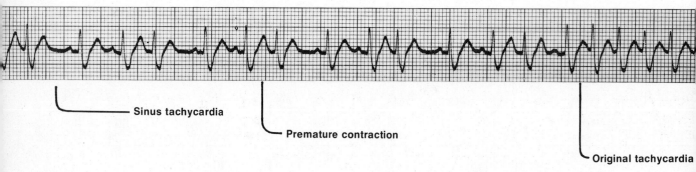

Sinus tachycardia

Premature contraction

Original tachycardia

The premature contraction is assumed to be of atrial origin, since the T wave of the beat before it is taller and more peaked than the T waves of isolated sinus beats, suggesting a superimposed P wave. Similar premature contractions are found elsewhere on the tracing. The presence of frequent atrial premature contractions immediately preceding the tachycardia under question suggests the probability of sustained atrial beats. Supporting the diagnosis of atrial tachycardia is the slightly sharper T wave configuration again appearing as if P waves were occurring simultaneously with the T waves of the previous beat.

SELF-EVALUATION: STAGE 2

Label each tracing completely: components, rate, rhythm(s).

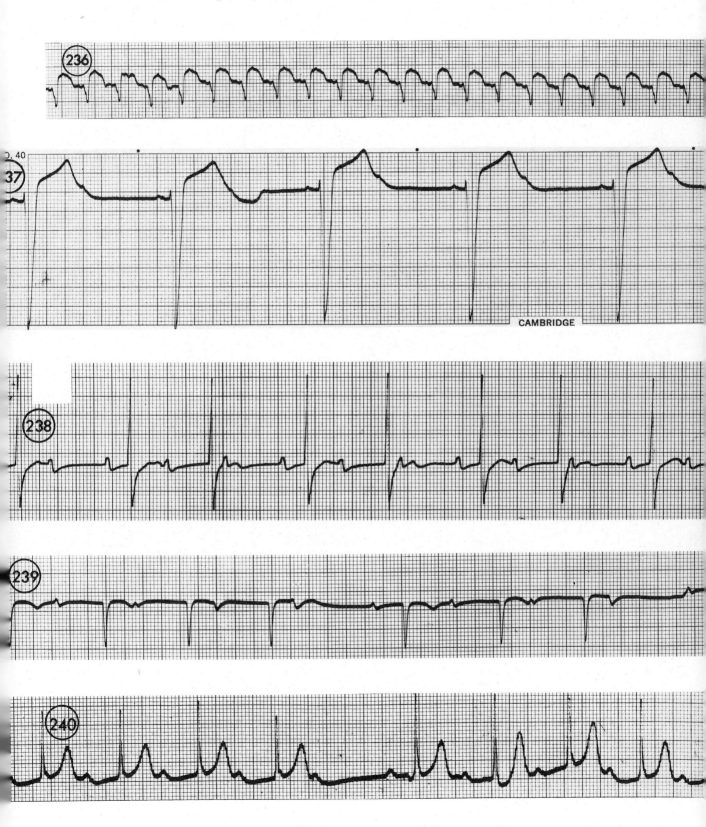

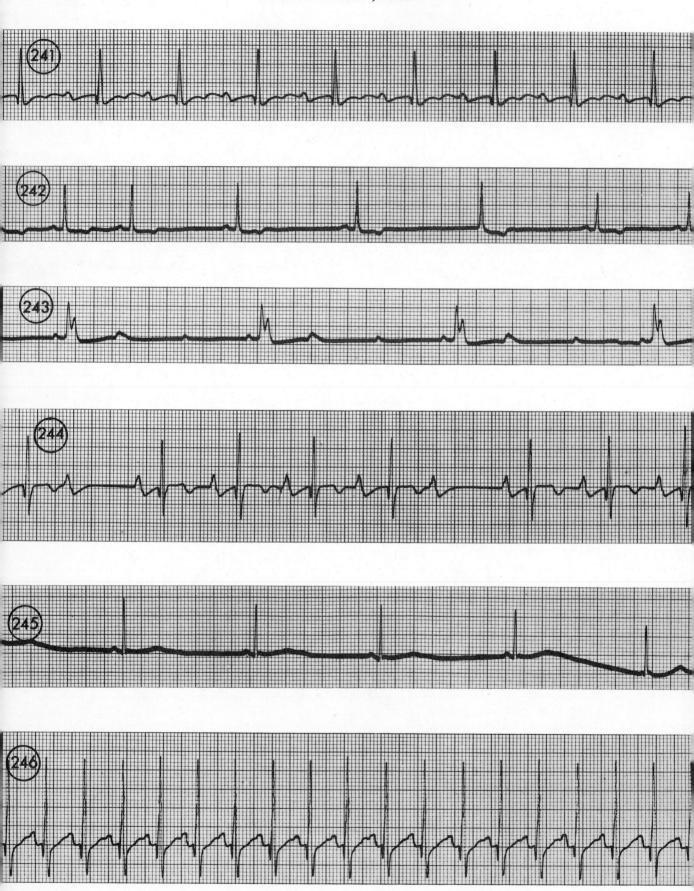

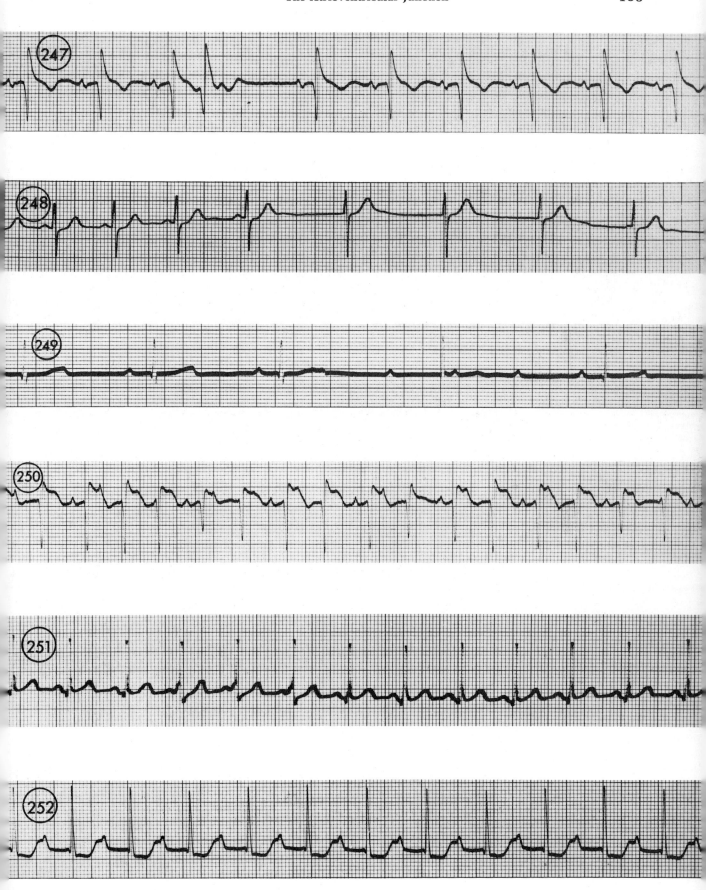

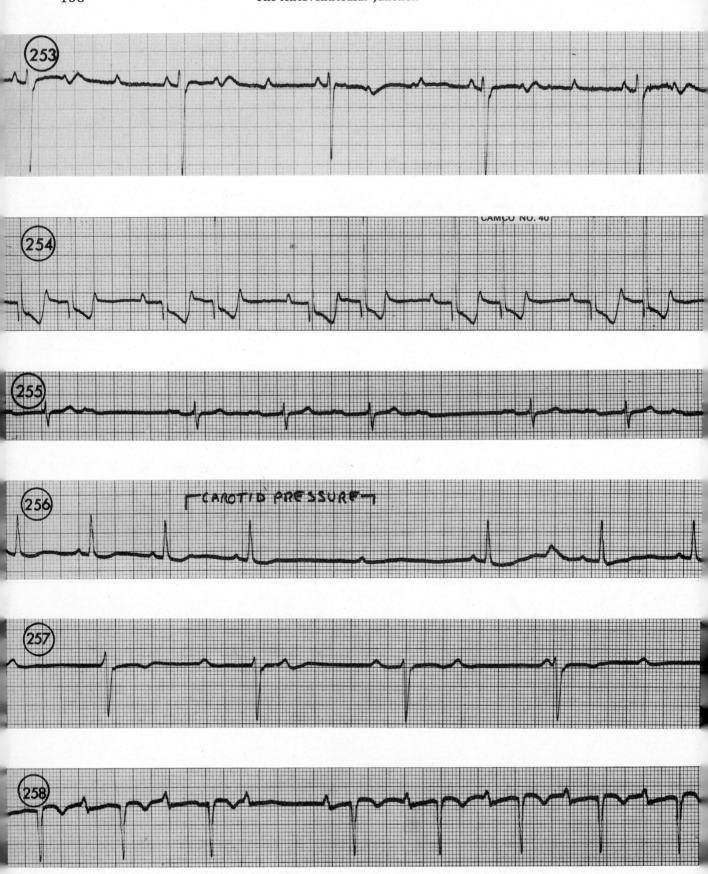

CAMCO NO. 40

CAROTID PRESSURE

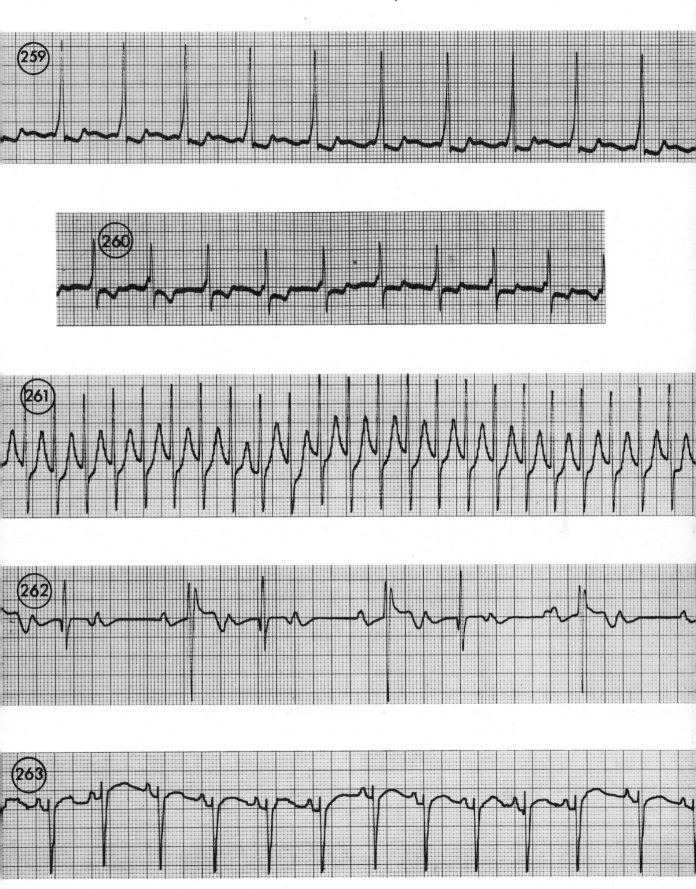

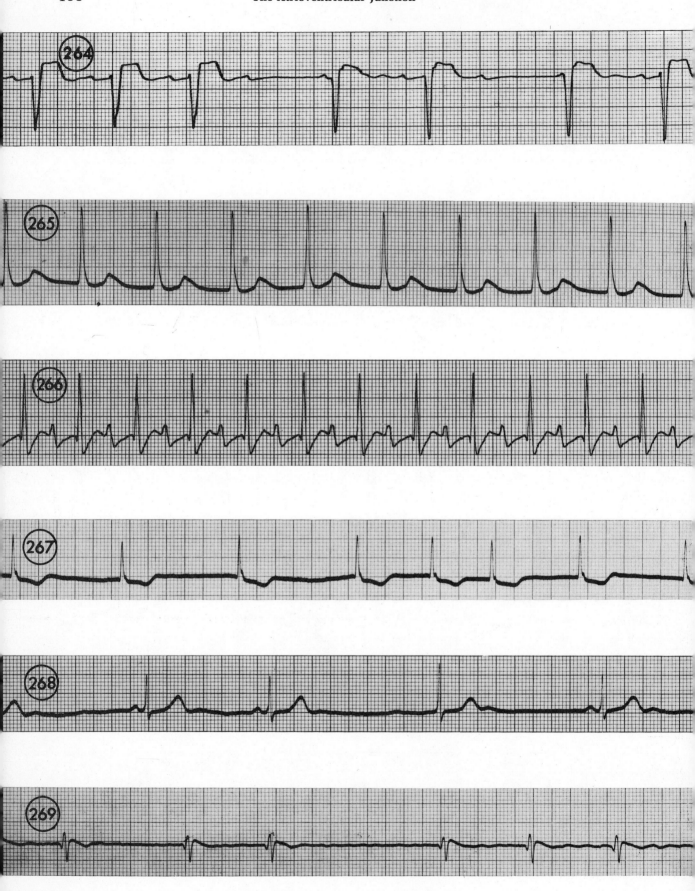

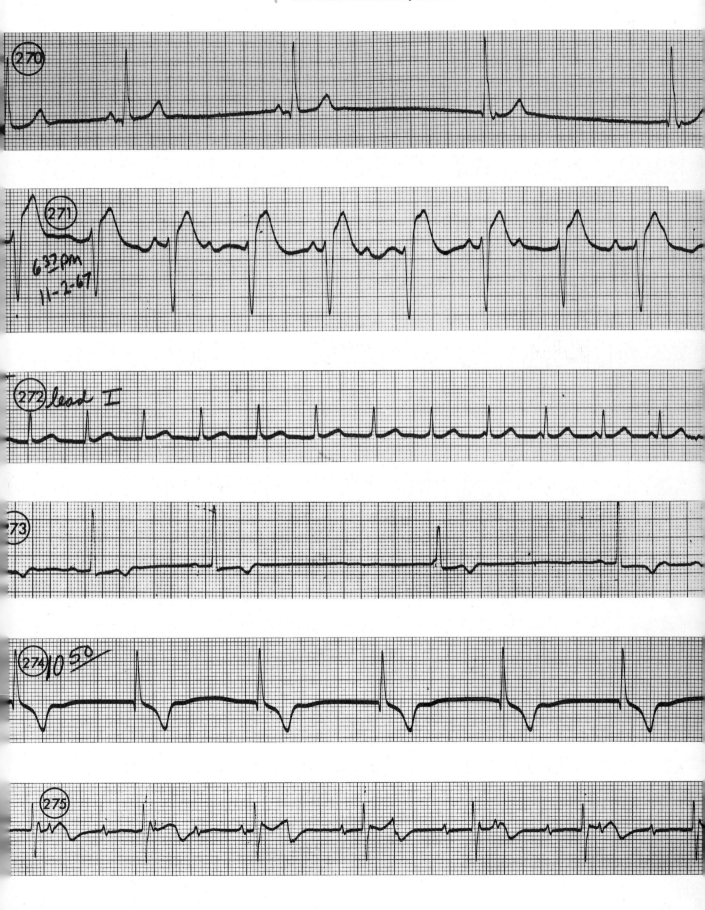

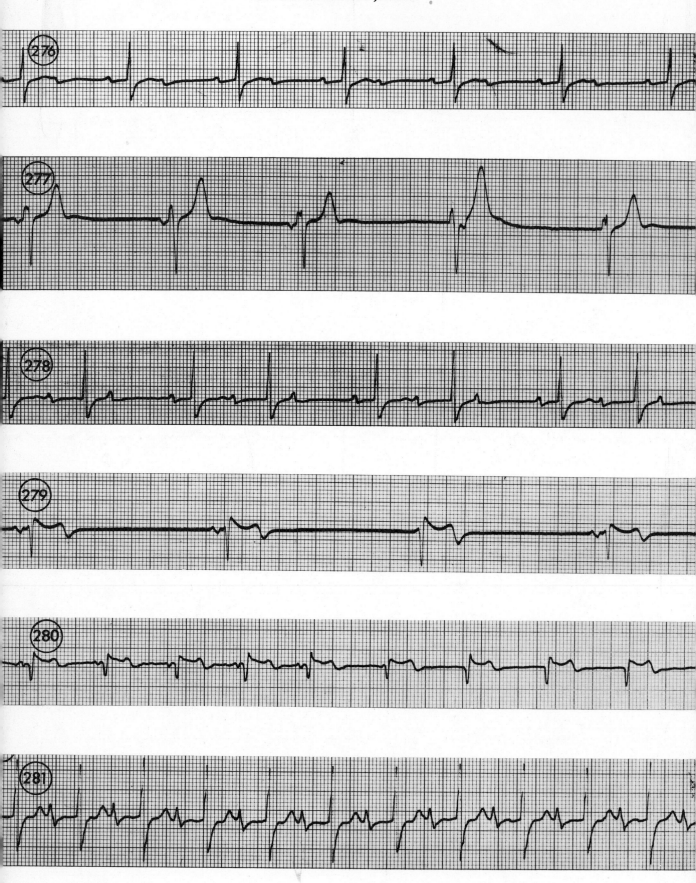

Chapter 7

THE BUNDLES

BUNDLE: IMPULSE CONDUCTION

Depression

RBBB = Right bundle branch block
LBBB = Left bundle branch block
LAH = Left anterior hemiblock
LPH = Left posterior hemiblock

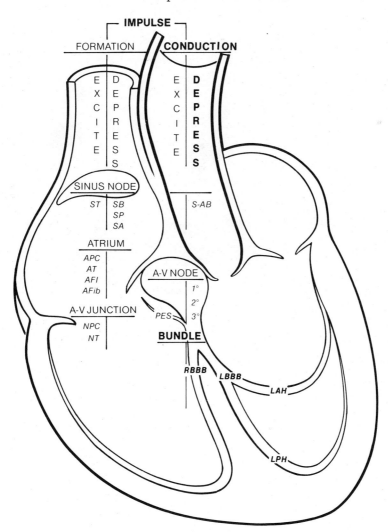

An impulse which passes through the A-V node may be significantly delayed or blocked entirely by a lesion in the common bundle or either of its branches. The resultant electrocardiographic changes help to identify the location of the depression of conduction velocity. The defect in impulse propagation may be due to a structural lesion (ischemic or inflammatory) or to a physiological delay.

Common Bundle Block

A lesion in the common bundle may totally disrupt impulse transmission from the A-V node into the ventricular conduction system. This is a form of third degree heart block and is indistinguishable by conventional electrocardiography from complete A-V block produced by a lesion within the A-V node itself. However, a conduction defect in the common bundle is more likely to be distal to potential A-V junction pacemaker tissue. A sustained ventricular beat will then be dependent upon impulses formed somewhere in the ventricles. Such **ventricular escape rhythms** will be described in the subsequent chapter on ventricular impulse formation.

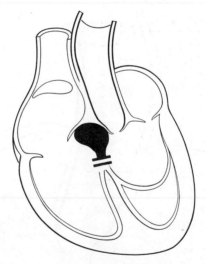

Common bundle block.

Right Bundle Branch Block

The term **right bundle branch block** is applied to conditions in which impulse conduction is blocked in only the right bundle. Impulses descend in the left bundle branch normally, and the left ventricle is depolarized in its usual sequence. The right ventricle is then depolarized by propagation of the impulse directly from the left ventricle. The wave is *not* transmitted along the usual Purkinje system, but rather through muscle by aberrant and slower conduction pathways.

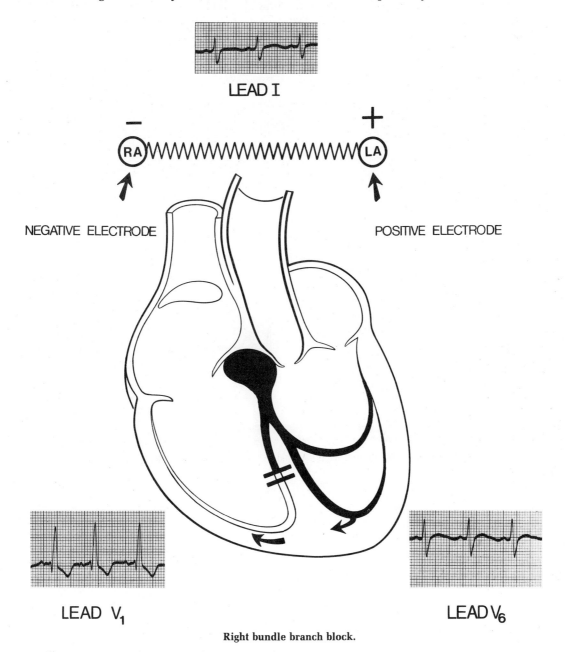

Right bundle branch block.

Sinus tachycardia with right bundle branch block is demonstrated in leads I, V_1, and V_6. Note the prolonged QRS complex duration, the wide S wave in leads I and V_6, and the wide R′ in lead V_1.

The initial portion of the QRS complex is unaffected in **right bundle block**, since the septum is stimulated in the normal sequence. However, the remainder of the QRS complex is widened and distorted by the conduction defect. The total QRS duration is 0.12 second or greater. Standard ECG leads have a characteristic pattern revealing the delayed and aberrant depolarization of the right ventricle. This late depolarization wave moves toward lead V_1, and a broad upward component (R') is formed. Leads with the positive electrode (lead I) away from the right ventricular depolarization wave direction have wide terminal downward components of QRS. Therefore, right bundle branch block can be identified by a QRS duration greater than 0.12 second and a wide S in leads I and V_6. A similar pattern is also generally present in the suggested monitoring lead.

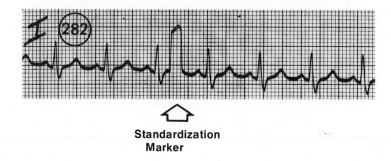

**Standardization
Marker**

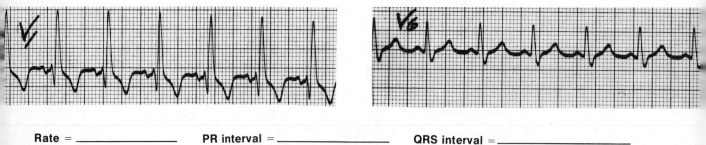

Rate = _____   PR interval = _____   QRS interval = _____

Right bundle branch block from selected leads of the standard electrocardiogram.

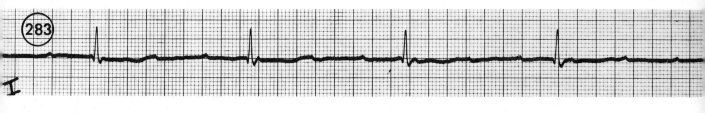

Sinus rate = _____   Ventricular rate = _____   QRS duration = _____

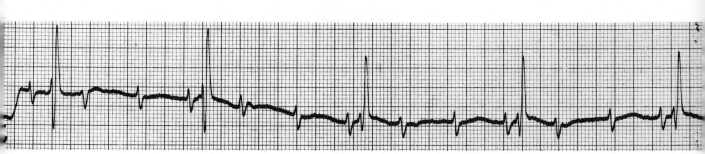

Compound arrhythmia (having more than one electrical disturbance) taken from leads I and V_1.

Interpretation:
1. Sinus tachycardia.
2. Complete A-V block.
3. Ventricular complexes have right bundle branch block pattern (i.e., prolonged QRS complex, wide S in lead I, wide R′ in lead V_1).

The presence of right bundle branch block in this rhythm indicates that the pacemaker driving the ventricles arises from A-V junctional tissue. It cannot be located in the atria, since the atria are under the control of the sinus pacemaker. The sequence of depolarization of the ventricles places the secondary pacemaker high in the ventricular conduction system near the A-V node. Thus, identification of a bundle branch block pattern is helpful in establishing the origin of ventricular beats.

The right bundle branch is relatively vulnerable to adverse physiological or pathological factors which may retard impulse conduction. Right bundle branch block occurs in many forms of heart disease and is sometimes present in individuals with no other cardiac abnormalities.

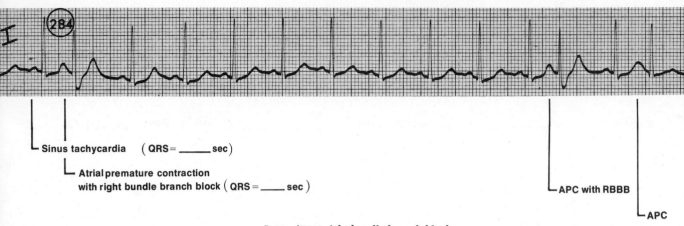

Sinus tachycardia   (QRS = _____ sec)

Atrial premature contraction
with right bundle branch block (QRS = _____ sec)

APC with RBBB

APC

Intermittent right bundle branch block.

In this tracing from lead I, premature contractions having aberrant ventricular conduction are evident. Note the first and second atrial premature contractions; each is characterized by the following:

1. Prolonged QRS complex.

2. Initial QRS complex similar to that of normally conducted beats, while the terminal portion consists of a widened S component.

3. Altered contours of ST segment and T wave.

Compare these forms with the third APC in which the QRS complex is similar to that of the sinus beats. This APC occurs at a slightly longer interval after the previous beat, which allows just enough additional time for the right bundle branch to recover and conduct the atrial impulse normally.

A premature beat may take place before full recovery of the conduction pathways from the previous beat (e.g., during the refractory period). A conduction defect, particularly right bundle branch block, is commonly associated with atrial and nodal premature contractions.

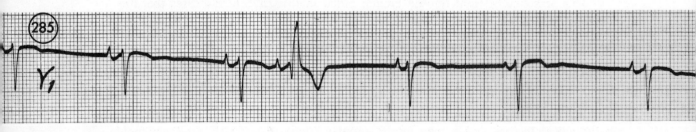

Rate = _____

Premature contraction with conduction defect.

Sinus bradycardia: Atrial premature contraction with right bundle branch block. Locate _____.

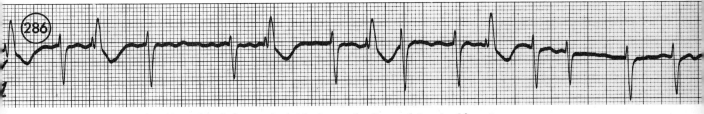

Normal and abnormal ventricular conduction as determined by rate.

Atrial fibrillation with intermittent right bundle branch block is evident. Locate the abnormally conducted ventricular beats _____.

The bundle branch block pattern appears with the more rapidly occurring beats, suggesting a relationship of bundle branch conduction to rate. Evidently, the earlier beats are formed while the right ventricular conduction fibers are still in a refractory state. This is analogous to the failure of conduction in the A-V node after some atrial premature contractions. Note the changes in ST segment and T wave configuration caused by the bundle branch conduction defect.

Right bundle branch block produced by deep breath holding (Valsalva maneuver) is revealed in the following tracings. Notice that the increased vagal tone has decreased conduction velocity in *both* the A-V node and the right bundle branch, producing transient lengthening or failure of conduction and bundle branch block.

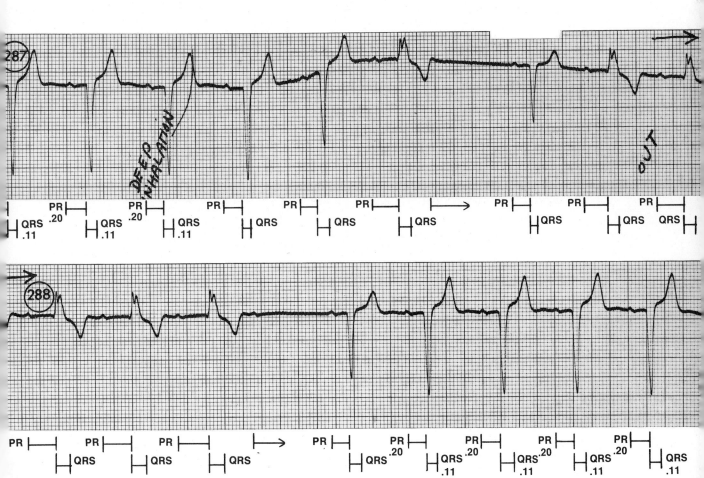

Note these effects with deep breath holding:
1. Slowing of the sinus rate.
2. Development of right bundle branch block.
3. Prolongation of A-V conduction; this is progressive and results in a sequence of second degree A-V blocks of the Wenckebach type.
4. Recovery of A-V and right bundle conduction.

The following tracing reveals intermittent right bundle branch block in the presence of atrial tachycardia with Wenckebach phenomenon and a regular 3:2 atrial/ventricular ratio. The arrhythmia is recorded from a special monitoring lead.

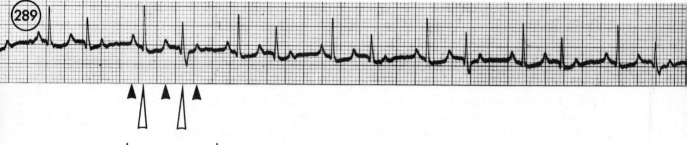

L─ Wenckebach ─J
cycle

1. Determine PR intervals.
2. Complete diagram.
3. Label all beats with RBBB _____, _____, _____, _____.

Each instance of right bundle branch block appears in the second beat of the three beat Wenckebach series. It is at this time that the ventricular conduction pathways have had the least time for recovery, and the impulse reaches the right bundle during its refractory period.

Left Bundle Branch Block

When pulses are delayed or blocked in the left bundle branch, another QRS form results. The conduction defect may be in the main stem, so that the entire left ventricle is activated by an impulse received through muscular transmission from the right bundle branch system. As the muscle mass on the left is much larger, the aberrant conduction pattern is very prominent in the ECG.

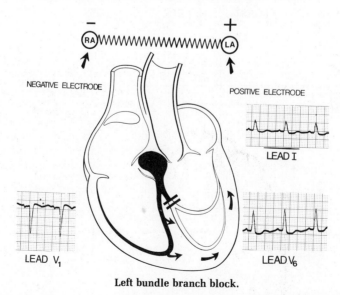

Left bundle branch block.

Left bundle branch block is most readily identified in leads I and V_6, in which the complexes are characteristically upright and broad with slurring of the terminal shape. The lead V_1 positive electrode is away from the direction of the major electrical forces so that a wide negative QRS complex is inscribed. The normally occurring small Q wave in leads I and V_6 is usually absent in left bundle branch block, demonstrating that even the initial electrical forces of ventricular depolarization, generated in the ventricular septum, are affected. Left bundle branch block is almost always an expression of some form of heart disease, usually ischemic, hypertensive, or valvular.

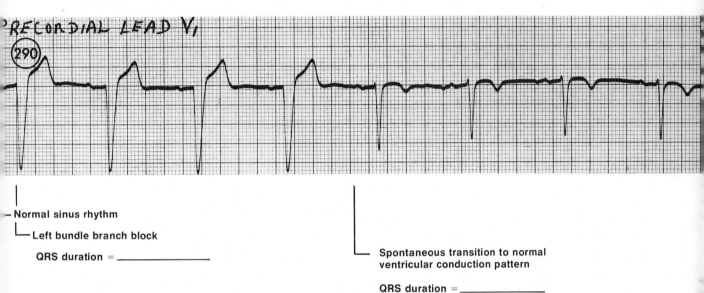

Normal sinus rhythm

Left bundle branch block

QRS duration = _____

Spontaneous transition to normal
ventricular conduction pattern

QRS duration = _____

Transient left bundle branch block.

Note the marked alteration in ST segment and T wave configuration produced by the conduction defect.

The suggested monitoring electrode placement, which is similar to lead I of the standard ECG, is usually sufficient to distinguish these major bundle branch block patterns.

QRS Complex Configuration from the Suggested Monitor Lead for Bundle Branch Block

	Initial Portion	*Terminal Portion*
RBBB:	Normal depolarization of ventricular septum: **Usually Small Q**	Delayed right ventricular depolarization: **Wide S**

RBBB

	Initial Portion	*Terminal Portion*
LBBB:	Reversed depolarization of ventricular septum: **Absent Q**	Delayed left ventricular depolarization: **Wide R**

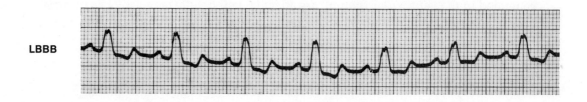

LBBB

The left bundle branch divides into the anterior (or superior) and posterior (or inferior) limbs, of which the latter is the larger. Conduction defects often occur in only one of these limbs (or fascicles), creating a **hemiblock.**

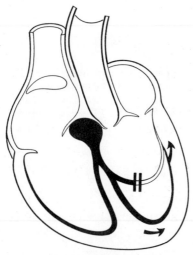

Left anterior hemiblock.

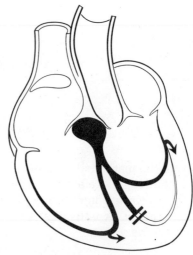

Left posterior hemiblock.

A **bifascicular block** (LAHb and LPHb) in effect produces a pattern indistinguishable from LBBB.

LAHb and RBBB could be considered other forms of bifascicular conduction defect. This combination is not uncommonly present in clinical practice.

The hemiblocks produce widened and distorted ventricular complexes on the electrocardiogram. However, their precise identification cannot be made from a single monitoring lead, and recognition of the various patterns is beyond the goal of this text. Impulse blockage may also occur in branches distal to the major limbs, producing changes in the QRS complex. These end-of-the-line disturbances in depolarization, as well as the hemiblocks, may be grouped as **intraventricular conduction defects.**

A trifascicular block consists of RBBB, LAHb, and LPHb. Actually, this is another form of complete A-V block, and the electrocardiographic pattern cannot be distinguished from that of a single lesion in the A-V node or common bundle.

The right bundle appears to be most susceptible to chemical and pathologic processes which adversely affect impulse conduction, and RBBB is the most frequent monofascicular defect seen clinically. The left anterior branch is somewhat less so. Left posterior bundle branch block, involving the largest fiber mass, is most resistant.

Persons with bifascicular blocks have a high incidence of progression into complete A-V block. This is particularly true if prolongation of the PR interval is also present. A patient who complains of periods of syncope, lightheadedness, or other manifestations of sudden circulatory depression and who, in addition, has multiple electrocardiographic conduction disorders should be suspected of having periods of complete A-V block.

An example of multiple conduction pathway defects can be seen in the case of a 56-year-old baker who had episodes of unexplained lightheadedness for several weeks with increasing frequency. A standard electrocardiogram revealed normal sinus rhythm with right bundle branch block and left anterior hemiblock. During the recording of lead V_1, an arrhythmia appeared which helped to elucidate the cause of the symptoms.

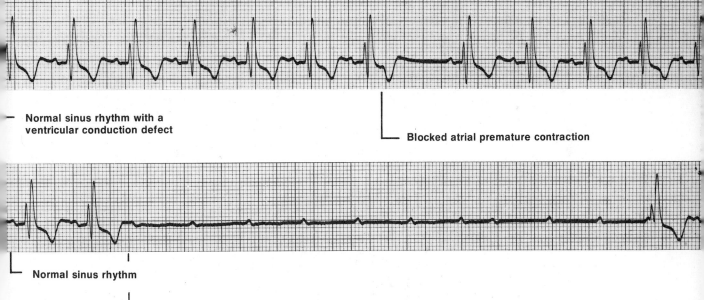

— Normal sinus rhythm with a
ventricular conduction defect

└── Blocked atrial premature contraction

└─ Normal sinus rhythm

└── Continued sinus rhythm with absence of ventricular response

During this time, the patient felt faint. A six-second period of ventricular asystole is ended with a nodal escape beat, after which the sinus rhythm is resumed. At this instant, the patient recovered fully.

Note that the PR interval of conducted beats is normal, suggesting that impulse transmission through the A-V node is unimpaired. As the patient was known to have complete block of two of the major bundle branches (bifascicular block), it was presumed that the third bundle (left posterior branch) was diseased and temporarily incapable of transmitting impulses, producing intermittent trifascicular block. A poorly functioning escape mechanism led to a period of symptomatic ventricular asystole.

Chapter 8

THE VENTRICLES

Tissue within the ventricles, like that in other areas of the heart, has the capacity to undergo spontaneous discharges. These may originate from the major intraventricular conduction fascicles or anywhere along the Purkinje system, including the terminal fibers intimately distributed among the myofibrils. There is some doubt that the myocardial cells themselves can generate impulses.

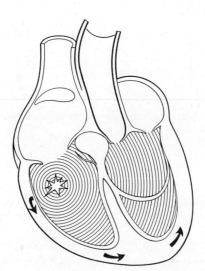

Ventricular impulse formation.

The natural rate of automaticity in a ventricular focus is relatively slow (20 to 50 per minute). Normally the potential pacemakers of the ventricles are continually suppressed by impulses emanating from the more rapid pacemakers—sinus, atrial, and A-V junctional.

Impulse formation may occur within the ventricles by two mechanisms:
1. *Escape:* response to depressed *impulse formation* above the ventricles, or depressed *impulse conduction* of impulses from above the ventricles.
2. *Excitation:* response to stimulation of automatic foci.

Ventricular Escape Beat

When the ventricles do not receive stimuli from above within a certain period of time, they normally respond by forming an impulse at some focus of automaticity. **Ventricular escape beats** appear when the sinus node impulse formation is severely retarded and escape beats are not generated within the atria or A-V junctional tissue. They may also occur if these supraventricular impulses do not proceed into the ventricles because of a conduction block.

An impulse originating from a focus within the ventricles and propagating throughout the ventricular mass does not travel along the normal conduction pathways. The wave of excitation spreads radially at relatively slow velocity. These factors produce a QRS complex which has:
1. *Altered form:* abnormal conduction pathway.
2. *Increased duration:* slowed conduction velocity.

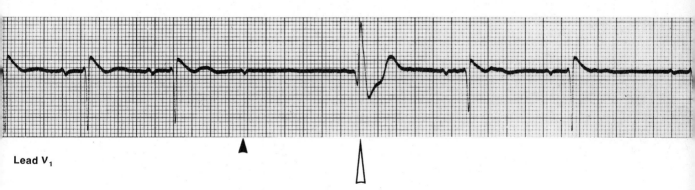

Lead V₁

Ventricular escape beat.

First degree A-V block (PR interval = 0.24 second) is evident. Following a nonconducted beat, there is a long pause, then a QRS complex having altered form and increased duration. This is a ventricular escape beat. Note that the initial as well as the terminal portions of the QRS complex differ from those of the normal beats. This beat does *not* have the recognizable pattern of a bundle branch block.

Ventricular escape beats interrupting sinus pauses.

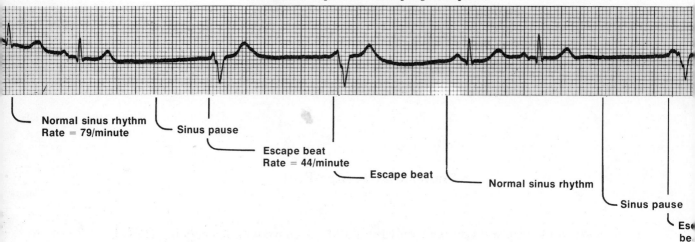

Normal sinus rhythm
Rate = 79/minute — Sinus pause — Escape beat Rate = 44/minute — Escape beat — Normal sinus rhythm — Sinus pause — Es... be...

Two consecutive escape beats appear following the first sinus pause. Each of these beats has a wide QRS complex with an anomalous form. The intrinsic rate of the beats is slow. These are ventricular escape beats.

After the second sinus pause, another ventricular escape beat occurs. This time, however, it is immediately preceded by a normal-appearing P wave. Because the escape beat is similar to those observed earlier and the duration between the P wave and the QRS complex is far shorter than a normal PR interval, it is assumed that these beats occurred almost simultaneously but from independent pacemakers (e.g., sinus and ventricular).

When paths of depolarization are altered, repolarization sequences are also altered. This usually results in changes in ST segment and T wave form.

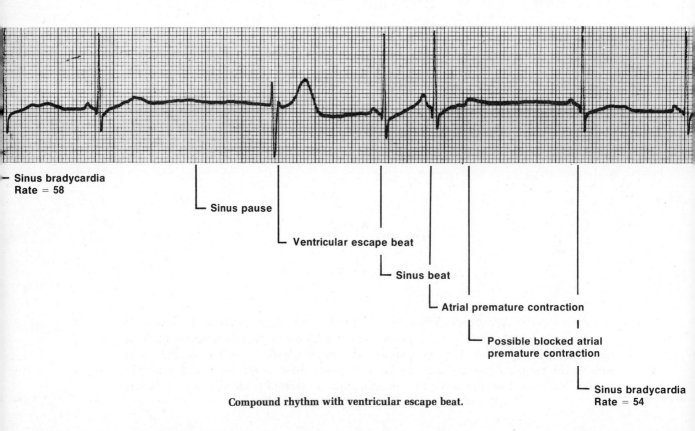

Sinus bradycardia
Rate = 58 — Sinus pause — Ventricular escape beat — Sinus beat — Atrial premature contraction — Possible blocked atrial premature contraction — Sinus bradycardia Rate = 54

Compound rhythm with ventricular escape beat.

The ventricular escape beat appears after a pause in the sinus pacemaker. The QRS complex of this beat is prolonged (0.12 second) and altered in configuration. Note particularly that it begins with an R deflection, in contrast with QRS complexes of supraventricular beats (sinus and atrial) which begin with a Q wave. Note also the change in the ST segment and T wave of this beat.

Another common feature of beats originating in the ventricles is the absence of retrograde conduction through the A-V node. Therefore, sinus activity and atrial activity are not disturbed, and P waves are chronologically independent of QRS complexes.

Sinus arrest in the absence of atrial or A-V junctional escape pacemakers or complete A-V block may lead to a ventricular escape rhythm. Thus, when all else fails to produce a heart beat, a latent pacemaker will hopefully be activated in the ventricles to prevent asystole. The **idioventricular rhythm** can be considered a normal response to depression in higher pacemakers or in impulse conduction from them.

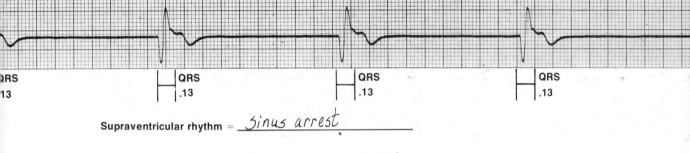

QRS .13   QRS .13   QRS .13   QRS .13

Supraventricular rhythm = *Sinus arrest*

Ventricular rhythm: Rate = *31*   QRS duration = *.13 sec.*

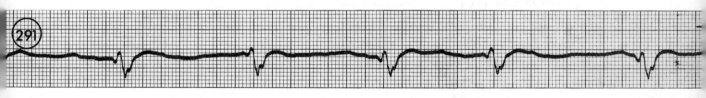

(291)

Supraventricular rhythm = *Atrial activity indistinct*

Ventricular rhythm: Rate = *43*   QRS duration = _____

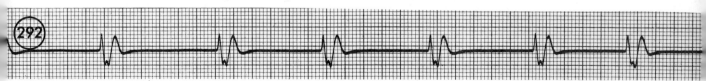

(292)

Supraventricular rhythm = _____

Ventricular rhythm: Rate = _____ QRS duration = _____

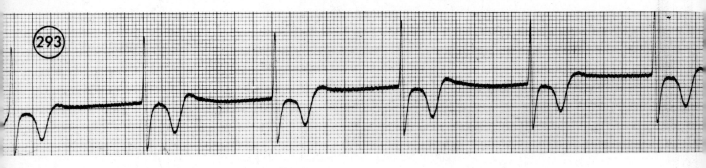

Supraventricular rhythm = _____

Ventricular rhythm: Rate = _____ QRS duration =_____

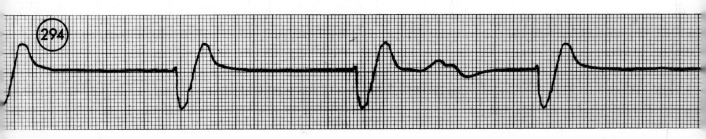

Supraventricular rhythm = _____

Ventricular rhythm: Rate = _____ QRS duration =_____

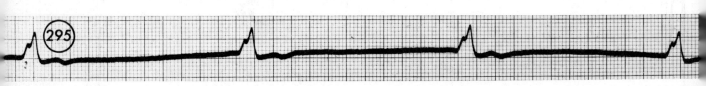

Supraventricular rhythm =_____

Ventricular rhythm: Rate = _____ QRS duration =_____

Complete A-V Block with Ventricular Pacemaker

Subsidiary pacemakers located within the ventricles may become activated in the presence of complete A-V block. The escape mechanism in this conduction defect is similar to that described with cessation of impulse formation at higher sites (e.g., sinus arrest). The escape or idioventricular rhythm is comparable to that of A-V nodal rhythms developing during complete A-V block, but the ventricular pacemaker tends to be slower and more irregular.

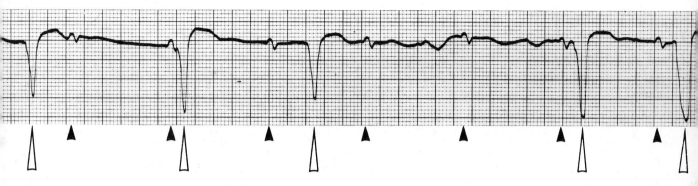

Sinus rhythm: Rate = 58   **Ventricular rhythm, extremely irregular: Rate = approximately 30**

Note that the sinus and ventricular rhythms are completely independent of each other. The ventricular contractions display delayed depolarization (0.16 second), and the cadence is erratic.

Examples of complete A-V block with ventricular pacemakers.

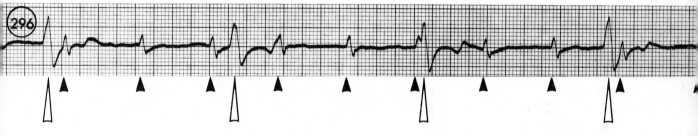

Sinus rhythm: Rate =_____   **Complete AV block (no sinus impulses are conducted to the ventricles)**

Ventricular rhythm: Rate =_____   **QRS complex duration =_____ seconds**

(QRS complex duration is estimated since the precise point at which ventricular depolarization ends cannot be ascertained.)

In the following example, the ventricular rhythm is completely regular.

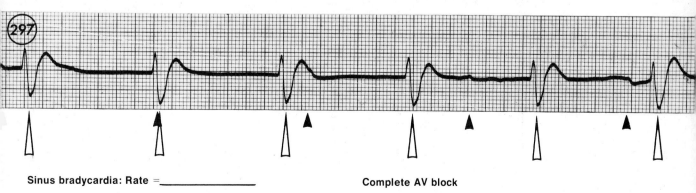

Sinus bradycardia: Rate =_____   **Complete AV block**

Ventricular rhythm: Rate =_____   **QRS duration =_____**

Label the following electrocardiograms completely and give a full interpretation of them. Include rates of supraventricular and ventricular rhythms. Determine QRS complex duration.

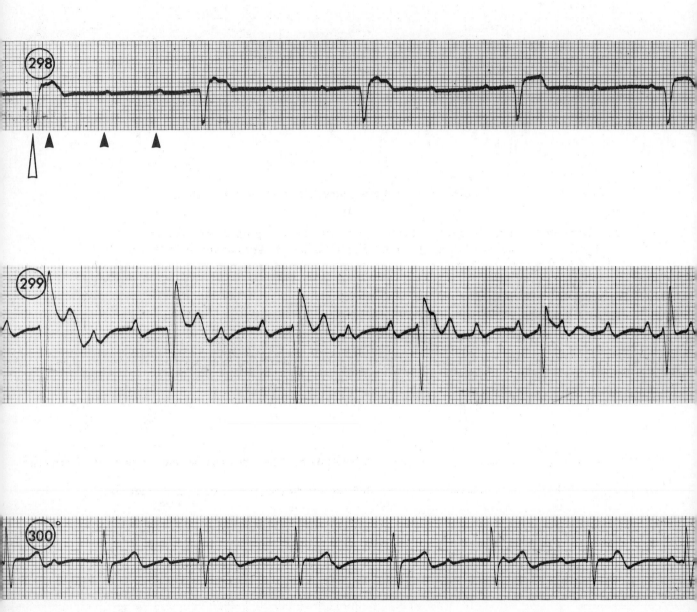

VENTRICLE: IMPULSE FORMATION

Excitation

VPC = Ventricular premature contraction
VT = Ventricular tachycardia
VFl = Ventricular flutter
VFib = Ventricular fibrillation

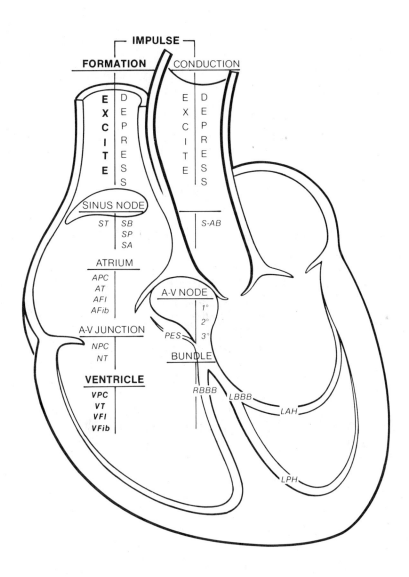

Ventricular Premature Contractions

Sympathetic nervous system stimuli or abnormal intrinsic excitability may induce premature firing of latent ventricular pacemakers. These beats are similar in form to ventricular escape beats from the same ectopic focus. However, they result from an accelerated spontaneous discharge rate rather than an escape response to depression of impulse formation or conduction velocity from usually dominant centers.

Excitation of a ventricular automatic site causes a beat distinguished by:

1. Prematurity (accelerated rate).
2. Wide, distorted QRS complex (aberrant depolarization wave).
3. Altered T wave form (aberrant repolarization sequences).
4. Failure of retrograde conduction into atria (sinoatrial activity is usually unaffected by ventricular impulses, and P wave cadence is not interrupted).

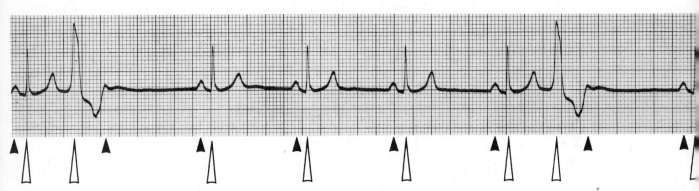

Normal sinus rhythm with ventricular premature contraction.

Note that the sinus cadence is *not* interrupted by the ventricular ectopic beat (check with calipers).

Ventricular premature contractions (VPC's) are occasionally present in normal individuals. They may be induced by sympathetic stimulation (adrenergic drugs, amphetamines, caffeine, emotional challenge) or by changes in the threshold of excitability in ventricular tissue (digitalis toxicity, hypoxia, anesthetic agents, myocardial injury).

In acute myocardial infarction, as many as 80 per cent of patients have ectopic ventricular beats. These may prove innocuous, or as shall be seen, may lead directly into more serious, and often fatal, arrhythmias.

A ventricular premature contraction may occur without interfering with the normal cardiac cycles. The extrasystole is in *fact* an "extra" contraction and is known as an **interpolated beat.** It is most likely to appear when the sinus rate is slow, allowing the ventricles to recover from the self-excited beat in time to respond to the next sinus impulse.

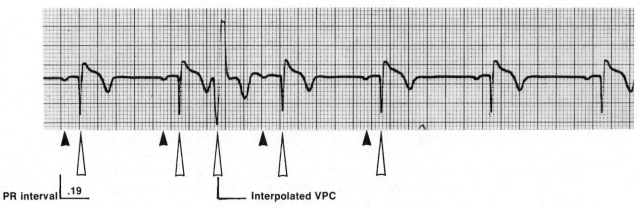

PR interval └─.19─┘   └──── Interpolated VPC

Interpolated ventricular premature contraction.

The ventricular premature contraction appears between two conducted sinus beats. There is no retrograde conduction from the ventricles to the atria, and the sinus rhythm is not interrupted. In addition, after the premature contraction and the subsequent sinus beat, the major conduction pathways have recovered enough to conduct the sinus impulse to the ventricles. Note, however, that the PR interval of the cardiac cycle which follows the premature contraction is somewhat prolonged. This indicates that the A-V node has not fully recovered, causing some decrease in the velocity of impulse conduction.

After most ventricular premature contractions, however, the conduction system is in a refractory state by the time the subsequent sinus beat reaches it, and the ventricles do not respond. The nonconducted P wave can often be identified. The relatively long interval detected between the premature contraction and the subsequent sinus beat is referred to as the **compensatory pause.** Note that no basic change in the cadence of the sinus rhythm occurs and that there is *no* extra (or additional) ventricular beat.

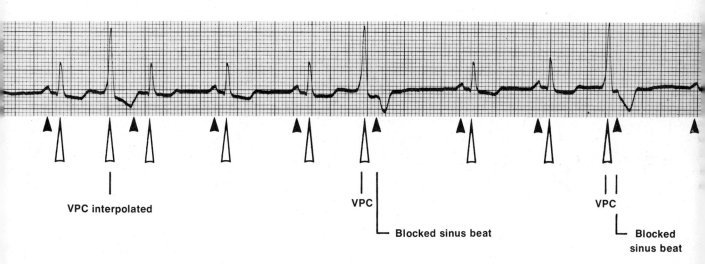

VPC interpolated

VPC

└ Blocked sinus beat

VPC

└ Blocked sinus beat

The first ventricular premature contraction does not prevent completion of the subsequent full cardiac cycle, although a slight delay in A-V conduction is present in this beat. This is, therefore, an interpolated beat.

Two ventricular premature contractions occur later in the tracing. These do not alter the cadence of the sinus rhythm (there is no retrograde conduction). However, the sinus beat following each of the premature contractions is blocked. In these cases, the A-V node has not sufficiently recovered to allow transmission of the normal sinus impulse to the ventricles.

The compensatory pause occurs when the sinus impulse following a premature contraction in the ventricles is blocked; it is that interval between the premature contraction and the subsequent normal ventricular contraction. The interval between the two normal beats which flank the premature contraction is twice the interval between two adjacent normal beats.

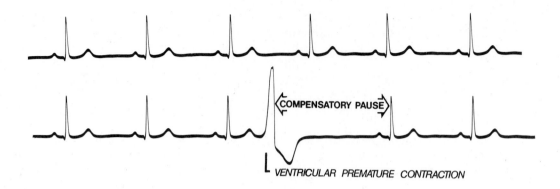

COMPENSATORY PAUSE

VENTRICULAR PREMATURE CONTRACTION

The ventricular premature contraction does not produce any change in the cadence of the sinus rhythm. Note that these simultaneously displayed rhythms remain in phase, even though the ectopic beat has occurred. The atrial beat following the ventricular premature contraction is blocked, resulting in a pause in ventricular contractions. The **compensatory pause** is so named because it results in resumption of the cadence without a "change in step."

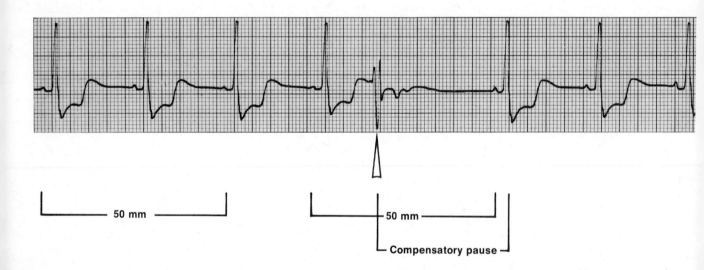

50 mm   50 mm

Compensatory pause

Contrast this long pause after ventricular premature contractions with premature impulses from the atria or A-V node. These depolarize the sinus node prematurely, which must then repolarize before generating another impulse. This resets the cadence of the sinus rhythm, and the next sinus discharge occurs at a regular interval. This relationship is known as a **noncompensatory pause.**

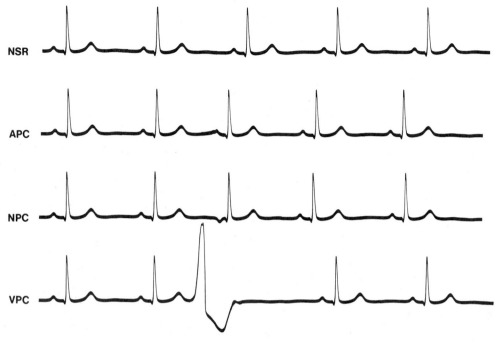

Compensatory and noncompensatory pauses.

Locate the atrial and nodal premature contractions of tracings No. 2 and No. 3, respectively. Note that there is a change in the cadence of the sinus rhythm following these ectopic beats. The next normal P wave usually occurs at a slightly delayed interval. The noncompensatory pause follows immediately after the premature contractions.

Now locate the ventricular premature contraction in tracing No. 4. This is followed by a blocked sinus beat, then resumption of normal sinus rhythm without any interruption of the sinus pacemaker cadence. The compensatory pause is usually much longer than the noncompensatory, particularly if the ectopic beat occurs early in the cycle, and the sinus cadence does not change.

In each of the following examples of ventricular premature contractions, label the premature contraction, the blocked sinus beat, and the compensatory pause.

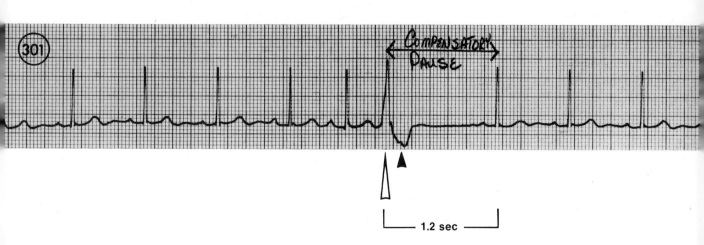

Label as preceding.

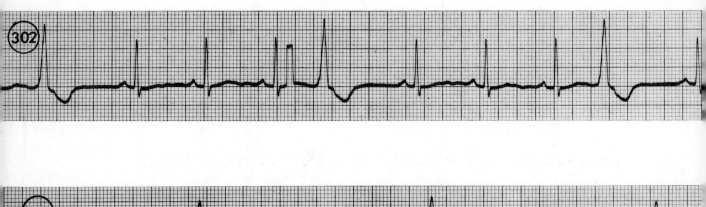

Ventricular premature contractions (VPC's) can be found in varying time relationships to the previous beat: early, intermediary, and late.

Early VPC

The ectopic QRS appears before the normal P wave of the next beat. (If this atrial wave is conducted, the VPC is termed "interpolated"; if it is not conducted, a compensatory pause occurs.)

Label the VPC, the nonconducted P wave, and the compensatory pause.

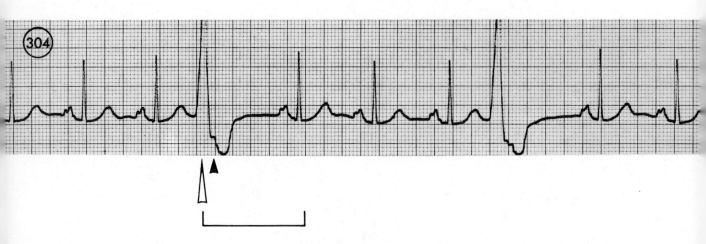

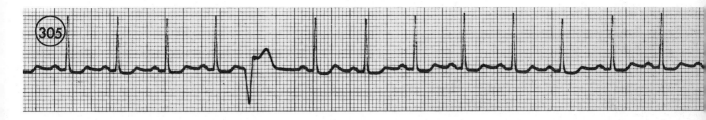

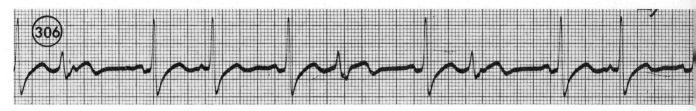

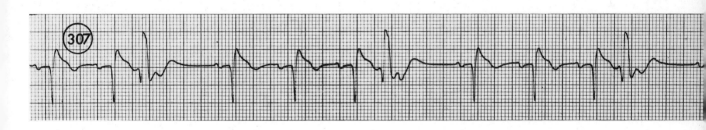

Special monitoring lead.

Note the right bundle branch block; the atrial premature contractions (locate
_____, _____); and the early ventricular premature contractions
(locate _____, _____, _____).

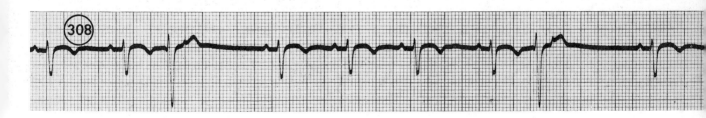

Intermediary VPC

An ectopic QRS is superimposed on the normal P wave. Only a part of the P wave
can usually be identified, if the wave is visible at all.

Label the VPC, the site of the anticipated P wave (estimated with calipers), and the compensatory pause.

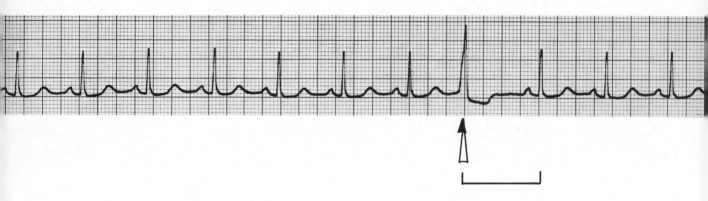

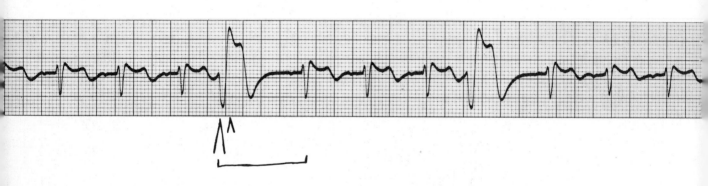

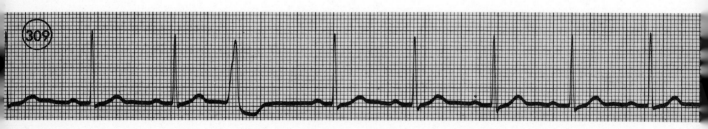

Late VPC

Ectopic QRS appears after the P wave. Sometimes only the initial portion of the P wave is formed when the VPC begins.

Label the VPC, the nonconducted P wave, and the compensatory pause.

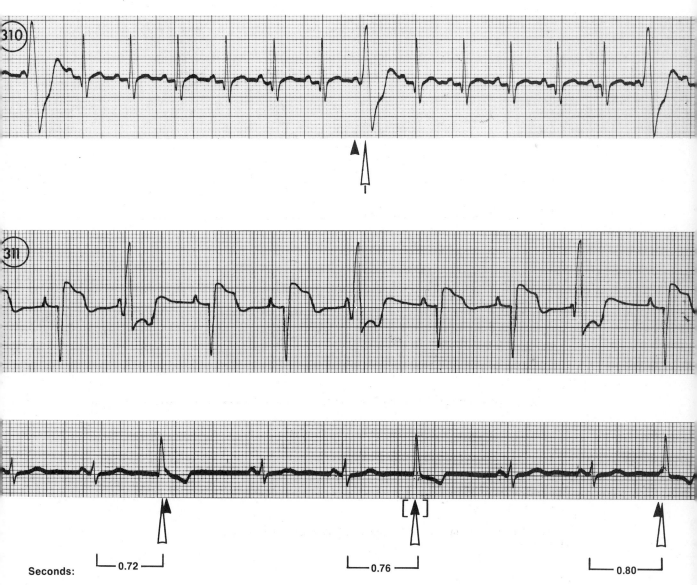

Comparison of ventricular premature contractions with varying degrees of prematurity.

Three ventricular premature contractions are found which occur with slightly increasing intervals after the respective normal beat. The P wave of the associated blocked sinus beat can be located after, during, and before the ectopic QRS complex according to the degree of prematurity.

The Ventricles

Ventricular Premature Contractions

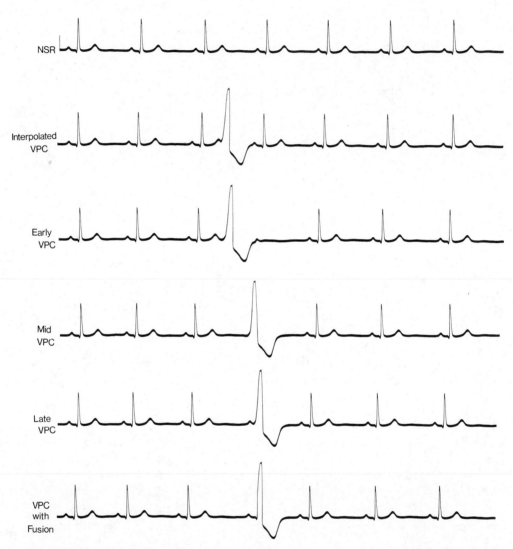

NSR

Interpolated
VPC

Early
VPC

Mid
VPC

Late
VPC

VPC
with
Fusion

Pictorial summary of ventricular premature contractions as they occur at various times in the cardiac cycle.

The Fusion Beat

A ventricular premature contraction may occur so late in the cycle that a normal sinus pacemaker or ectopic atrial or A-V nodal pacemaker impulse has already penetrated the A-V node and started to depolarize the ventricles. Before this is completed, however, the ventricular ectopic focus fires at a more distant site and initiates a wave of depolarization. These two waves, one proceeding downward in a normal direction and the other moving toward the atria, collide. Thus a QRS complex is inscribed representing ventricular depolarization initially from a supraventricular focus and concluding with depolarization activity from an ectopic ventricular focus. Such a combination of depolarization forces is known as a **fusion beat.**

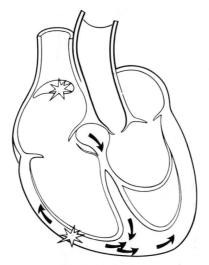

The fusion beat.

A cardiac contraction is formed from two impulses, one from the sinus node and one from the ventricle. The resultant waves of depolarization fuse to produce a complex cardiac cycle.

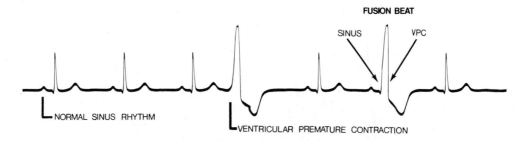

The fusion beat in this illustration begins with a normal sinus complex, then takes on the form of a ventricular premature contraction. This ventricular extrasystole occurs much later in the cardiac cycle than the previous one.

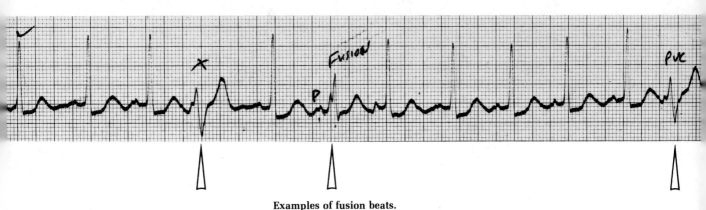

Examples of fusion beats.

Compare ventricular premature contractions. Each appears after a P wave has already begun to form. The second premature contraction occurs so late that the preceding P wave is completely inscribed. There follows an isoelectric period and the beginning of a QRS complex which is similar to that of the normal beats. Then the QRS complex takes on the form of the premature contractions. This beat represents the fusion of normal ventricular depolarization with depolarization of ectopic origin.

Ventricular premature contractions may occur in definite patterns, for which there is specific terminology.

Ventricular Bigeminy

This consists of premature ventricular beats alternating with supraventricular beats (sinus, atrial, or nodal origin) in a regular repetitive sequence.

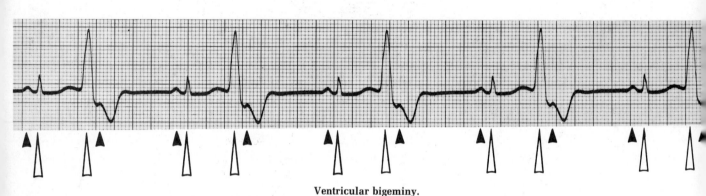

Ventricular bigeminy.

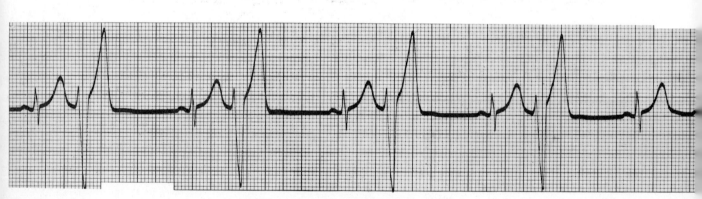

Transient ventricular bigeminy.

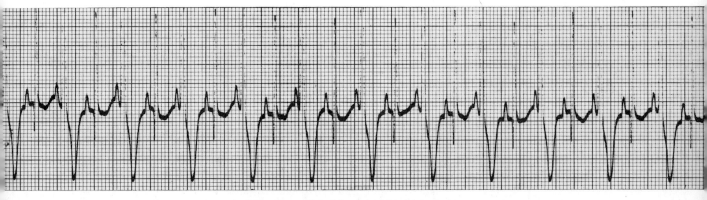

Atrial tachycardia with ventricular bigeminy.

This tracing was taken from a 13-year-old beagle, Candy. Late ventricular premature contractions in consistent bigeminal pattern appear after completion of atrial depolarization.

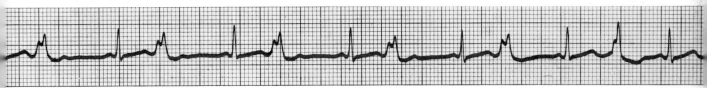

Bigeminal pattern in lead I.

This appears to be ventricular bigeminy. However, the premature contractions have the pattern of left bundle branch block. Therefore, it is assumed that the ectopic site is above the ventricles and in the A-V junctional tissue or common bundle.

Ventricular Trigeminy

This consists of two ventricular premature contractions following each supraventricular beat in a recurring pattern.

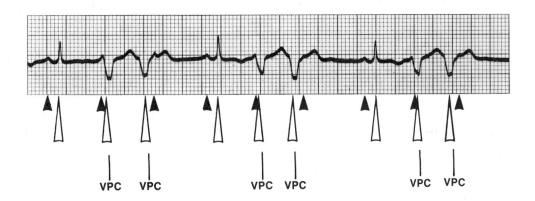

Unifocal

When ventricular premature contractions appear uniform in configuration and duration, it is assumed that they originate from a single excited ventricular site.

Identify the basic rhythm and rate. Locate the VPC's and compare.

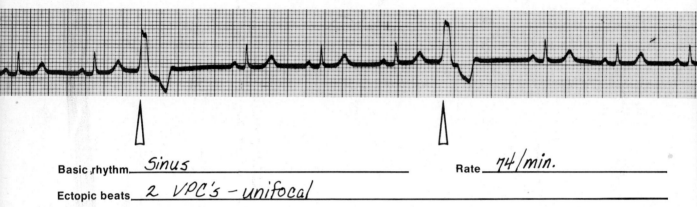

Basic rhythm___*Sinus*___   Rate___*74/min.*___

Ectopic beats___*2 VPC's – unifocal*___

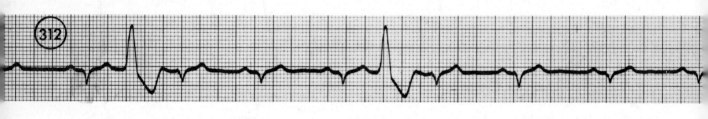

Basic rhythm_____   Rate_____

Ectopic beats_____

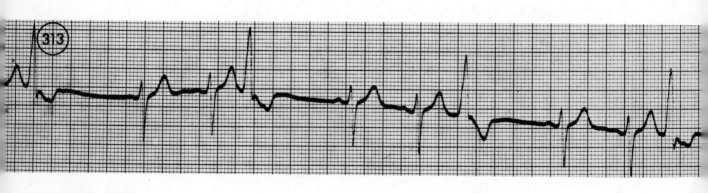

Basic rhythm_____   Rate_____

Ectopic beats_____

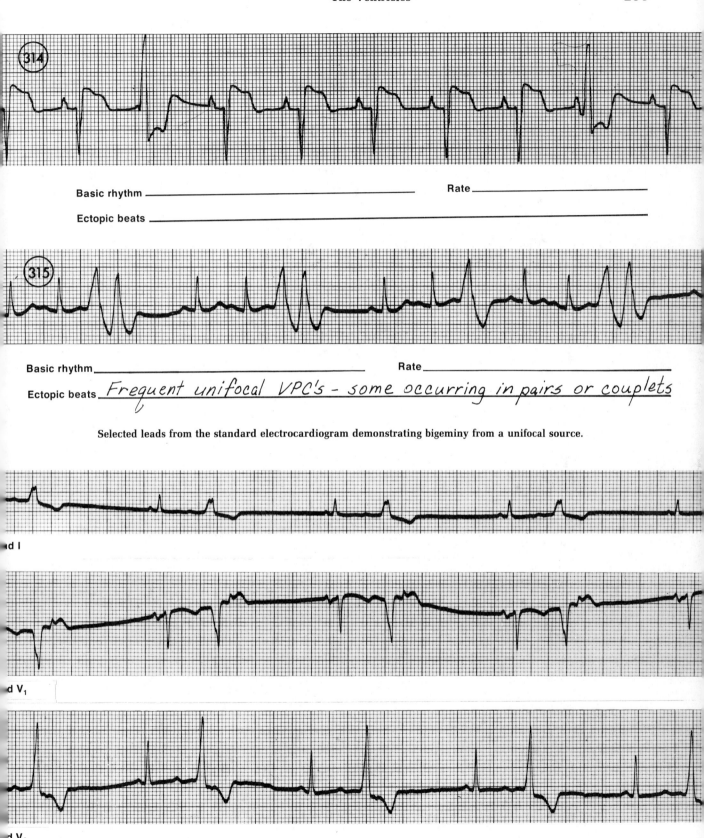

Basic rhythm _____ Rate _____

Ectopic beats _____

Basic rhythm _____ Rate _____

Ectopic beats *Frequent unifocal VPC's - some occurring in pairs or couplets*

Selected leads from the standard electrocardiogram demonstrating bigeminy from a unifocal source.

d I

d V₁

d V₆

When ventricular premature contractions in all three leads are compared, the
pattern of left bundle branch block can be identified. The site of origin of these

ectopic beats is most likely in the mainstem ventricular conduction tract. Retrograde atrial depolarization does not occur, and compensatory pauses are present after the ectopic beats.

Multifocal

When impulses are generated from more than one site in the ventricles, the resultant ectopic beats are referred to as **multifocal.** Ventricular premature contractions of multifocal origin display variations in timing, contour, and duration of QRS complexes. These reflect differences in the sequence of depolarization.

In the following electrocardiograms, interpret the basic rhythm and rate. Locate ventricular premature contractions and compare coupling intervals, configuration, and duration. Can groups or families of similar ventricular premature contractions be found in the same strip?

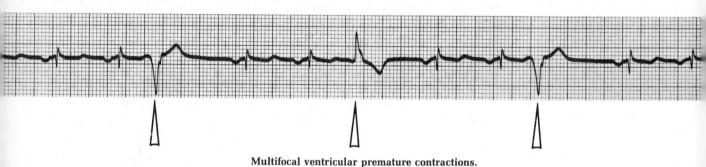

Multifocal ventricular premature contractions.

Note that the first and third ventricular premature contractions are similar and are, therefore, from the same site of origin.

Complete the interpretation:

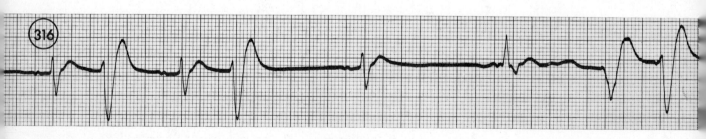

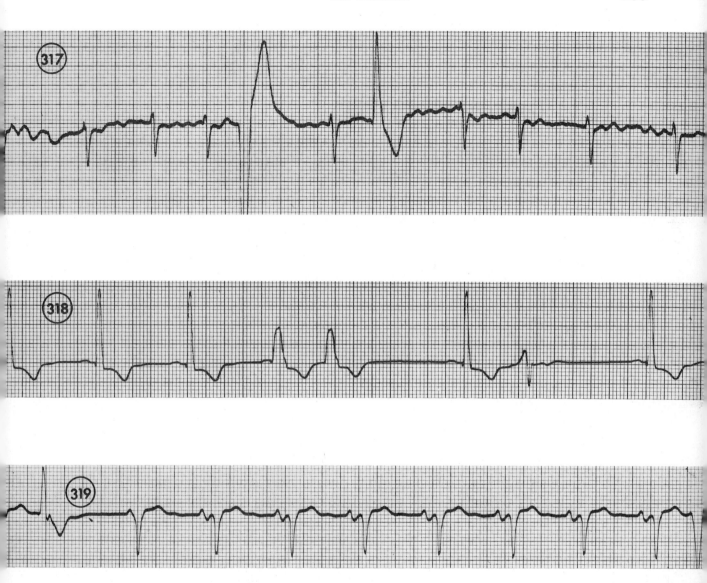

Fixed Coupling

Ventricular premature contractions appearing at a constant interval after the previous cardiac cycle are said to have **fixed coupling.**

Determine the basic rhythm and rate. Locate the VPC's and compare. Measure the interval between the beginning of normal QRS and the beginning of QRS-VPC.

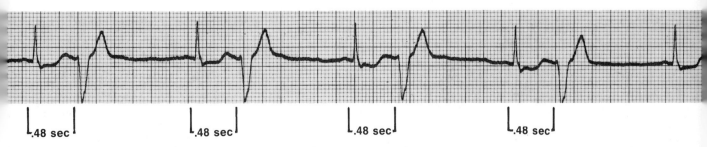

Normal sinus rhythm (presuming a nonconducted P wave unidentifiable in the T-VPC) with ventricular bigeminy of unifocal origin and with fixed coupling is evident.

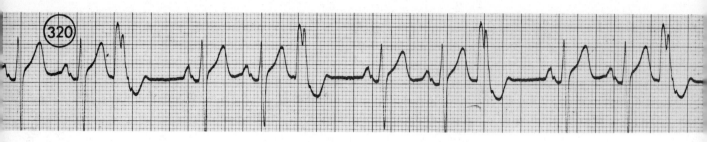

Is this ventricular trigeminy?

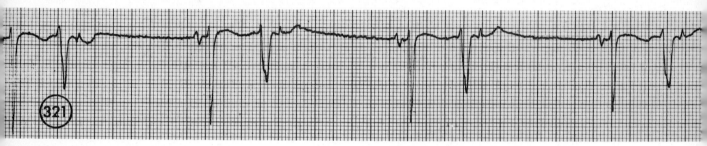

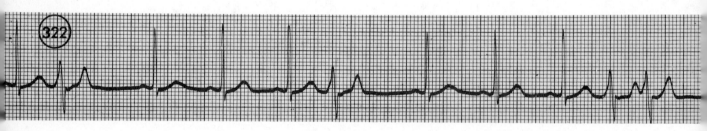

Variable Coupling

Ventricular premature contractions may occur with varying time relationship to the preceding normal beats. This situation is usually more ominous than fixed coupling, as will be described further.

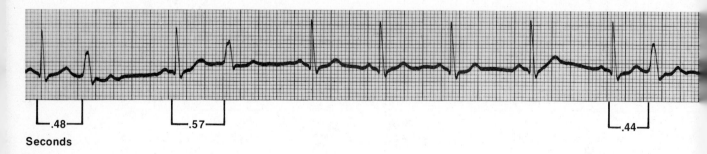

└ .48 ┘   └ .57 ┘   └ .44 ┘

Seconds

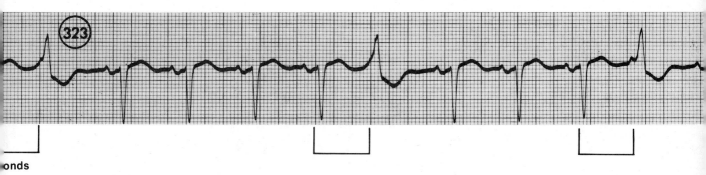

Unifocal ventricular premature contractions occur late in the cardiac cycle with slight variations in the coupling intervals. The changes in the initial portions of the ectopic QRS complexes are caused by superimposition of non conducted P waves with small differences in time relationships.

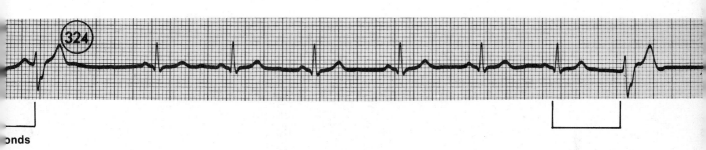

Examples of various forms of ventricular premature contractions follow. Label the basic rhythm and rate. Identify ventricular premature contractions and describe them fully.

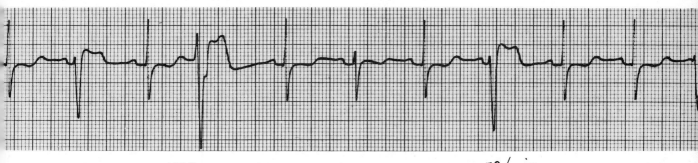

Basic rhythm _NSR_____   Rate _78/min._____

Ectopic beats _VPC's - multifocal; variable coupling_____

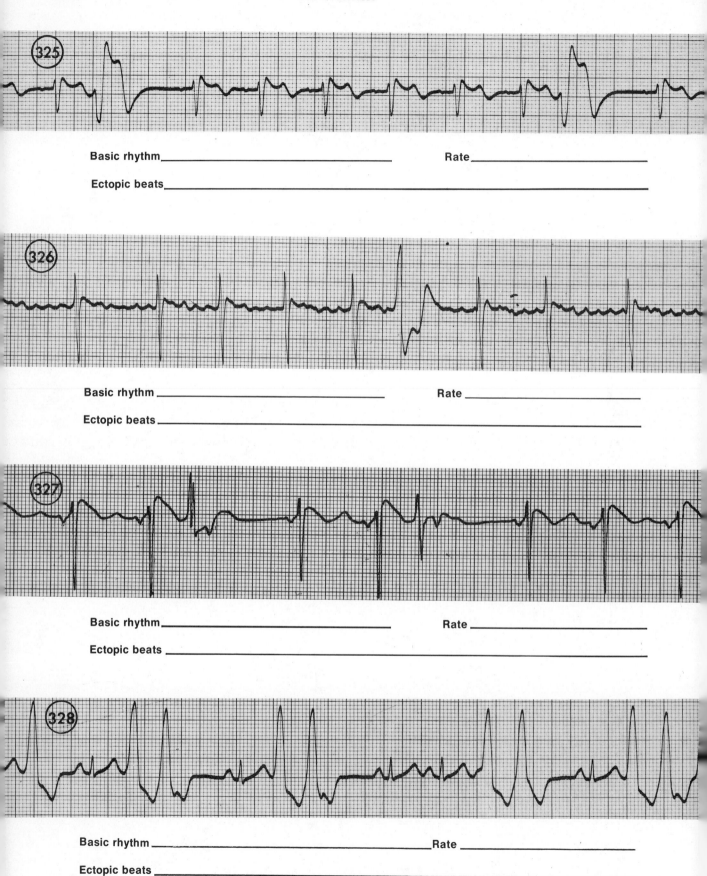

325

Basic rhythm_____   Rate_____

Ectopic beats_____

326

Basic rhythm _____   Rate _____

Ectopic beats _____

327

Basic rhythm_____   Rate_____

Ectopic beats_____

328

Basic rhythm _____Rate _____

Ectopic beats _____

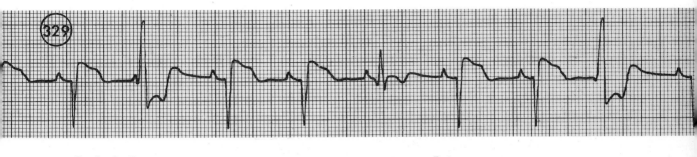

Basic rhythm _____ **Rate** _____

Ectopic beats _____

Serial tracings of a 66-year-old man with a recent subendocardial infarction demonstrating an untoward drug effect follow.

10:30 AM: The patient is admitted to the Coronary Care Unit.

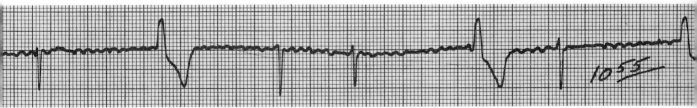

Atrial fibrillation with moderate ventricular rate response.

10:55 AM: The ventricular rate has slowed, and escape beats of ventricular origin have appeared. The ectopic beats only occur following a long delay in the normally conducted beats.

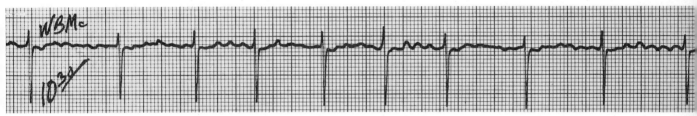

11:12 AM: A sustained ectopic ventricular rhythm has replaced the usual response to atrial fibrillation. Note that the ectopic rhythm appeared after a pause in conducted beats and was slower than the preceding rhythm. At this point, the clinician elected to control the ectopic beats with a depressor agent.

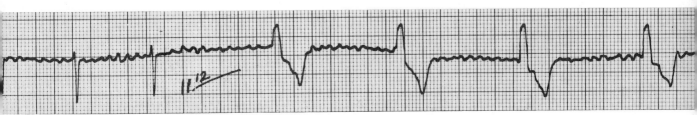

11:15 AM: Lidocaine, 80 mg, was given by intravenous injection.

11:22 AM: Ventricular escape beats have been eliminated. However, there are now long pauses between some ventricular beats, all of which are conducted from the atria. The drug has suppressed the ventricular escape mechanism which had previously protected the heart against excessive ventricular slowing.

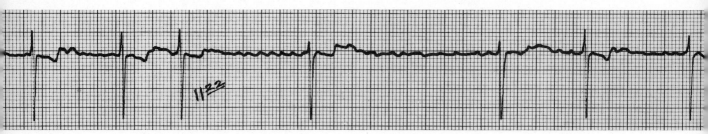

Theory of Re-Entry Beats

Premature contractions have usually been attributed to **excitation** of impulse **formation.** However, an alternate explanation holds that they may be produced by **depression** of impulse **conduction.** There is considerable and growing experimental evidence to support this concept.

The myocardium may contain islets of tissue which have a longer refractory period or slower conduction velocity than the surrounding tissue. As a depolarizing wave front passes such an islet, it may leave behind a localized eddy of electrical activity. The impulse, which is thus delayed, later emerges from the islet to re-enter the surrounding tissue at a time when it has already recovered from the original wave and is again excitable. Thus a new depolarizing wave is initiated, generating a premature contraction, referred to as a re-entry beat. (See illustrations at top of following page.)

Drugs which suppress ectopic beats may operate by altering the refractory period or the conduction velocity or both within small areas of affected tissue. It is not possible to distinguish between beats produced by a re-entry and those produced by an automatic mechanism. However, some authorities state that premature contractions having fixed coupling intervals are more likely to represent the re-entry phenomenon.

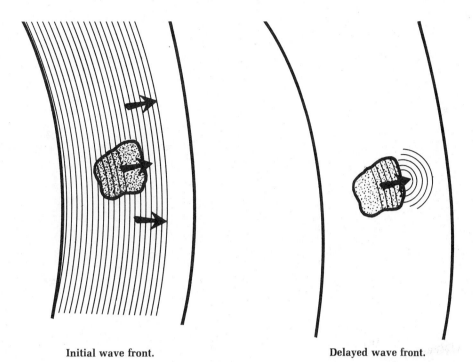

Initial wave front.   Delayed wave front.

Parasystole

Careful analysis of ventricular premature contractions sometimes discloses unifocal complexes which have varying coupling but which have themselves a regular cadence. Such a constantly recurring ectopic beat is known as **parasystole.** Its detection requires comparative interval measurement with ruler or calipers and usually a long tracing. Parasystole is established by an active focus of automaticity, usually in the ventricle, which operates independently of the dominant pacemaker. The rhythmic discharges are somehow not affected by the propagation of the primary impulse. It is as though electrical activity were prevented from entering the area of automaticity, while an impulse discharged by it will exit for further propagation. This could be considered a unidirectional (input) block at a small site of impulse-forming tissue. The ventricular focus sometimes fires during the refractory period of a supraventricular beat, and no parasystolic beat occurs, but the parasystolic rhythm is thereafter resumed without a change in cadence.

PARASYSTOLE

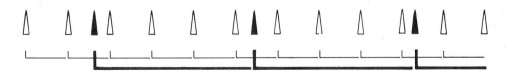

Open symbols—dominant rhythm

Closed symbols—parasystolic rhythm

Graphic representation of a parasystolic rhythm.

Note that both the dominant and parasystolic rhythms have separate and independent cadences.

Parasystole is evident in a 25-year-old woman medical student in good general health and without symptoms or findings of a cardiac disorder except for occasional palpitations often associated with anxiety, drinking coffee, or smoking.

Lead II, resting supine

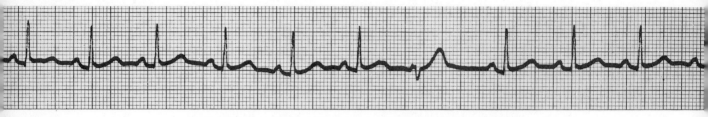

Normal sinus rhythm with one late ventricular premature contraction.

This was the only ectopic beat occurring during two minutes of continuous recording.

Immediately after smoking half a cigarette rapidly, ventricular premature contractions become much more frequent.

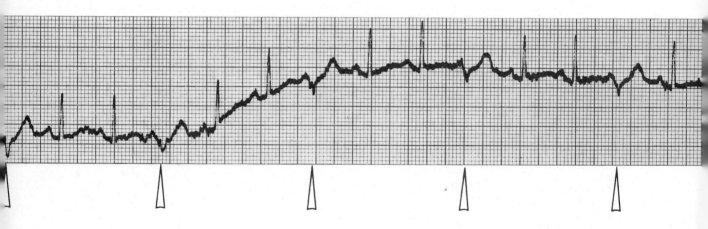

Note that the ectopic beats themselves appear in a perfectly regular cadence and that the coupling interval with normal beats is not fixed. It appears that an impulse-forming center in the ventricles has been activated, producing an entirely independent and slower rhythm than that of the sinus node.

A break in the parasystolic rhythm now occurs.

Lead I

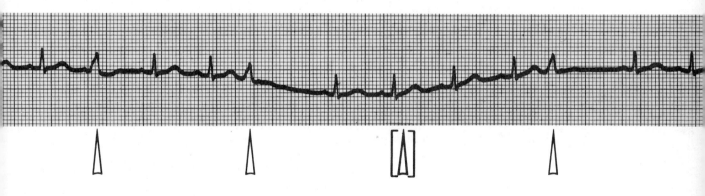

The QRS complex symbol with brackets indicates the site where a parasystolic beat would occur if the regular cadence were not interrupted. Even though no ectopic beat appears at this point, the subsequent ventricular premature contraction occurs at a predicted, measured interval. It is assumed that the parasystolic center fired, but the impulse came so soon after the previous normal beat that no ectopic contraction was generated. In other words, the ventricles were refractory to the parasystolic impulse at this time.

Two consecutive blocked parasystolic impulses can be measured out.

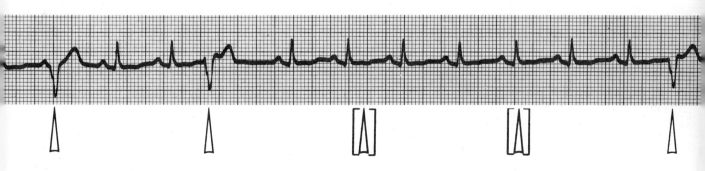

In this tracing, the interval between one set of ventricular premature contractions is exactly three times the basic parasystolic interval. Again, measured parasystolic impulses fall very soon after a normal beat, and no ectopic contraction results. Note also the marked variability in the sinus beat–ventricular beat coupling intervals. This is characteristic of a parasystolic rhythm.

Parasystole is usually a benign condition. While the arrhythmia is quite uncommon, diligent search for it is warranted in all records with frequent ectopic beats.

Ventricular Tachycardia

An excited site of automaticity within the ventricles may discharge a series of impulses. These occur at a more rapid rate than the normal ventricular impulse-forming rate of 20 to 50 per minute. This rhythm of excitation is known as **ventricular tachycardia.** Some authorities use the term *accelerated ventricular rhythm* if the rate of ventricular beats is greater than 50 per minute but less than the dominant supraventricular pacemaker rate.

Individual beats in ventricular tachycardia have the characteristics of ventricular extrasystoles; QRS complexes reveal slowed depolarization and anomalous conduction pathways and repolarization patterns.

Ventricular tachycardia is almost always a sign of serious underlying heart disease. It may occur in brief or sustained paroxysms with spontaneous remission. It may be the prelude to a potentially lethal arrhythmia.

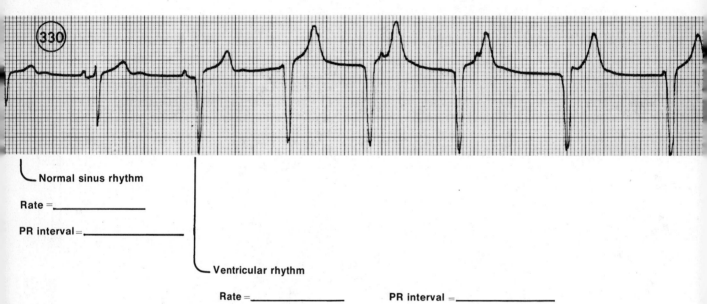

Normal sinus rhythm

Rate =_____

PR interval =_____

Ventricular rhythm

Rate =_____   PR interval =_____

Normal sinus rhythm is replaced by a rhythm consisting of:

1. A-V dissociation.

2. Ventricular complexes which are changed in form or abnormally wide.

3. A pacemaker driving the ventricles which is more rapid than the sinus pacemaker.

In the third ventricular contraction, observe that the PR interval is slightly shorter than in the sinus beats before it. The QRS complex of this beat is similar to those which follow without association with the sinus pacemaker. It is therefore presumed that this third sinus impulse is not conducted to the ventricles but rather that a late ventricular premature contraction has occurred, the first of a succession of ventricular beats appearing in a somewhat irregular cadence. There is no retrograde conduction, and atrial and ventricular rhythms are completely independent. This arrhythmia is a form of A-V dissociation produced by sustained excitation of a ventricular pacemaker. Since the rate is more rapid than is seen in ventricular escape rhythms (20 to 50 beats per minute), the terms accelerated ventricular rhythm or ventricular tachycardia are applicable.

No criteria for preference of either term has been generally accepted. As an arbitrary guide, it is suggested that **accelerated ventricular rhythm** be used when the rate is faster than 50 per minute but less than 100. The term **ventricular tachycardia** is preferred when the rate is more rapid than 100.

The term A-V dissociation has come to include many forms of differential atrioventricular beating, and dozens of names have been introduced to define them. Unfortunately, no standard classification exists, and the vocabulary of these arrhythmias has become rather confusing. Specific descriptive terminology will be applied here.

Ventricular excitation is evident in a 52-year-old swimming coach with an acute myocardial infarction. Ectopic beats occur in both isolated and sustained episodes.

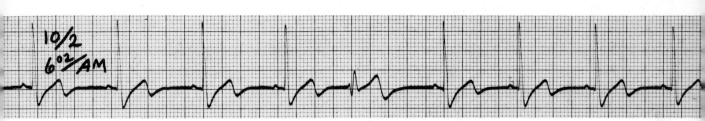

Normal sinus rhythm with a premature beat which has a prolonged QRS complex of abnormal form and a compensatory pause appears. Therefore, this ectopic beat is a ventricular premature contraction.

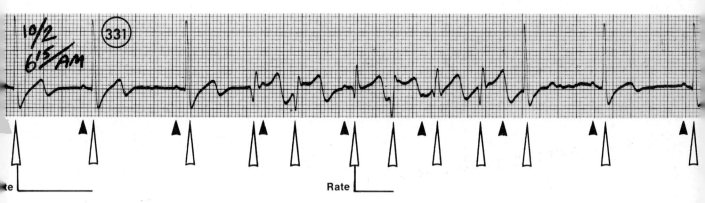

Following the third sinus beat, a premature contraction occurs with some characteristics of the ectopic beat in the first tracing. Five similar beats then appear in rapid succession, during which P waves can be measured out. This is an episode of ventricular tachycardia with dissociation of atrial and ventricular rhythms. Normal sinus rhythm is thereafter resumed.

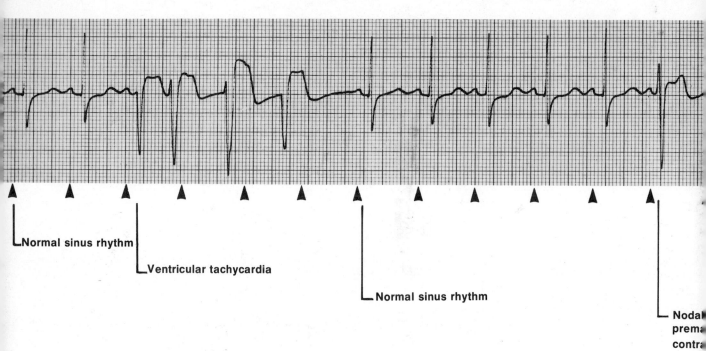

Normal sinus rhythm

Ventricular tachycardia

Normal sinus rhythm

Nodal
prema
contra

Episode of ventricular tachycardia recorded from a monitoring lead in a patient with suspected acute myocardial infarction.

During the brief episode of tachycardia, atrial activity can be measured out and is unaffected. The ventricular cadence is irregular and the QRS complexes widened and abnormal in shape. T waves have also become misshapen. These findings are characteristic of ventricular tachycardia.

Recurring paroxysmal ventricular tachycardia is evident in a 52-year-old woman without other manifestations of heart disease. This patient complained of a frequent fluttering sensation in her chest but otherwise had no symptoms.

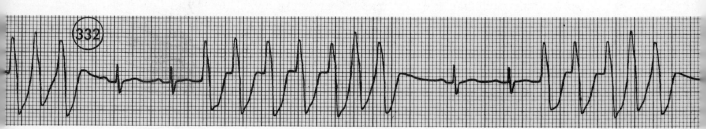

Determine the most rapid rate in this tachyarrhythmia.

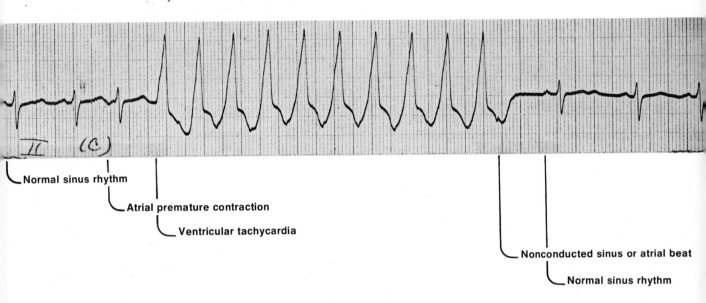

Normal sinus rhythm

Atrial premature contraction

Ventricular tachycardia

Nonconducted sinus or atrial beat

Normal sinus rhythm

Apparent P waves can be measured out with calipers during the period of ventricular tachycardia. As these beats occur at regular intervals and at a considerably more rapid rate than the sinus beats, atrial tachycardia is probably also present. This phenomenon is often referred to as a **double tachycardia.**

The next series of electrocardiograms illustrates transient periods of ventricular tachycardia.

1. Determine the basic rhythm and rate.
2. Mark isolated ventricular premature contractions, if present.
3. Identify and bracket periods of ventricular tachycardia.
4. Using calipers, locate and mark P waves, if possible, through the periods of ventricular tachycardia.

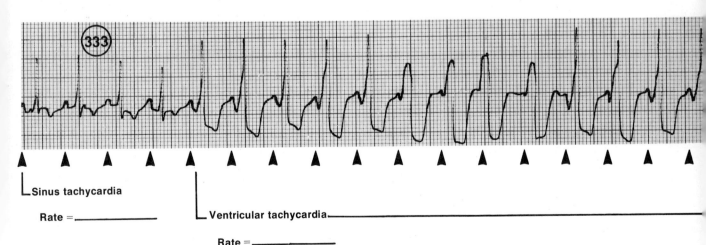

Sinus tachycardia

Rate = _____

Ventricular tachycardia

Rate = _____

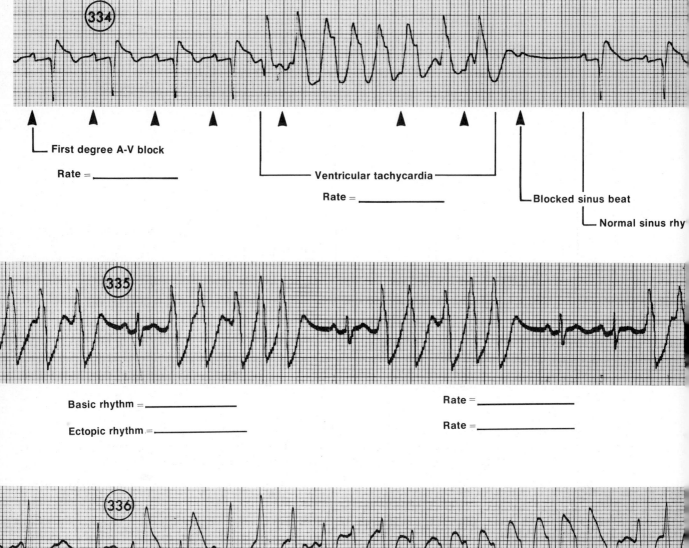

First degree A-V block

Rate = _____

Ventricular tachycardia

Rate = _____

Blocked sinus beat

Normal sinus rhy

Basic rhythm = _____

Ectopic rhythm = _____

Rate = _____

Rate = _____

Basic rhythm = _____

Ectopic rhythm = _____

Rate = _____

Rate = _____

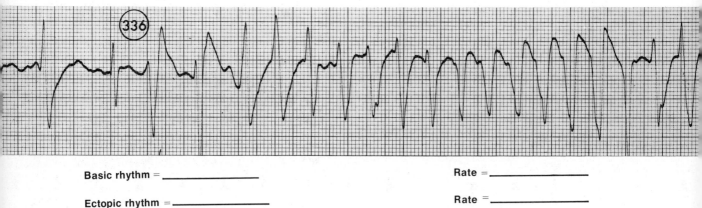

Atrial activity is more difficult to detect in the rapid ventricular rates. Calipers will help. Note how P waves, even though obscure, can be identified by the distortion imposed on various components. As the ventricular rate becomes faster, P waves may only be distinguishable by rhythmic changes in QRS-T or the baseline. This change may, in fact, be a major clue for identifying a rhythm as ventricular tachycardia.

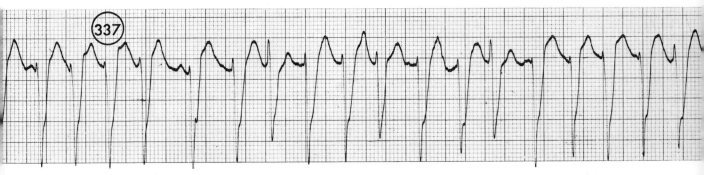

Ventricular tachycardia: Rate = _____

P waves seem to be visible in various places throughout the tracing, but these can be plotted out only roughly with calipers. The highly variable contour of the baseline is evidence of atrial activity out of phase with the ventricular rhythm.
Measure out and mark P waves where possible.

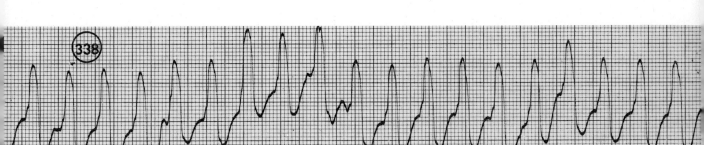

Ectopic rhythm_____   **Rate**_____

At very rapid rates in ventricular tachycardia, the following features are usually present:

1. QRS complexes and T waves tend to vary in contour and in amplitude. This is in part due to unidentifiable but superimposed atrial beats which are dissociated from the ventricular beats. In addition, the sequences of depolarization and repolarization tend to be more variable from a rapid ventricular focus than with normal electrical activation.
2. Ventricular beats tend to be irregular, although this is not necessarily true.
3. QRS complexes merge directly with T waves, so that it becomes difficult or impossible to separate clearly the phases of depolarization and repolarization.
4. QRS complexes become broader and less well organized as the rate increases.

Look for these features in the following examples of ventricular tachycardia.

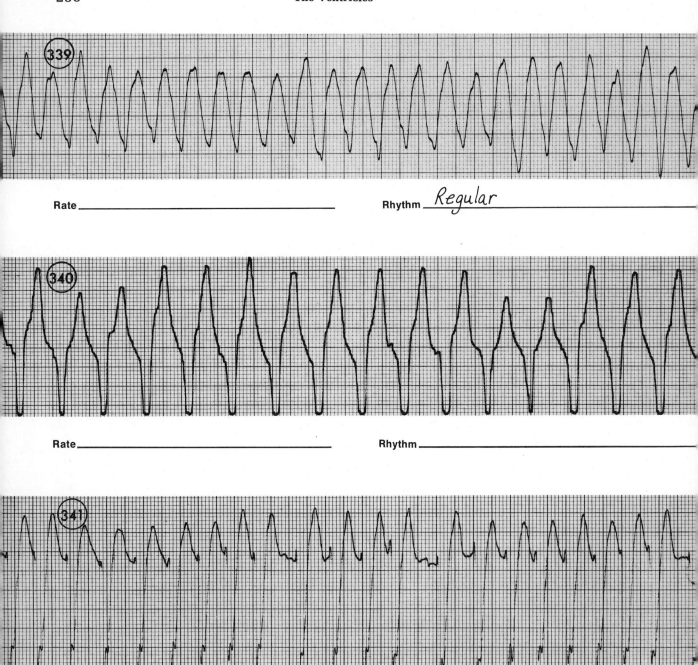

Rate _____   Rhythm _Regular_____

Rate _____   Rhythm _____

Rate _____   Rhythm _____

Ventricular tachycardia can produce cardiac contractions with such rapidity that the cardiac chambers do not have time to fill adequately during the intervals between contractions. This causes a diminution in the blood volume ejected with each contraction. Any gradation of low cardiac output may be associated with these arrhythmias, depending upon the rate and the condition of the heart. The manifestations range from no symptoms or mild anxiety to lightheadedness or severe circulatory collapse and coma.

Label the tracings completely; indicate atrial activity when possible.

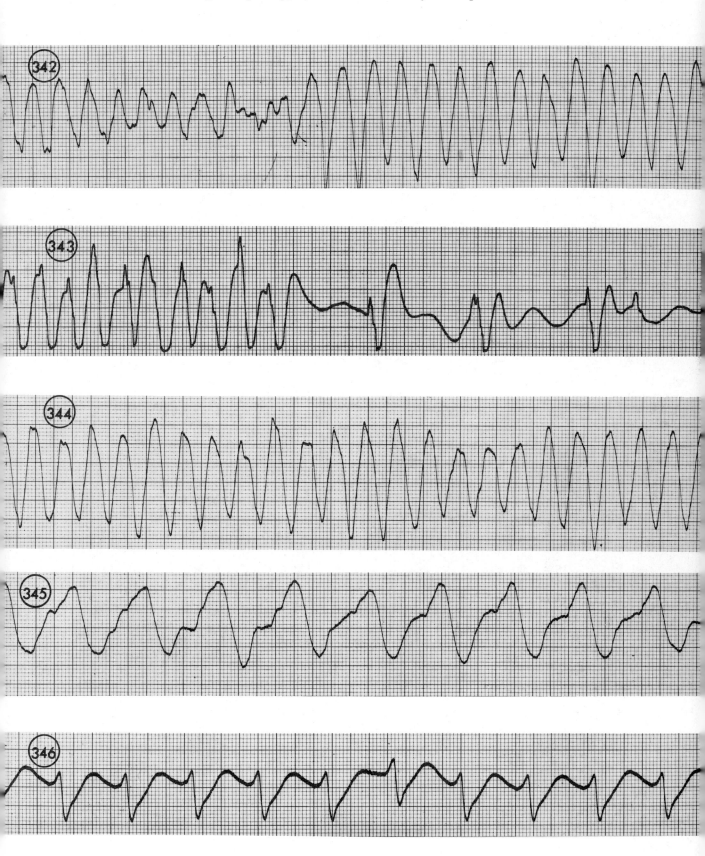

Ventricular Flutter

When ventricular excitability causes an extremely rapid rate, the QRS complexes tend to merge with T waves, producing a continuous, wavy pattern with no clear separation between cardiac cycles. This pattern has been termed **ventricular flutter.** Its mechanism is similar to that of atrial flutter, but in atrial flutter, the ventricles are protected to a degree against excessively frequent stimulation by physiological A-V block. In ventricular flutter, the ventricles contract so rapidly that there is inadequate time for chamber filling. Stroke ejection volume is inadequate, and circulatory failure ensues.

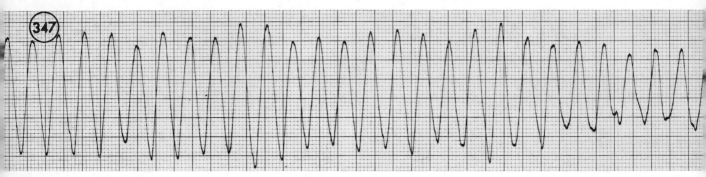

Rate = _____

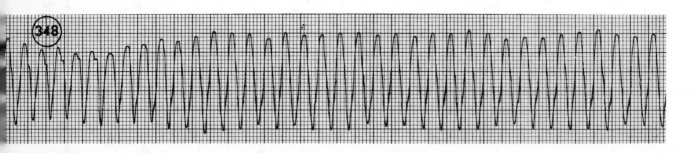

Rate = _____

Examples of ventricular flutter.

Ventricular tachycardia and flutter may be complications of acute myocardial ischemia or infarction. Excessive adrenergic stimulation, such as administration of the catecholamine drugs, or severe exercise can produce these arrhythmias. They may also be manifestations of advanced toxicity due to digitalis. In each case, these disturbances of ventricular automaticity represent a more serious degree of excitation than ventricular premature contractions. The sustained arrhythmias may, in fact, be initiated by a ventricular premature contraction occurring during an extremely sensitive period of a cardiac cycle known as the **vulnerable period.**

The Vulnerable Period

Toward the final phase of repolarization, the heart becomes supersensitive to stimulation. The ventricles may respond to excitation at this time by developing tachycardia or fibrillation. This increased state of excitability or *vulnerable period* occurs near the peak of the T wave on the ECG. Ventricular premature contractions which appear during this phase of repolarization of the previous beat are especially dangerous because of this brief period of vulnerability.

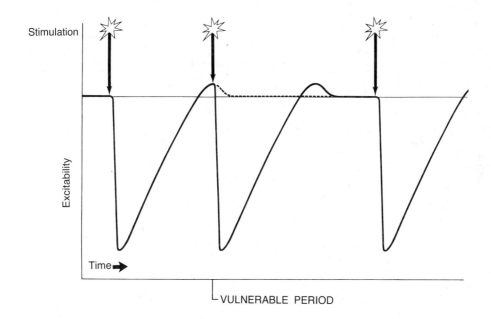

A threshold stimulus activates a resting cell which undergoes depolarization, then repolarization. As the cell returns to the resting state, it overshoots the normal level of excitability. During this brief phase of hyperexcitability, the vulnerable period, the cell is relatively unstable and may respond to a stimulus of less than threshold intensity. Repetitive spontaneous firing may then follow.

The following sequence was taken from a standard electrocardiogram on the general medical-surgical ward. The patient was admitted for evaluation of ill-defined chest discomfort.

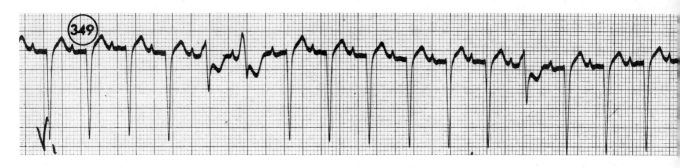

Locate the VPC's _____, _____, _____.

Precordial lead V_1 reveals sinus tachycardia with frequent unifocal ventricular premature contractions occurring late in the cardiac cycle. Two extrasystoles appear in tandem, although these do not appear to threaten the basic rhythm since they do not fall close to the expected vulnerable period. However, note the unexpected in the following tracing.

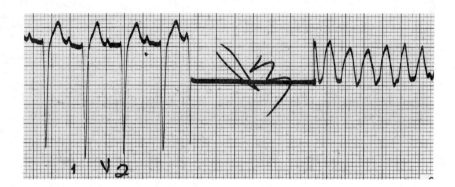

While switching from precordial lead V_2 to V_3, the ECG technician noted a sudden change in the patient's affect and then recorded ventricular tachycardia. Further recording was not possible because of the patient's violent movements which preceded cardiovascular collapse and coma, from which the patient could not be revived. Presumably an innocent VPC fell at a period of ventricular vulnerability and induced a lethal arrhythmia.

Drug and Electric Shock Therapy

Drugs which depress ventricular impulse formation may effectively control ventricular ectopic rhythms. Quinidine, procainamide (Pronestyl), and propranolol (Inderal) have been used extensively and effectively in treatment.

These suppressing drugs may also decrease sinus and atrial impulse formation, alter conduction time in the A-V node and Purkinje system, lessen myocardial contractile force, and lower blood pressure. Awareness of these potential alterations is critical when the agents are used.

Lidocaine (Xylocaine) is commonly used for suppression of ventricular extrasystoles. It can be given as an infusion, the concentration and rate of infusion determined by the cardiac response. This drug is quite selective in its effect on ventricular extrasystoles, since it usually has little effect in reducing atrial excitation, cardiac contractility, A-V nodal conduction, and blood pressure. It acts rapidly, and its effects disappear rapidly when the drug is discontinued. For these reasons, lidocaine approaches the ideal agent for use in the Cardiac Care Unit.

Concentrated lidocaine may be given intravenously when frequent ventricular premature contractions and ventricular tachycardia suddenly appear. Suppression of the ectopic excitability usually occurs within a minute or two, and control can be thereafter maintained with intravenous infusion of the diluted agent. Lidocaine, incidentally, seldom has any beneficial effect in treating atrial tachyarrhythmias.

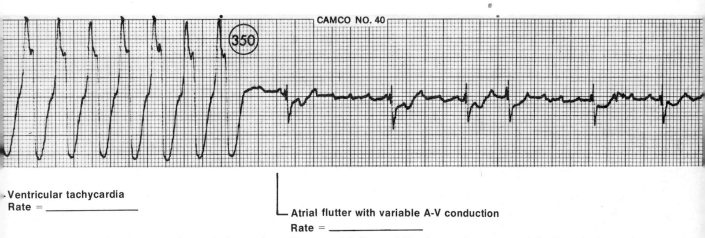

- Ventricular tachycardia
Rate = _____

Atrial flutter with variable A-V conduction
Rate = _____

Conversion of ventricular tachycardia to atrial flutter following an intravenous injection of lidocaine.

Continuous tracings from a 62-year-old teacher taken 1½ hours after admission to the CCU demonstrate the effect of lidocaine on VPC's.

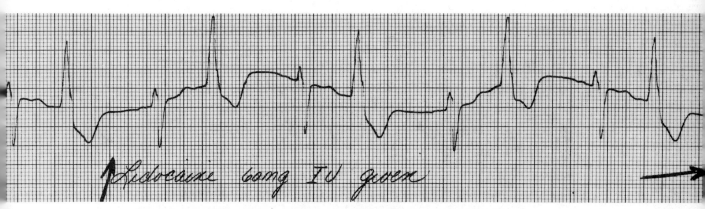

Lidocaine 60mg IV given

Sinus rhythm with an intraventricular conduction defect and ventricular bigeminy.

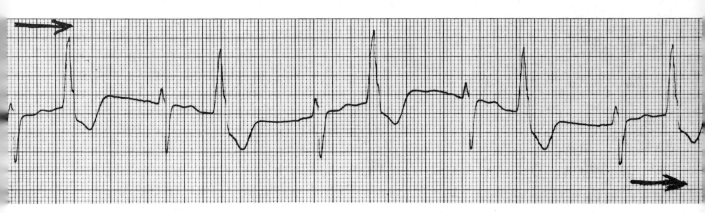

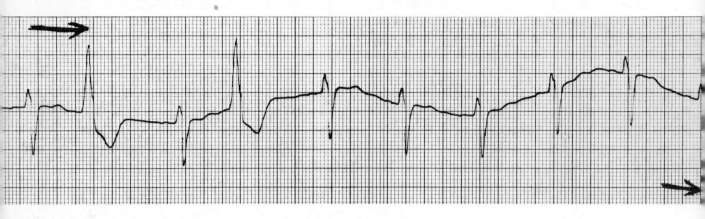

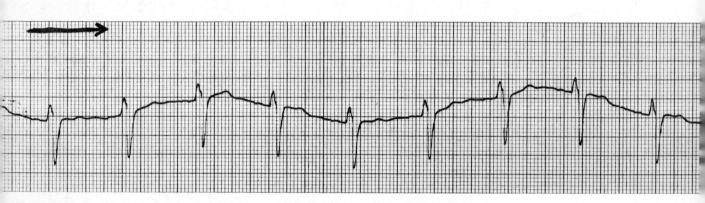

Suppression of ventricular premature contractions is evident within half a minute after the injection of lidocaine.

Electric shock technique is frequently effective in converting ventricular tachycardia. With a monitored patient, this arrhythmia should be recognized immediately at its onset and precordial shock applied within the minute. Conversion to a stable supraventricular rhythm is usually accomplished in patients with acute myocardial infarction when ventricular tachycardia is so treated within this time. However, this opportunity diminishes significantly with every moment's delay.

A helpful rule in deciding whether to use a drug or electrical means to treat ventricular tachycardia depends on the condition of the patient. If he remains alert and has at least a fair blood pressure or strong peripheral pulses, a quick-acting suppressor drug such as lidocaine can be given initially. If, instead, the patient becomes obtunded and has signs of circulatory failure, precordial shock is the better first approach.

The following sequential arrhythmias were treated with pharmacologic and electrical agents. These represent selective tracings from a monitoring lead in the Cardiac Care Unit. The patient is a 44-year-old construction laborer with a diagnosis of acute myocardial infarction.

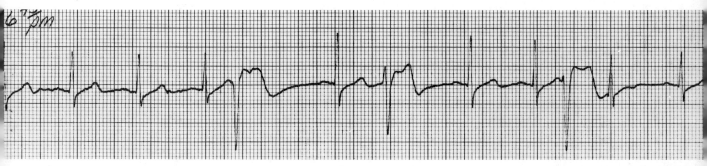

Moderately frequent ventricular premature contractions from different foci are present. These have a varying coupling interval, and two begin just after the peak of the T wave of the preceding beat.

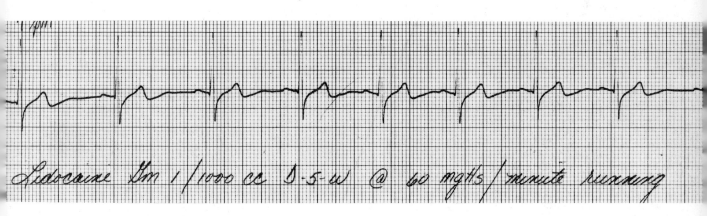

An infusion of lidocaine was started with satisfactory initial suppression of VPC's.

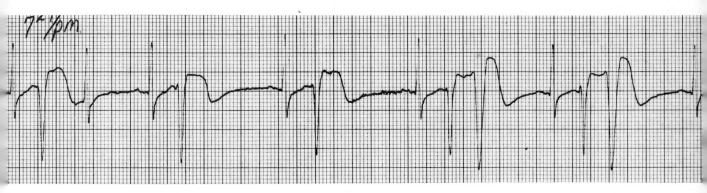

Suddenly VPC's recurred, some in couplets. Many continue to appear near the vulnerable period.

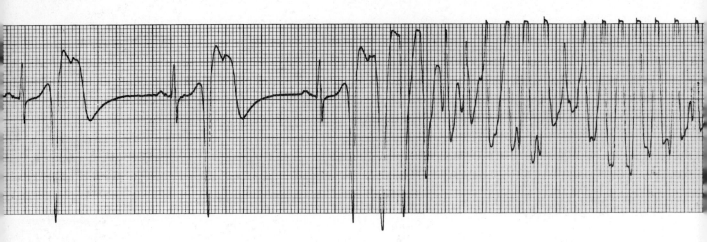

Before the rate of lidocaine infusion could be increased, a VPC falling during the vulnerable period initiated ventricular tachycardia of approximately 250 per minute. The patient immediately became extremely restless, then convulsed.

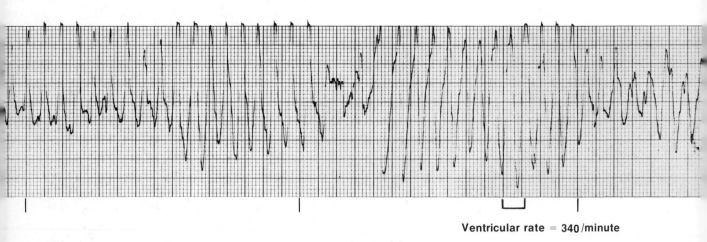

Ventricular rate = 340 /minute

This degree of ventricular tachycardia is often referred to as ventricular flutter.

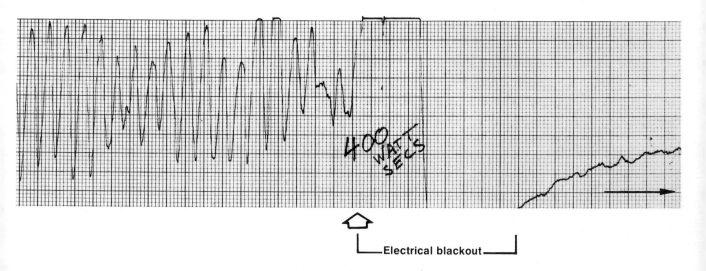

Electrical blackout

Anterior-posterior direct current (DC) shock of 400 watts per second was applied to the chest, followed by severe ventricular depression.

Notice the sequential rhythms now developed in the following continuous recordings.

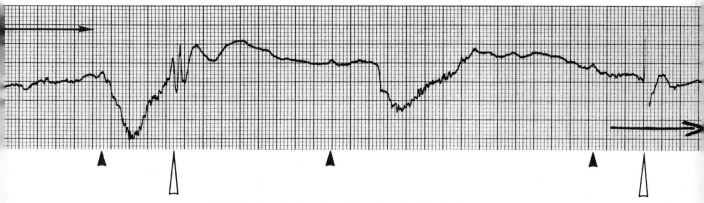

Blocked sinus beats and multifocal ventricular beats.

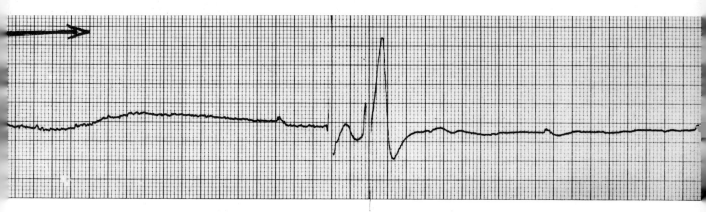

The period of extreme cardiac depression is now followed by a period of marked electrical irritability.

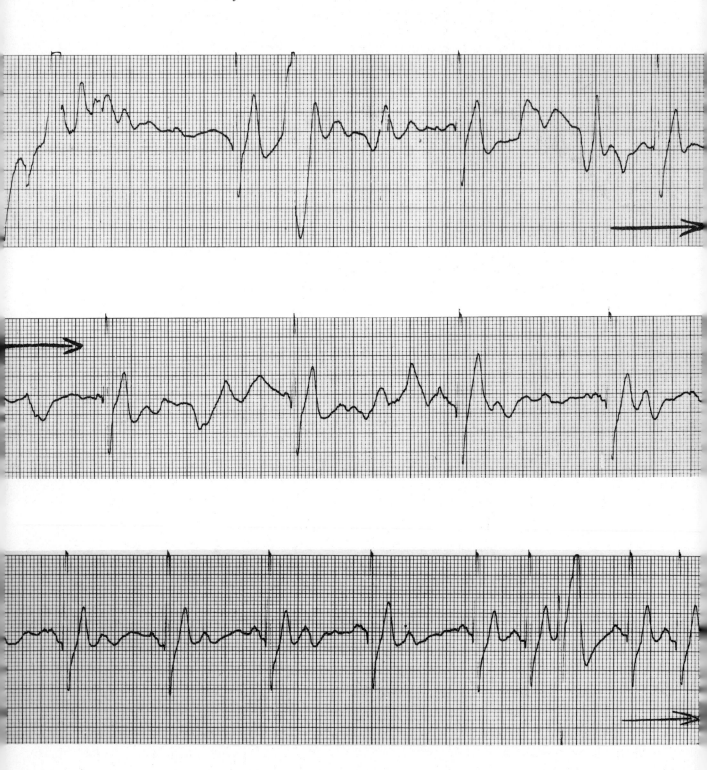

Severe A-V nodal depression (represented by 2:1 block) is superseded by complete A-V nodal conduction.

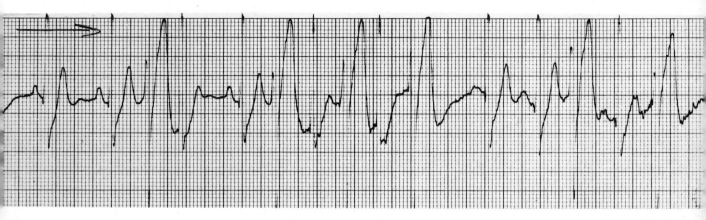

Gradually, spontaneous and effective ventricular beats were restored, although frequent VPC's were present. The patient regained full sensorium within a few minutes. Control of VPC's was obtained with higher concentrations of lidocaine.

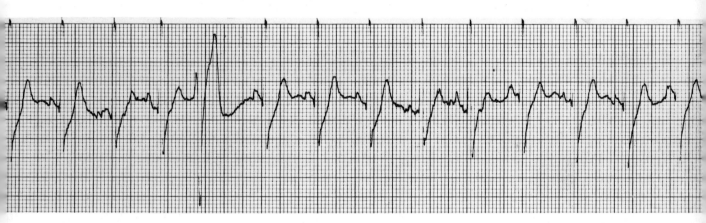

In subsequent days, VPC's became less frequent and appeared considerably later than in the vulnerable period. Gradually, the lidocaine concentration was decreased; the drug was then discontinued altogether, with subsidence of ectopic beats.

Ventricular Fibrillation

Sustained ventricular tachycardia and flutter lead inexorably to diminished myocardial performance and erratic electrical behavior. QRS complexes become widened and more variable in contour as progressive hypoxia and circulatory failure from the tachycardia affect the metabolism of the heart itself. The next stage in the deteriorating situation is **ventricular fibrillation,** in which ventricular impulses are formed too rapidly to be propagated in an orderly sequence. The condition is similar to that of atrial fibrillation in that countless minute portions of the muscle are in various states of depolarization and refractoriness. In this case, however, the primary pump is disabled. There is no pulse or heart sounds, and circulatory flow is negligible. If the heart could be viewed directly, one would see disjointed shimmering of the ventricular surface instead of a vigorous, coordinated systole.

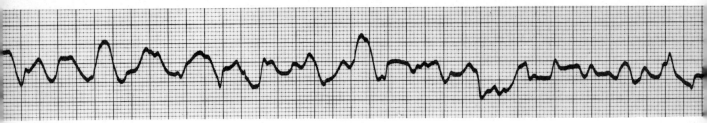

Ventricular fibrillation.

Note the irregular, widened QRS complexes of poor definition.

In the following examples, advanced electrical disorder of the ventricles is demonstrated. In some tracings, intermediary stages between ventricular tachycardia–flutter and fibrillation are present.

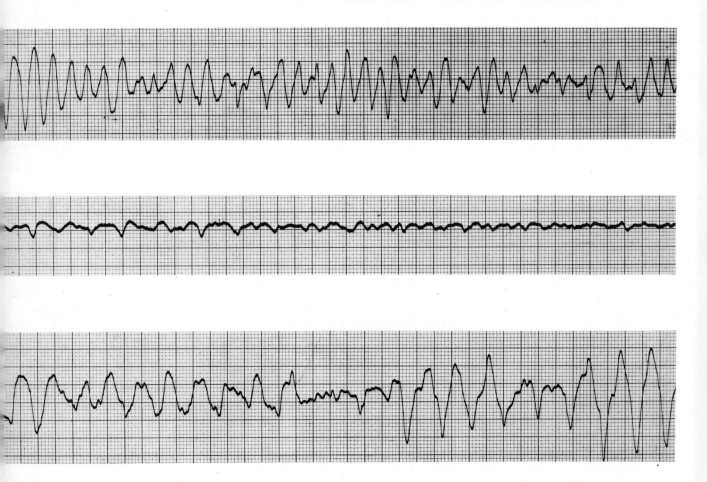

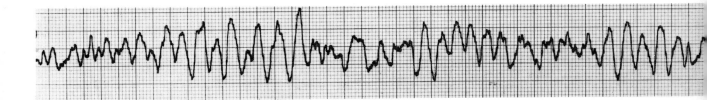

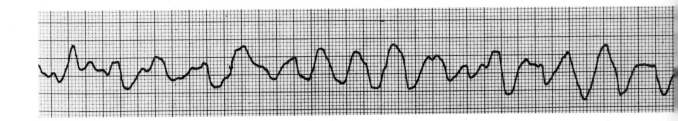

Seizurelike movements and loss of consciousness occur within several seconds after the onset of ventricular fibrillation. Survival depends upon prompt restoration of organized ventricular contractions. This sometimes happens spontaneously, but pharmacologic or electrical treatment is generally required. When applied early enough, treatment is often effective.

Electric shock treatment is often successful in converting ventricular fibrillation to a higher order of rhythm, providing it is administered within a minute or two. A longer delay, particularly if cardiac massage and assisted ventilation is not given or is inefficient, is associated with severe metabolic complications, and the chances for rhythm conversion decrease rapidly.

As there are no distinct complexes in ventricular fibrillation, the electrocardioverting instrument cannot be synchronized with the cardiac activity. Therefore, the automatic synchronization control cannot be used. Instead, the operator must turn the control knob to **defibrillate** (or the equivalent terminology, as used by various manufacturers).

Ventricular fibrillation is treated electrically in a 57-year-old police sergeant two hours after onset of chest pain. Acute myocardial infarction is documented by standard electrocardiogram. The initial tracing was taken from a special monitoring lead.

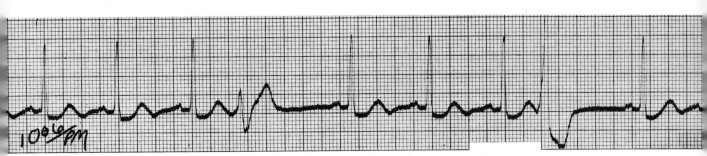

Normal sinus rhythm with multifocal premature contractions.

The following tracing was initiated by an automatic alarm–write-out system.

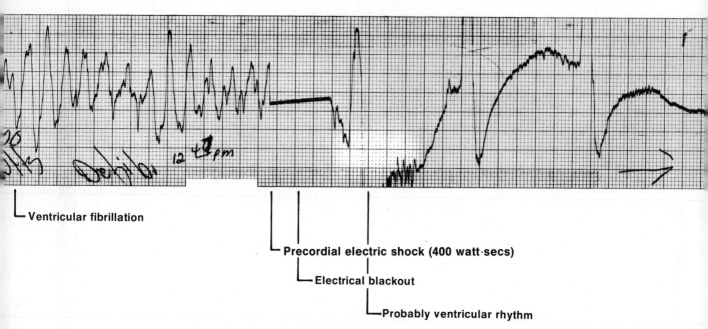

Ventricular fibrillation

Precordial electric shock (400 watt·secs)

Electrical blackout

Probably ventricular rhythm

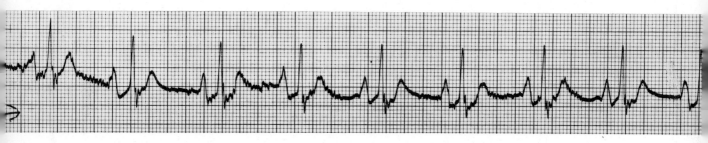

Normal sinus rhythm is resumed with prolongation of PR intervals initially and with an intraventricular conduction defect.

Ventricular Tachyarrhythmias

Rhythms of ventricular excitation are the most common immediate cause of death in acute myocardial infarction. There is a steadily growing body of information indicating that this mechanism is by far the most frequent fatal event in the United States. The significance of this is underscored by considering that the infarction may not cause great damage to the myocardium itself and that the arrhythmia may be easily controlled if properly treated.

Awareness of the frequency with which ventricular premature contractions occur in acute myocardial infarction and of their role in precipitating lethal arrhythmias has been a principle factor in development of the Cardiac Care Unit. Emphasis has shifted from cardiac resuscitation to prevention of cardiac emergencies through control of the rhythm.

VENTRICLE: IMPULSE FORMATION

Depression

VB = Ventricular bradycardia
VP = Ventricular pause
VA = Ventricular arrest

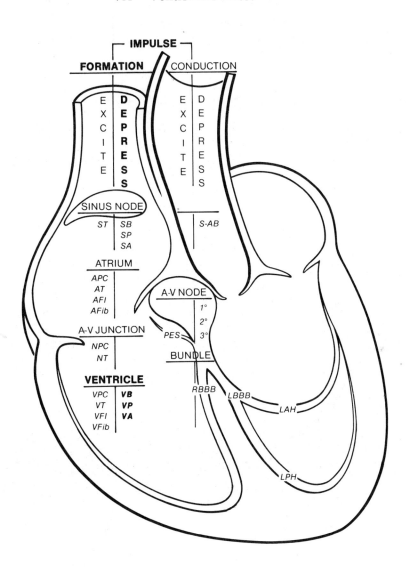

Ventricular Bradycardia

The natural propensity of the unstimulated ventricles to beat at 20 to 50 times a minute may be severely depressed by metabolic or ischemic disease, resulting in **ventricular bradycardia.** While this term is not often used in electrocardiography, it is appropriate and implies that supraventricular impulses are absent or not conducted and that impulse formation within the ventricles is depressed. The idioventricular rate is extremely slow, producing symptoms and signs of advanced cardiac output failure. The rhythm is usually irregular. General cardiac depression is frequently further reflected by markedly delayed ventricular depolarization with wide, varying QRS complexes. Diminished myocardial contractile force often accompanies the condition, to compound the circulatory problems.

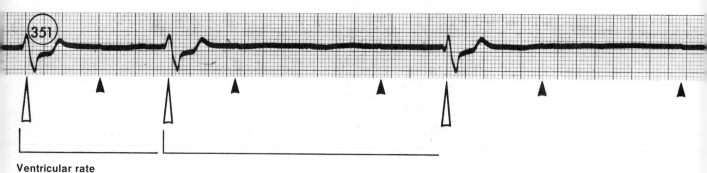

Ventricular rate

Complete A-V block with ventricular bradycardia.

At this stage, vigorous and concerted measures are required to restore adequate cardiac output, including increasing the rate of the heart beat and myocardial strength. A stimulatory agent, such as isoproterenol, may affect both. In addition, contributing factors, such as hypoxia and acidosis, must be treated.

In each of these examples of ventricular bradycardia, record the rate from beat to beat. Note the great variability in the cadence of impulse formation in these depressed states. Also note the extreme lengthening of ventricular depolarization in many instances, indicating marked depression of intraventricular conduction as well. Designate whether the VB is unifocal or multifocal.

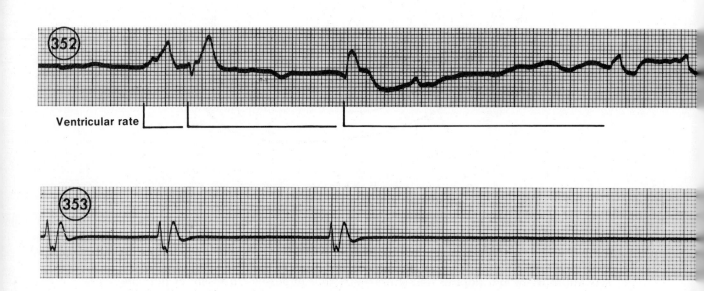

Ventricular rate

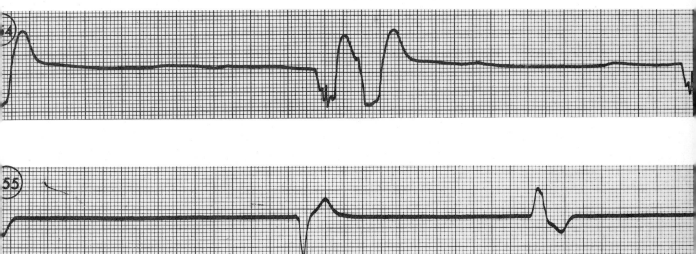

Progressive and fatal cardiac depression in a 48-year-old male admitted to the Cardiac Care Unit is evident in the following series. The patient sustained an acute myocardial infarction, complicated by an episode of atrial excitation.

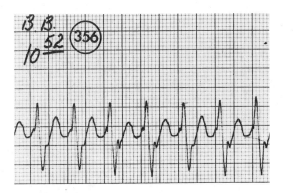

10:52: Atrial tachycardia with _____ : _____

A-V block and interventricular conduction

defect: QRS interval = _____

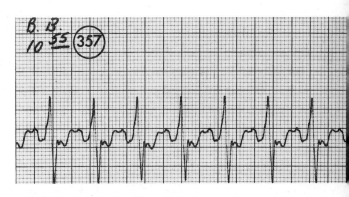

10:55: Atrial tachycardia with _____ : _____

A-V block and interventricular conduction

defect: QRS interval = _____

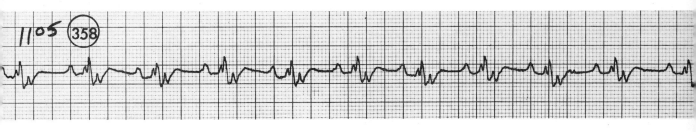

1:05: Normal sinus rhythm: Rate = _____

urther depression of conduction velocity: QRS interval = _____

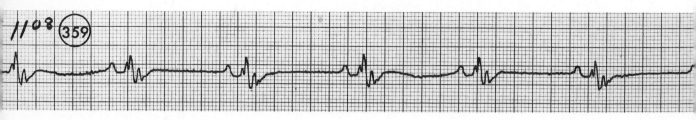

11:08: Sinus bradycardia: Rate = _____

Depression of sinus impulse formation

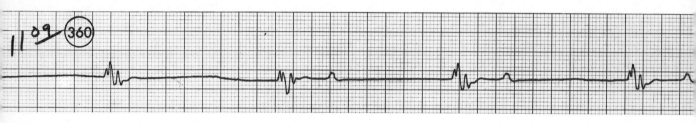

11:09: Sinus bradycardia: Rate = _____

Further depression of sinus impulse formation and depression of A-V conduction

producing complete A-V block and ventricular bradycardia: Rate = _____

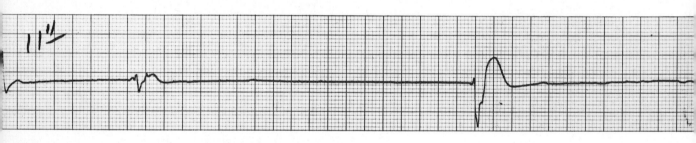

11:11 Depression of A-V junctional and ventricular pacemakers

Ventricular bradycardia with multifocal ventricular beats

Cardiostimulatory drugs, cardiac massage, and assisted ventilation failed to change this rapidly progressive sequence. Ruptured ventricular myocardium was identified on autopsy.

Ventricular Arrest

Cardiac arrest is the agonal state. The ventricles do not respond to stimuli, nor do they initiate contractions. Permanent tissue damage, particularly in the brain, will occur within a few minutes of its onset. Recovery may not be achieved, even with the most energetic and well-directed resuscitative measures, but it is sometimes possible with cardiac massage, assisted ventilation, and cardiac stimulatory drugs, plus correction of provocative causes.

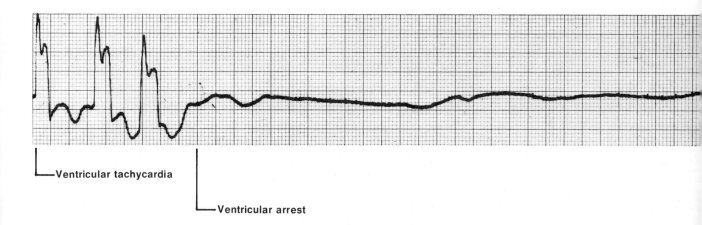

—Ventricular tachycardia

—Ventricular arrest

The following cardiac arrest sequence is from a 78-year-old woman with diffuse ischemic heart disease and refractory congestive heart failure. Progressive depression of ventricular impulse formation and conduction velocity is demonstrated in serial electrocardiograms.

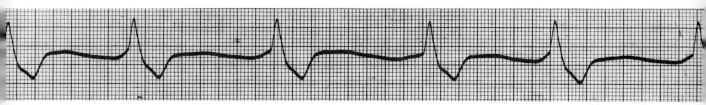

Ventricular rhythm: Rate = 40.

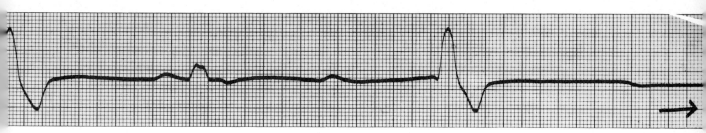

Ventricular bradycardia

The rate, initially 28, slows to 20. Changes in ventricular depolarization appear with variation in QRS complex form (multifocal beats) and further prolongation in QRS duration.

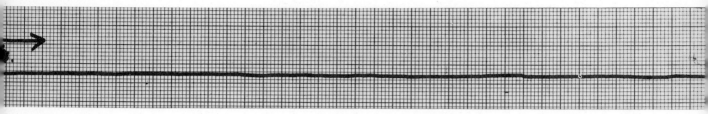

Ventricular arrest or standstill

There is no electrocardiographic evidence of cardiac activity.

SELF-EVALUATION: STAGE 3

Give a complete interpretation of the following electrocardiograms.

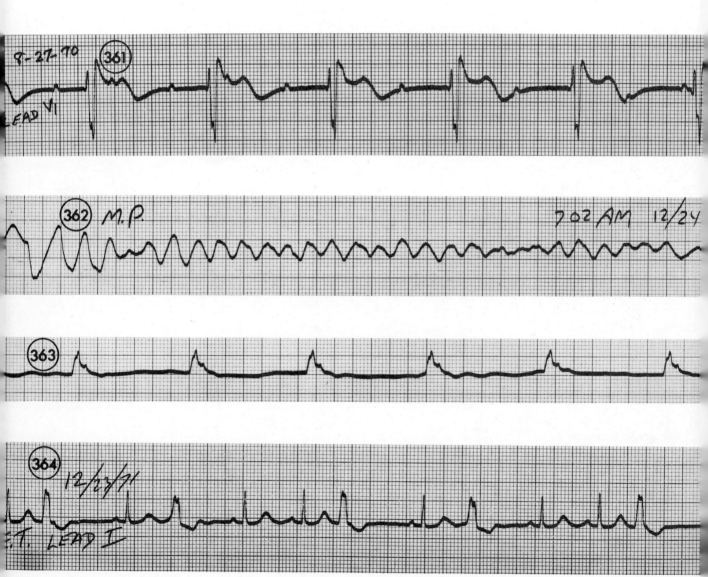

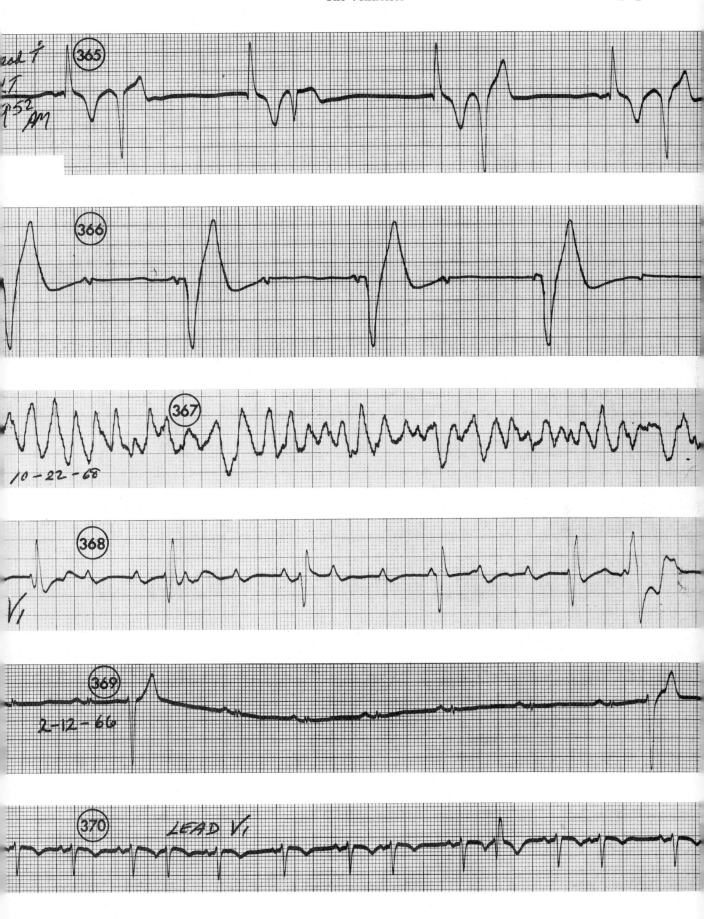

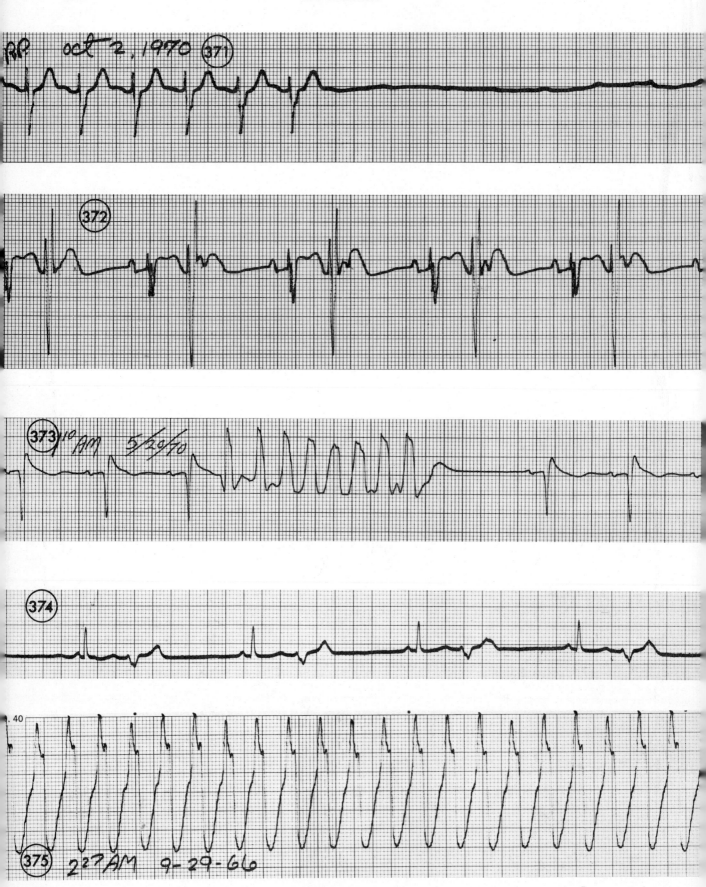

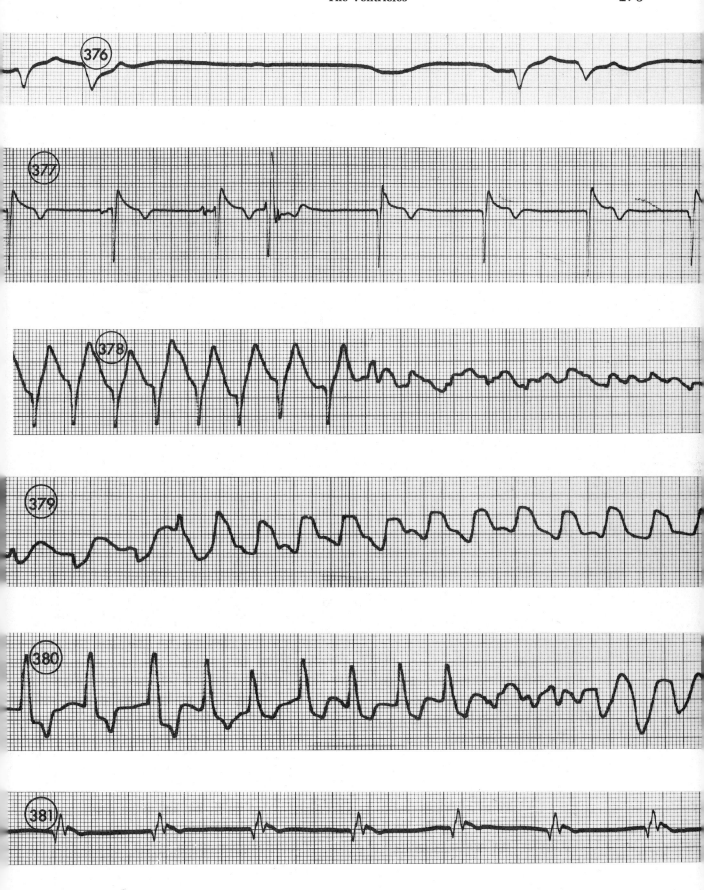

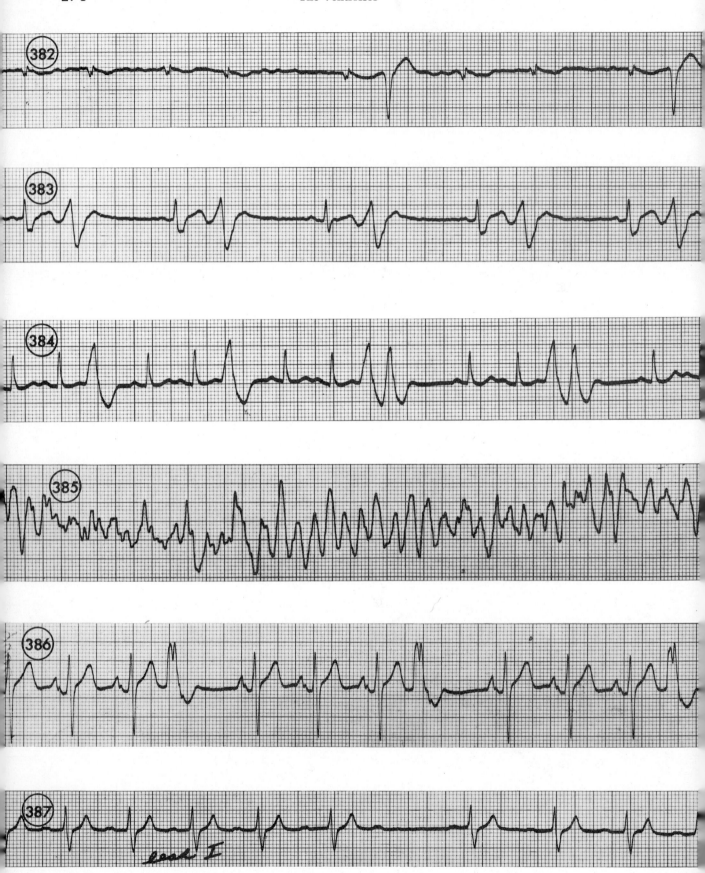

lead I

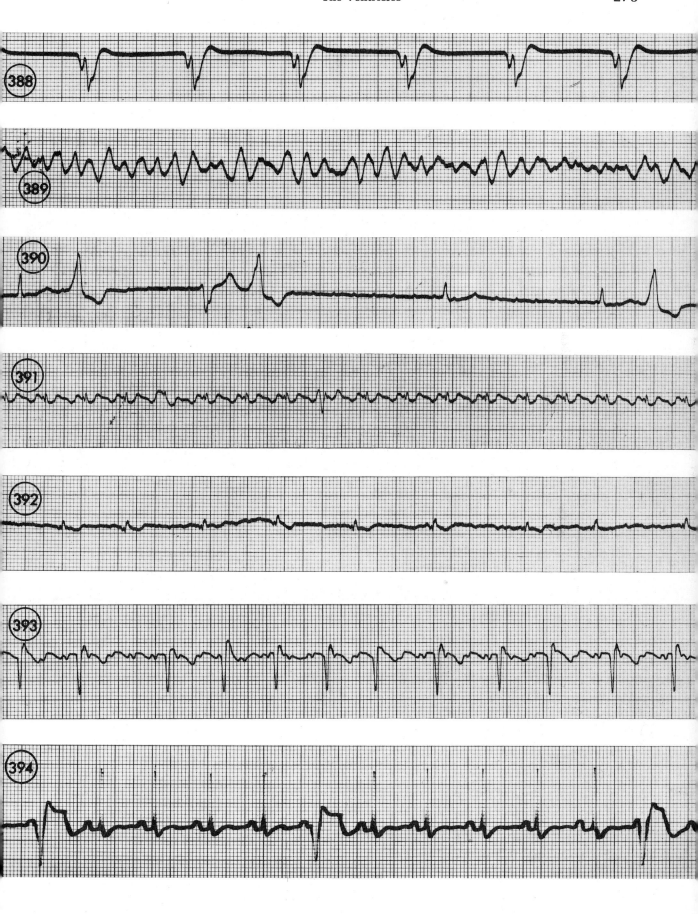

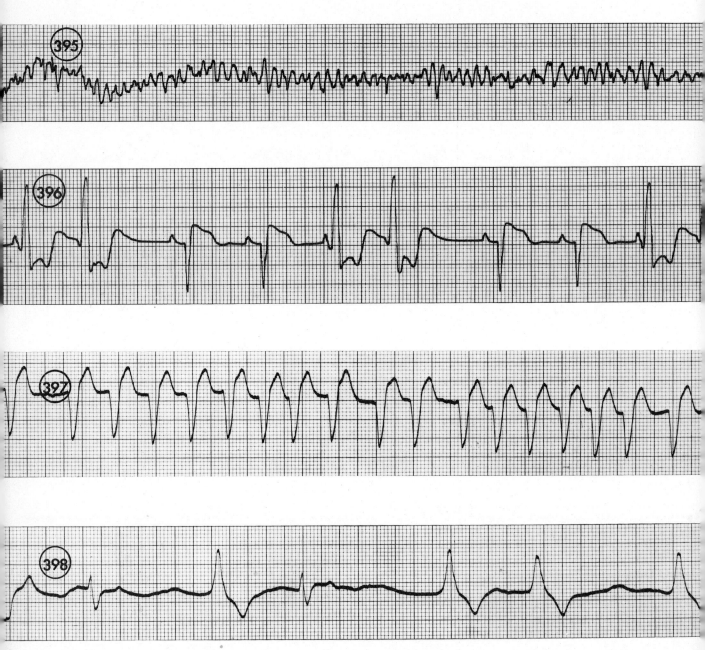

Chapter 9
THE ELECTRONIC PACEMAKER

ELECTRONIC: IMPULSE FORMATION

Excitation

EPM = Electronic pacemaker
= Symbol for electronic pacemaker impulse

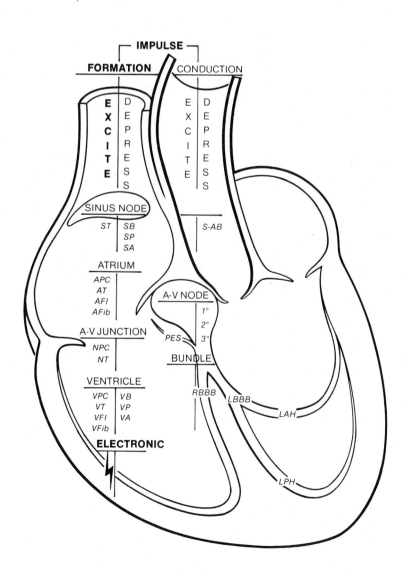

The electronic pacemaker is a battery-powered device which generates a series of timed electrical discharges. It is used to initiate depolarization of excitable cardiac tissue, thus operating as an artificial impulse formation source. The electronic pacemaker is currently widely used to provide an artificial cardiac rhythm when abnormalities of the impulse formation or conduction systems result in excessive slowing of the ventricular rate.

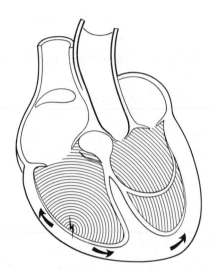

Electronic pacemaker.

The electronic pacemaker consists of a *power unit* which emits periodic electrical impulses, as well as a pair of insulated wires which terminate in electrode tips. These electrodes form the positive and negative poles of an electrical circuit. At least one of the electrodes is placed in direct contact with the heart. Two approaches are available for inserting the electronic pacemaker—the **transthoracic** and the **transvenous** methods.

The Transthoracic Method

The power unit is implanted into a subcutaneous pocket made in the wall of the chest or abdomen. Wires lead from the power unit through the chest wall, pleura, and pericardium to electrodes which are sutured onto the external surface of the heart. This method requires a thoracotomy; it is used for permanent cardiac pacing.

Transthoracic Method

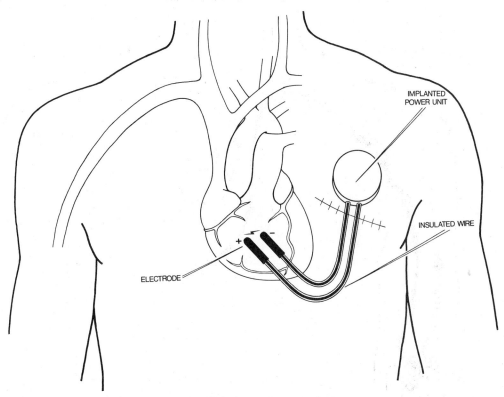

Epicardial electronic pacemaker.

The Transvenous Method

For *temporary* pacing, a power unit is used which remains external to the body. A pacing wire is inserted into a vein (brachial, jugular, or subclavian) and advanced until the electrode tip is in the apex of the right ventricle. The external end is connected to the negative terminal of the power unit. A second wire is connected to the positive terminal, and its other end is sutured into the skin to complete the electrical circuit. (See illustration at top of following page.)

The temporary electronic pacemaker method necessitates only the minor procedure of venipuncture or venous cut-down. The insertion and positioning can be made rapidly so that it is a useful method for arrhythmia problems requiring urgent treatment. It is also convenient for controlling an unstable rhythm which might be transitory while evaluating the necessity for a permanent electronic pacemaker.

For *permanent* pacing, the power unit is implanted underneath the skin, usually in the anterolateral chest. Wires lead from it subcutaneously to the shoulder or neck where they enter a major vein. This method for permanent use, unlike the transthoracic method, has the practical advantage of not necessitating a thoracotomy. Several modifications of this basic design are now available. (See illustration at bottom of following page.)

In both types of transvenous pacing, an electrode is in direct proximity with the endocardium. The electrode is not securely attached to the inner surface of the heart and may move out of position, causing failure of ventricular stimulation. This contrasts with the electrode of the transthoracic method which is sutured to the epicardial surface and is, therefore, not susceptible to displacement.

Transvenous Method

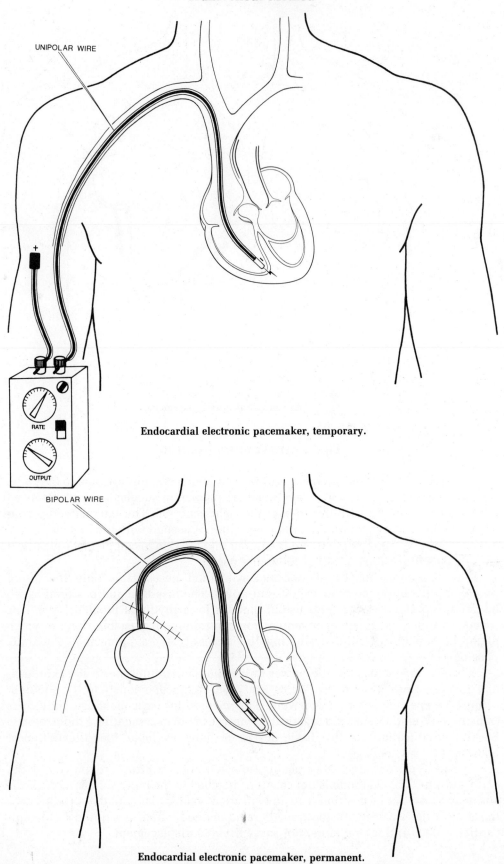

UNIPOLAR WIRE

RATE

OUTPUT

Endocardial electronic pacemaker, temporary.

BIPOLAR WIRE

Endocardial electronic pacemaker, permanent.

ELECTRONIC PACEMAKER RHYTHM

Impulses from an electronic pacemaker are easily identified in the electrocardiogram. They are inscribed so rapidly that they appear as sharp, spikelike deflections.

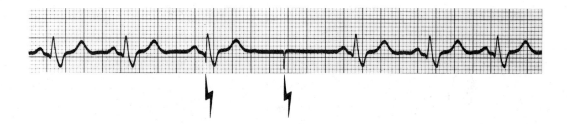

During a sinus pause, a sharp deflection interrupts the baseline. This is produced by a discharge from an electronic pacemaker. Close inspection of the cardiac cycle immediately prior to this reveals a similar spike falling in the early portion of the QRS component. In this example, the artificial impulses are isolated events and do not affect the basic rhythm.

Ventricular depolarization is initiated by the impulse from the electrode in contact with the endo- or epicardial surface of the ventricle. The wave front spreads through the ventricles in the same manner as spontaneous ectopic impulses from that site. Thus the QRS complex is prolonged and atypically shaped and the ST segment and T wave altered in form.

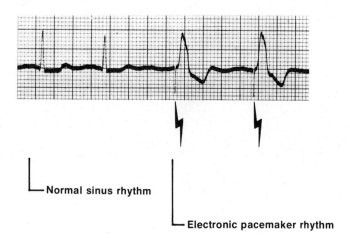

Normal sinus rhythm

Electronic pacemaker rhythm

Selected leads from the standard electrocardiogram demonstrate an electronic pacemaker rhythm. Each ventricular complex is initiated by an electronic stimulus occurring at a rate of exactly 74 per minute. Note that the direction and amplitude of the electronic pacemaker artifact varies in the different leads (see following page).

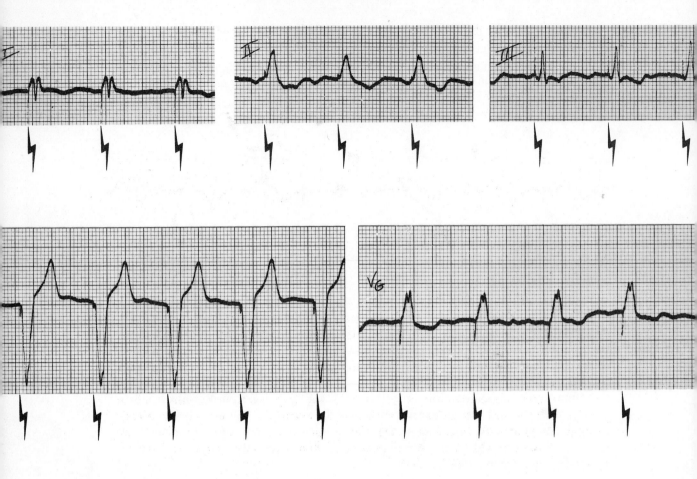

Following are examples of electronic pacemaker rhythm. Label each electronic stimulation artifact which initiates a ventricular contraction. Note the precise regularity of the rate (check with calipers).

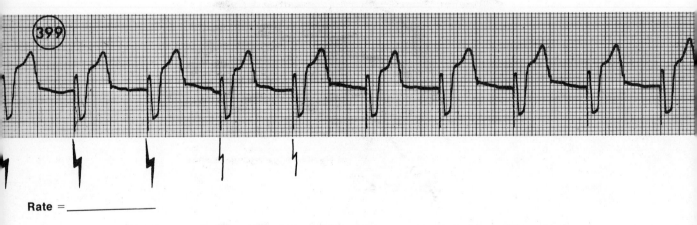

Rate = _____

Complete the diagram.

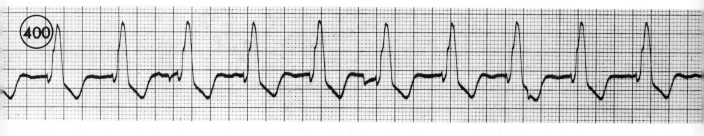

te = _____

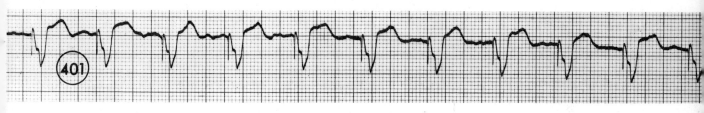

Rate = _____

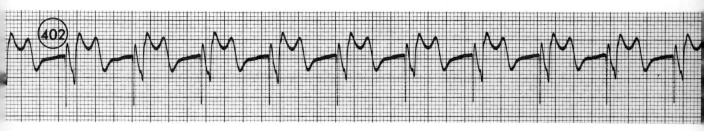

Rate = _____

The electronic pacemaker rhythm has the following electrocardiographic characteristics:

1. The rate has a clocklike, precise regularity.
2. The QRS complex immediately follows the pacemaker spike.
3. The QRS complex is prolonged.
4. The QRS complex, ST segment, and T wave vary in shape from normally stimulated beats.

Cardiac depolarization induced by an electronic stimulus is referred to as **capture. Complete capture** occurs when every artificial stimulus initiates a beat. In the following electronic pacemaker rhythm with complete ventricular capture, identify the above features.

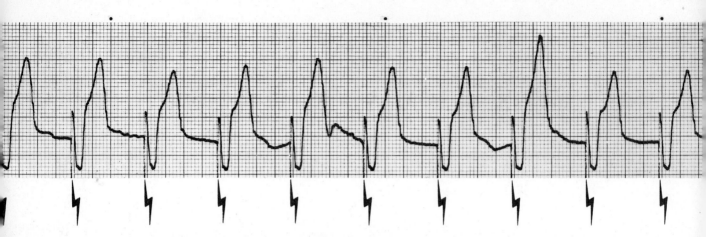

1. Pacemaker spikes appear with precise regularity at 75 per minute (verify exact uniformity of intervals with calipers).
2. Ventricular depolarization begins immediately after the pacemaker stimulus.
3. Each pacemaker stimulus leads to ventricular capture.
4. The QRS complex is prolonged (0.16 second).

In the following electrocardiograms, diagram the electronic pacemaker spikes and determine the rate and regularity of rhythm. Does complete ventricular capture occur?

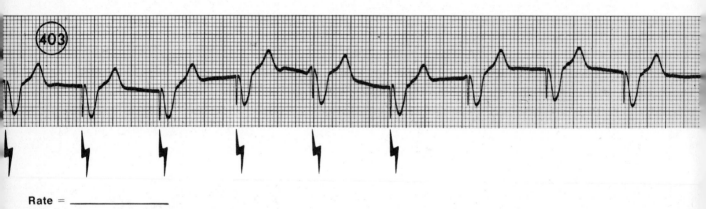

Rate = _____

Complete the symbols.

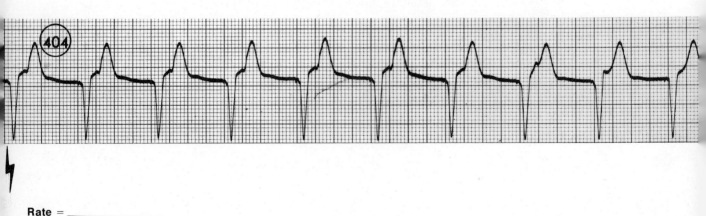

Rate = _____

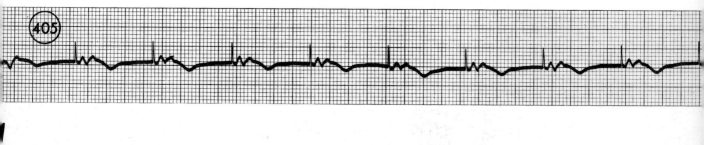

ate = _____

The electronic pacemaker is used to treat a variety of arrhythmias which involve depression of impulse formation in the sinus node and sites of potential escape rhythms or of impulse conduction in the A-V node and major ventricular pathways. The basic arrhythmia should be included in the descriptive interpretation of an electronic pacemaker rhythm. The following examples demonstrate several variations.

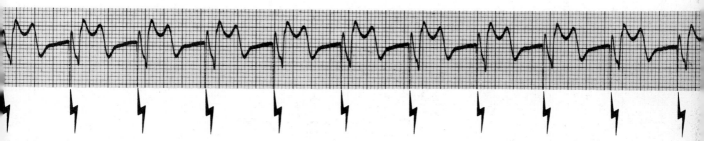

Electronic pacemaker rhythm: Rate = 80

No atrial activity is visible.

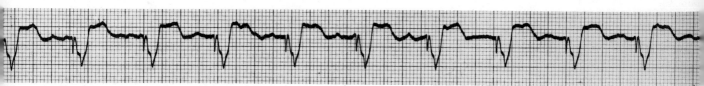

Electronic pacemaker rhythm: Rate = 77

The pattern of atrial fibrillation is present. Since no ventricular beats are recorded which may have been stimulated from atrial activity, either complete A-V block is present, or the potential ventricular rate response to atrial impulses is slower than that of the electronic pacemaker.

In the following examples of complete A-V block, independent atrial and electronic pacemaker rhythms can be clearly discerned. Calipers are helpful in locating P waves.

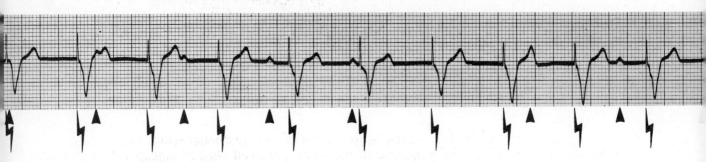

Sinus rhythm: Rate = 60

Complete A-V block (no sinus beats are conducted to the ventricles)

Electronic pacemaker rhythm: Rate = 77

Denote the P waves and electronic pacemaker spikes in the following electrocardiograms.

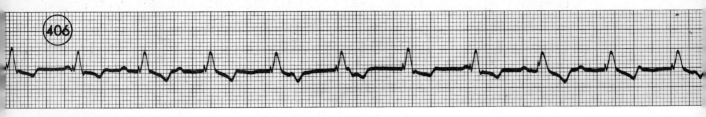

Sinus rate = _____

Electronic pacemaker rate = _____

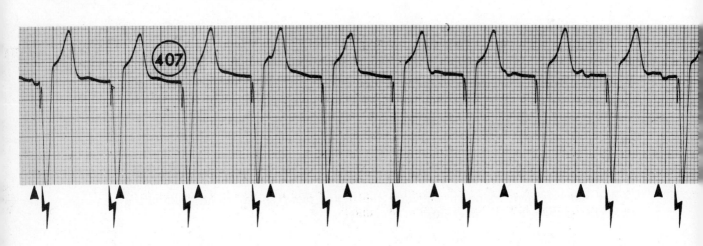

Sinus rhythm: **Rate =** _____

Basic arrhythmia _____

Electronic pacemaker rhythm: **Rate =** _____

Give complete descriptive interpretations of the following electrocardiograms.

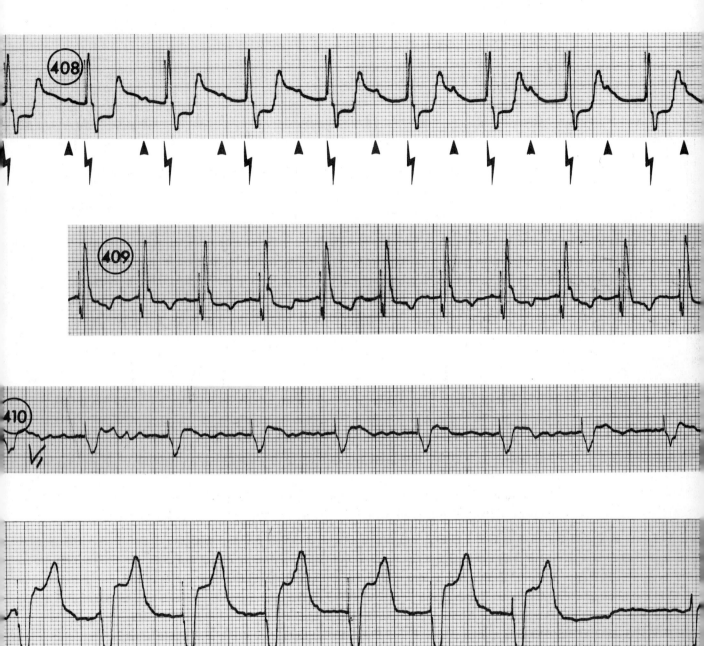

Identification of basic arrhythmia on cessation of electronic pacemaker activity.

After turning off the external electronic pacemaker power unit, the pattern of atrial fibrillation is evident. Following a two-second pause, a supraventricular beat appears. It is not possible to positively identify this as a conducted beat from the atria or as an A-V nodal escape beat.

An escape mechanism appears during the momentary cessation of electronic pacemaker activity.

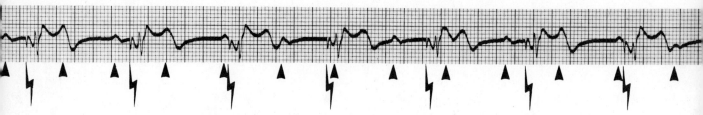

Sinus rhythm with complete A-V block; electronic pacemaker with complete ventricular capture.

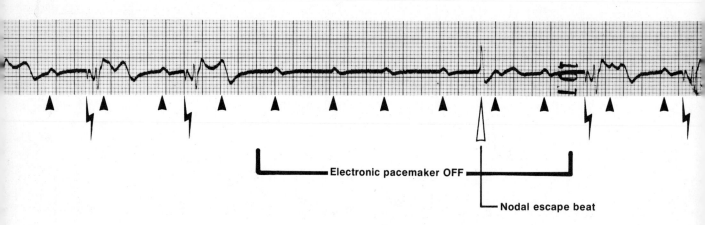

On temporary loss of electronic pacemaker power, a period of ventricular asystole appears. This is interrupted by a nodal escape beat. On restarting the electronic pacemaker, ventricular capture is once again achieved.

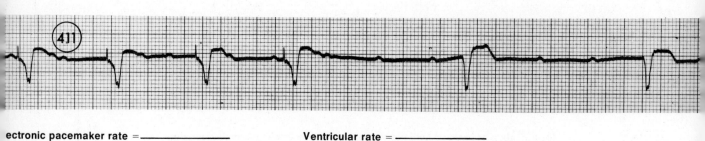

ectronic pacemaker rate = _____   Ventricular rate = _____

Transition from electronic pacemaker rhythm to a ventricular rhythm.

Sudden loss of function of an electronic pacemaker with complete A-V block and ventricular escape rhythm is revealed.

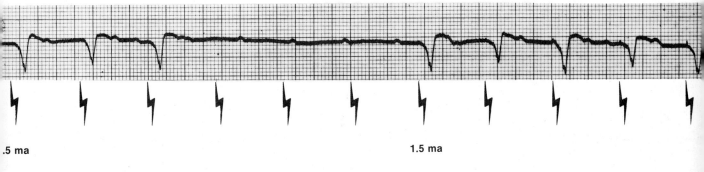

.5 ma   1.5 ma

A   B   C

Ventricular capture regained with increasing electronic pacemaker power output.

A. Energy output at 0.5 milliamp.
B. Loss of ventricular capture exposing sinus rhythm with complete A-V block and ventricular arrest. Pacemaker spikes are barely visible at this output level.
C. On increasing output to 1.5 milliamps, complete ventricular capture is restored.
    Note that the pacemaker spike amplitude has increased and is now obvious.

Failure of Electronic Pacemaker Capture

The electronic pacemaker may fire, but the impulse does not initiate depolarization. Failure of ventricular capture is recognized by the appearance of an electronic pacemaker spike in which there is no ventricular response.

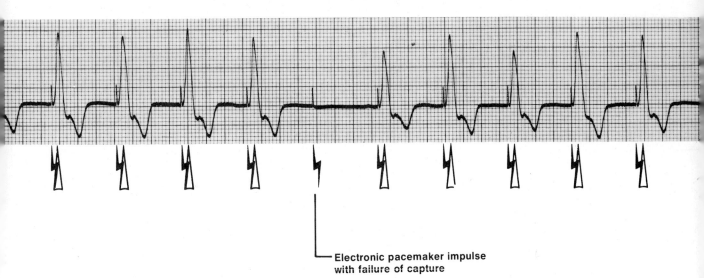

Electronic pacemaker impulse
with failure of capture

The electronic pacemaker spike not followed by a ventricular complex represents failure of stimulation. Satisfactory control of the ventricular rhythm is elsewhere observed.

Complete A-V block with electronic pacemaker and intermittent failure of ventricular capture is evident in the following tracing. Identify the noncapture impulse.

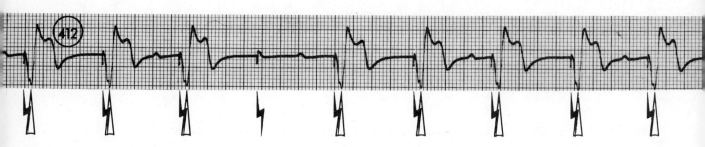

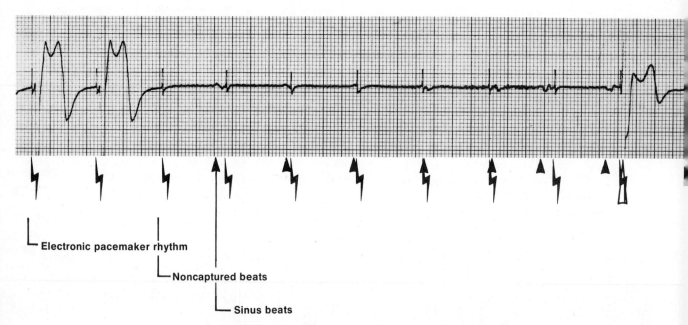

Electronic pacemaker rhythm

Noncaptured beats

Sinus beats

Sustained failure of ventricular capture by electronic stimulation.

After ventricular stimulation, the electronic pacemaker ceases to capture the ventricles. Complete A-V block becomes apparent with a 5.6-second period of ventricular asystole. Spontaneous beats then emerge in which the PR intervals are identical. These probably are sinus beats with aberrant ventricular conduction (as opposed to ventricular escape beats). Noncapturing electronic pacemaker artifacts can be found during this sinus rhythm.

Treatment of complete A-V block with a temporary transvenous electronic pacemaker requires adjustments in the controls of the power unit. The patient is a 78-year-old woman with a three-day history of marked weakness, instability on standing, and slow pulse.

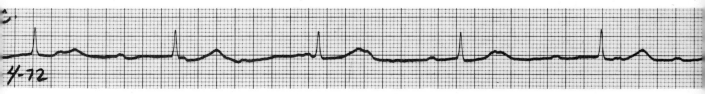

Interpretation: Complete A-V block with nodal rhythm

Electrocardiogram, Lead I, on admission.

The following tracings were taken from a monitoring lead after insertion of a wire electrode into the right ventricle through the left subclavian vein. The wire and a second wire attached to the skin were connected to the two poles of an external electronic pacemaker power unit.

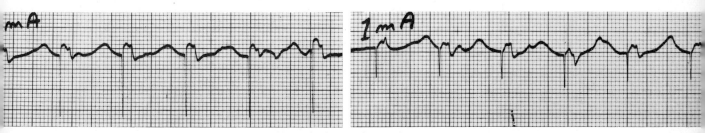

Adjustments in power output.

At 2 milliamps, complete ventricular capture occurs. (A milliampere is one thousandth of an ampere, a unit of electrical force.)

The electronic pacemaker continues to stimulate the ventricle, even when the power is reduced to 1 milliamp. Note the decrease in amplitude of the EPM impulse spike.

When the power output was reduced to 0.5 milliamp, the electronic pacemaker impulse was no longer strong enough to initiate depolarization. Failure to capture resulted, with a period of ventricular asystole.

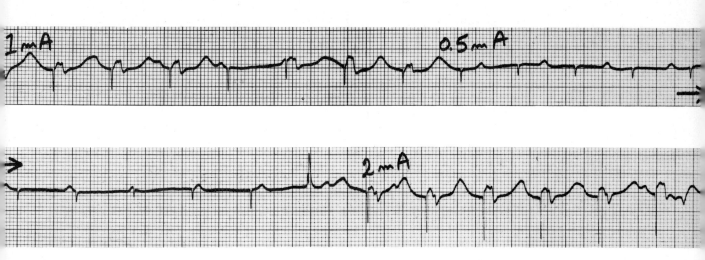

The 7-second episode of ventricular asystole is interrupted by a spontaneous nodal escape beat which is superimposed upon a noneffective electronic pacemaker spike. When the power output is increased, ventricular capture is once again achieved with the electronic pacemaker.

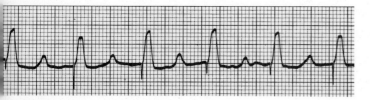 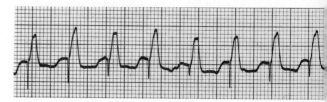

Electronic pacemaker rate = 83

EPM rate increased to 140 by manual control dial

Adjustment of rate:

Fixed Mode Electronic Pacemaker

The **fixed mode** electronic pacemaker emits periodic impulses regardless of the cardiac activity. The pacemaker spike will continue to appear even though a spontaneous cardiac beat is present. Observe this in the next electrocardiogram.

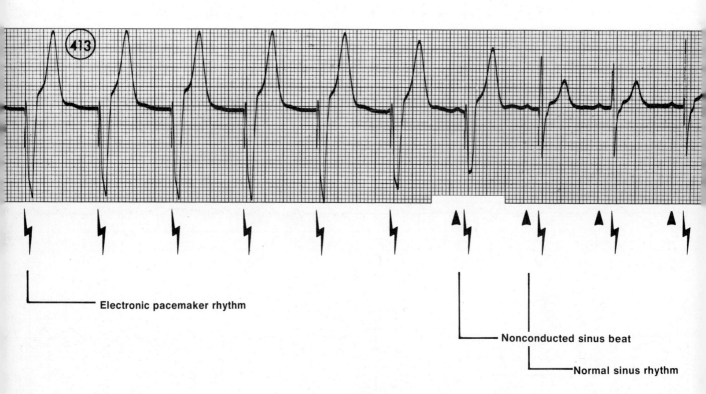

Electronic pacemaker rhythm

Nonconducted sinus beat

Normal sinus rhythm

A sinus beat emerges during an electronic pacemaker rhythm, but no ventricular stimulation results. Subsequent sinus beats are conducted, and normal sinus rhythm supervenes. The sinus rate _____ is slightly more rapid than the electronic pacemaker rate _____. The spikes can be found with careful caliper measurement to be moving further and further into subsequent QRS complexes of the spontaneous beats.

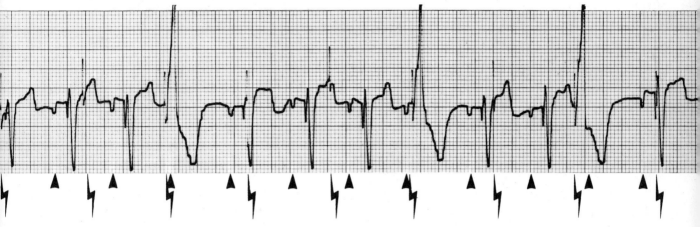

Competitive rhythm control between sinus and electronic pacemakers.

Normal sinus rhythm and electronic pacemaker activity are evident throughout the tracing. Some of the artificial impulses induce ventricular beats while others do not. It is also noted that sinus impulses fail to capture the ventricles when they occur soon after an electronically stimulated ventricular beat. It can be seen that the ventricular rhythm control is shared by both the spontaneous and the artificial impulse-forming sources.

A disadvantage of the fixed mode electronic pacemaker is the potential for inducing tachycardia in the presence of additional impulse formation from spontaneous sources. For example, if ectopic ventricular beats occur or if the conduction system recovers from complete A-V block while an electronic pacemaker is operative, the ventricles respond to more than one pacemaker. When this is sustained, serious tachyarrhythmias may result.

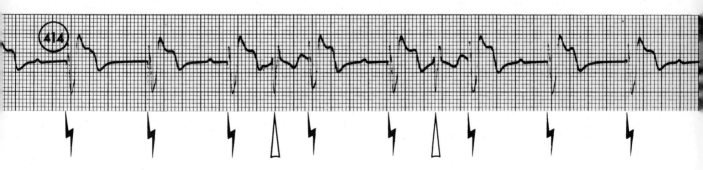

Lead V₁:

Complete A-V block with an electronic pacemaker rhythm in the presence of spontaneous ectopic beats.

Identify the spontaneous ventricular contractions. What pattern do these have? Note that these beats momentarily double the rate of the ventricles.

Sustained tachycardia produced by the additive effects of spontaneous impulse formation and a fixed mode electronic pacemaker can be treated by turning off the latter (if the power unit is external), removing it (if internal), or administering drugs which suppress the spontaneous beats.

Demand Mode Electronic Pacemaker

The **demand mode** electronic pacemaker has been developed to eliminate the hazard of additive (spontaneous plus electronic) rhythms. This unit has the capability of changing impulse emission from *operating* to *standby* when spontaneous ventricular beats occur. When the spontaneous ventricular rate slows beyond a certain level, the electronic impulse-forming mechanism once again becomes operative. In this regard, the electronic pacemaker has an escape impulse formation function and provides sustained pacemaker activity when spontaneous ventricular activity suppression is prolonged.

A sensory device is incorporated into the power unit of the demand mode pacemaker which is sensitive to small electrical currents. Stimuli generated by every heart beat are conveyed to the sensor component through the electrode-wire lead. These stimuli inhibit the discharge of impulses from the power unit. If a stimulus is not detected by the sensor within a specific time interval, the inhibition is released, and an electronic impulse is emitted. If spontaneous ventricular activity remains suppressed, the electronic pacemaker will establish a sustained rhythm at a constant rate.

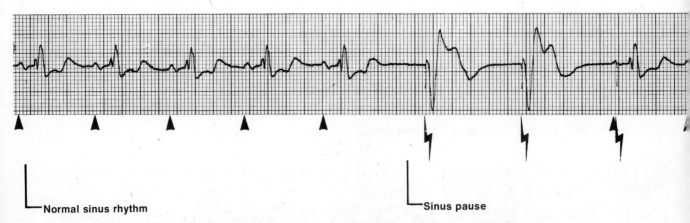

Normal sinus rhythm   Sinus pause

Activation of a demand mode electronic pacemaker with sinus rhythm slowing.

With slowing of the sinus rate, an electronic rhythm with a rate of 59 appears. After two electronically stimulated beats, the sinus rate speeds up to 76, and a sinus impulse once again controls the ventricular rhythm. Note that at this transition an electronic pacemaker spike occurs simultaneously with the P wave, but the resulting QRS complex is of the sinus-stimulated type. In this beat, the impulse from the sinus node wins the race.

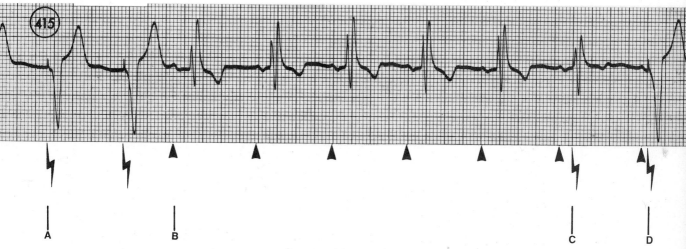

Spontaneous and demand mode electronic pacemaker rhythms as functions of rate.

A. Electronic pacemaker rhythm: Rate = _____.
B. Normal sinus rhythm with right bundle branch block. Carefully determine rate of each cardiac cycle, using the **one beat ruler.**
C. An electronic pacemaker spike appears at the beginning of the QRS complex. However, the QRS form is similar to that of the sinus beats (right bundle branch block pattern). This is, therefore, also a sinus beat. The electronic impulse does not induce a response.
D. An electronic pacemaker spike with ventricular capture occurs.

This example demonstrates the interplay of spontaneous and demand mode electronic pacemakers. With the appearance of a sinus rhythm, the electronic pacemaker stops firing. It is noted that the sinus rate is almost identical to that set for the electronic pacemaker rate. When the sinus rate slows to a critical point (in this case, slowing to a very slight degree), the electronic pacemaker impulse formation mechanism is again activated. The first artificial impulse on reactivation occurs after ventricular depolarization from the sinus beat has already started, and no stimulation results. This is *not* a *failure* of capture because of a defect in the power unit or electrode placement, but rather a feature of timing in relationship to the naturally occurring cardiac cycle. In the last beat of the tracing, the artificial impulse occurs toward the end of the P wave, before ventricular depolarization could begin from the atrial impulse. Instead, the ventricles respond to the electronic pacemaker impulse.

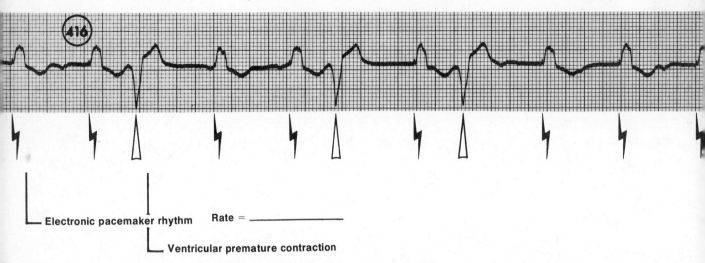

Electronic pacemaker rhythm   Rate = _____

Ventricular premature contraction

Demand mode electronic pacemaker with spontaneous premature beats.

Using calipers to compare intervals between electronic pacemaker beats, note the delay in cadence produced by the first premature ventricular contraction. After the delay, the electronic pacemaker commences to fire at the original rate. Subsequent ventricular premature contractions continue to interrupt the precise regularity of the artificial impulses.

This electrocardiogram illustrates the normally functioning systems of the demand mode electronic pacemaker. The power unit emits impulses at regular intervals, and each induces a ventricular response. The sensor component detects spontaneous ventricular activity on a beat-by-beat basis and shuts off the power unit emissions temporarily after each ventricular premature contraction.

Demand mode electronic pacemaker sensor function is demonstrated with changes in the sinus rate. In each of the following examples, a sinus rhythm appears at a faster rate than that of the electronic pacemaker, and the sinus impulse takes over control of the ventricles. Note the cessation of electronic pacemaker spikes at the appropriate time, indicating normal sensor and turn-off functions of the power unit. In all examples, rate changes were induced by sudden standing or mild exercise. The first two tracings were taken from patients with bifascicular conduction defects (right bundle branch block and left anterior hemiblock with intermittent complete A-V block).

Determine the electronic pacemaker and sinus rates in each example. Give complete interpretations.

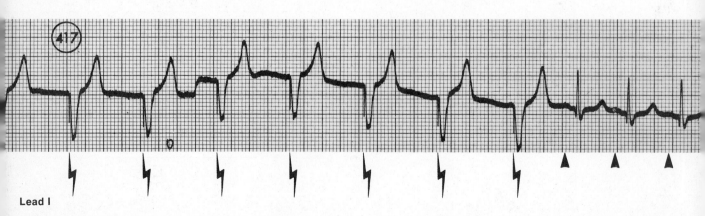

Lead I

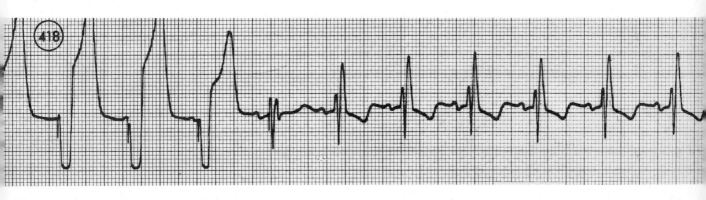

ad V₁

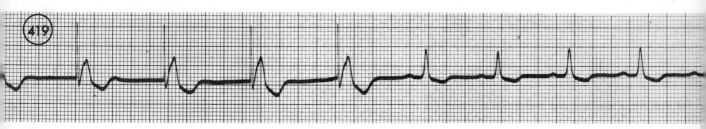

itoring lead

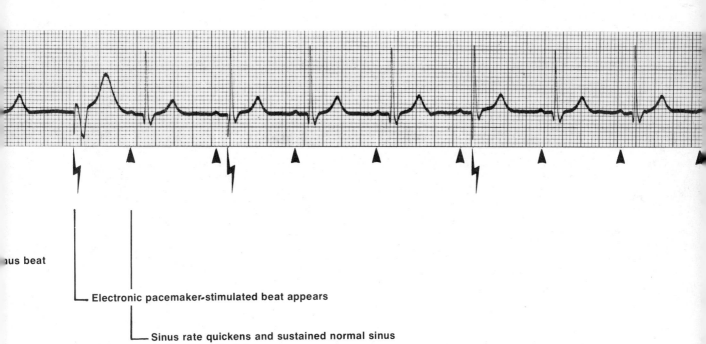

us beat

└── Electronic pacemaker-stimulated beat appears

    └── Sinus rate quickens and sustained normal sinus
       rhythm supervenes

   Demand mode electronic pacemaker with intermittent pacing activity.

   Two additional electronic pacemaker spikes are seen, but these occur just after
ventricular depolarization has started from the sinus impulse, and no electronic

pacemaker stimulation results. This tracing demonstrates activation of the power unit on demand (during excessive slowing of the ventricular rate) and shut-off during periods of faster spontaneous beating.

When a demand mode electronic pacemaker is in place but a sustained spontaneous rhythm causes continuous inhibition of power unit firing, special but simple tests may be used to determine if the sensor and firing systems are operable. A method of slowing the cardiac rate to less than the set rate of the electronic pacemaker will achieve this. Sufficient slowing is often accomplished by deep breath holding, the Valsalva maneuver, or carotid pressure.

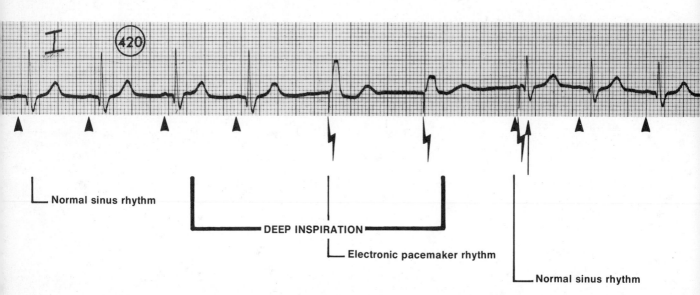

Appearance of an electronic pacemaker rhythm during slowing of the sinus rate.

The tracing begins with normal sinus rhythm and right bundle branch block. On vagal stimulation produced by deep breath holding, the sinus rate decreases, and an electronic pacemaker rhythm supervenes. This is sustained until the deep breath is released and until the sinus rate increases to the point at which it takes over control of the ventricles and the electronic firing stops. This tracing demonstrates satisfactory functioning of both the firing and sensor systems of the electronic pacemaker. Note the transition designated by the arrow. Which pacemaker stimulates the ventricles?

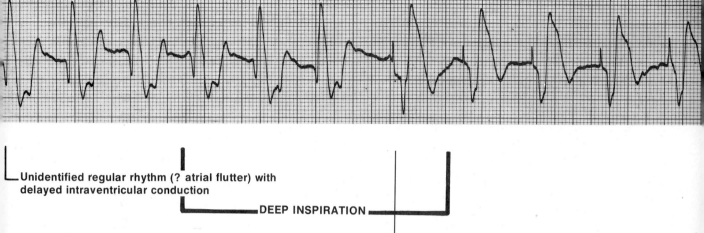

Unidentified regular rhythm (? atrial flutter) with
delayed intraventricular conduction

DEEP INSPIRATION

Electronic pacemaker rhythm

Testing of demand pacemaker sensor system in presence of spontaneous rhythm.

In this test, both the sensor and the ventricular stimulation mechanisms are demonstrated to be functioning satisfactorily.

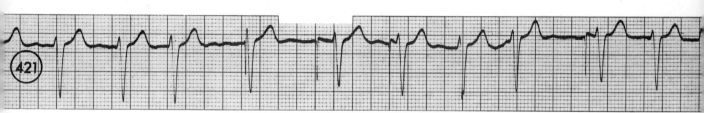

Activation of electronic impulse with failure of capture.

Atrial fibrillation is evident. During slowing of the ventricular rate response, impulses from a demand mode electronic pacemaker appear, but these do not capture the ventricles.

Locate all electronic pacemaker spikes. Note that successive electronic impulses occur at a constant rate. This tracing illustrates a well-functioning sensor system and impulse-generating mechanism but failure of ventricular stimulation.

Both the fixed mode and the demand mode pacemakers generate emissions at a constant rate. The appellation "fixed rate" pacemaker is confusing, since both this and the demand modes generate impulses at a constant or fixed rate. The basic difference is that the fixed pacemaker operates continuously, while the demand pacemaker can turn the impulse formation mechanism on and off in response to competing cardiac activity.

Both fixed and demand mode electronic pacemakers are available for external and implanted power units. The demand mode system is the more commonly used.

Synchronous Mode Electronic Pacemaker

An electronic pacemaker with rate variability is also manufactured. It employs an electrode sensor in the right atrium from which each atrial beat is relayed to the power unit. This induces emission of an impulse from the power unit to the heart, which in turn stimulates the ventricles. Thus a mechanism is provided in which, even in complete A-V block, the sinus node controls the ventricular rate. This modification of the electronic pacemaker has the advantage of allowing physiological pulse rate adjustments, such as speeding during exercise and slowing during rest. The synchronous mode electronic pacemaker will automatically convert to a fixed mode if the right atrial sensor system, for any reason, becomes inoperative.

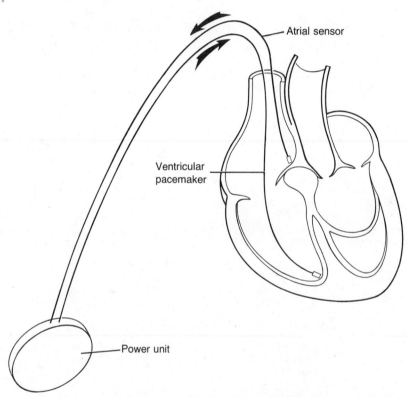

Synchronous mode electronic pacemaker.

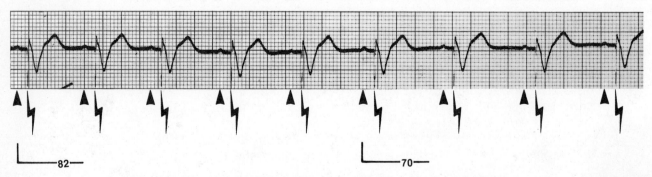

Sinus rhythm with synchronized ventricular electronic pacemaker response.

Note that an electronic pacemaker spike follows each sinus beat at a constant interval despite changes in the sinus rate. Thus the rate of the ventricles is controlled by the sinus node, even though direct stimulation of the ventricles results from electronic impulses.

The electronic pacemaker is designed to emit impulses at a given rate for many months. However, as batteries decay beyond a critical level, there is a tendency for the power unit to change the rate before impulse formation ceases completely. Usually, the rate change prior to complete failure is a decrease in speed. Occasionally the rate will speed up and may become extremely rapid. This latter condition, which represents an emergency situation, is referred to as a **runaway** pacemaker.

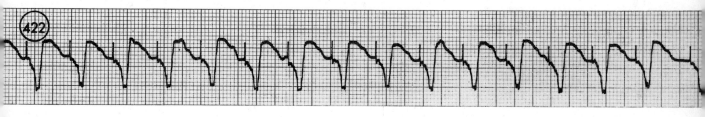

ate = _____

Runaway electronic pacemaker rhythm recorded from a patient having the power unit for 17½ months.

A variation of three or more beats per minute from the original setting is a sign of impending power failure. For this reason, very accurate pulse rates must be determined in periodic evaluations of an electronic pacemaker.

The description of an electronic pacemaker rhythm should include the following details:
1. Basic intrinsic rhythm (e.g., sinus rhythm with complete A-V block, sinus arrest).
2. Electronic pacemaker
   a. rate.
   d. ventricular capture (e.g., complete, intermittent, or absent).
   c. type (e.g., fixed, demand, or synchronous).
3. Ectopic impulse formation (e.g., premature contractions, fusion beats).

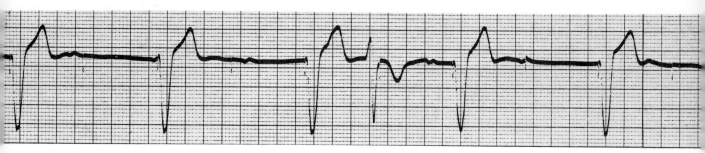

Interpretation of a sample electrocardiogram:
1. Sinus rhythm: Rate = 68.
   Complete A-V block.

 2. Electronic pacemaker rhythm: Rate = 72.
  Fixed mode (note continued firing without cadence change after a ventricular premature contraction).
  Intermittent ventricular capture by electronic stimuli.
 3. Ventricular premature contraction.

The next series of tracings illustrates many rhythm problems occurring within a relatively brief period. They were recorded from a 66-year-old man who received a permanent transvenous electronic pacemaker on the previous day. Write a complete rhythm interpretation for each tracing.

3/8/72 — 8:15 AM: The following three continuous strips are from the standard electrocardiogram taken on the first postoperative day. Until this time, no defect in the pulse rate had been detected since implantation of the electronic pacemaker. During the recording, the patient developed a period of lightheadedness and apprehension.

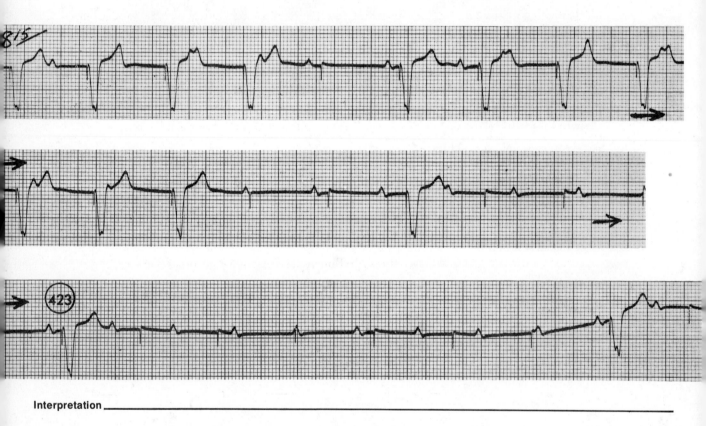

Interpretation _____

8:27 AM: The patient no longer had symptoms when lying supine but experienced lightheadedness upon sitting up.

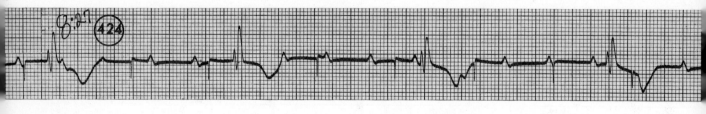

Interpretation _____

8:33 AM: Isoproterenol infusion was started: 1 mg/1000 cc 5 per cent D/W at 50 drops per minute.

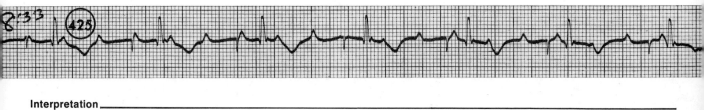

Interpretation_____

8:47 AM: The patient can tolerate sitting upright without symptoms. However, he now complains of palpitations.

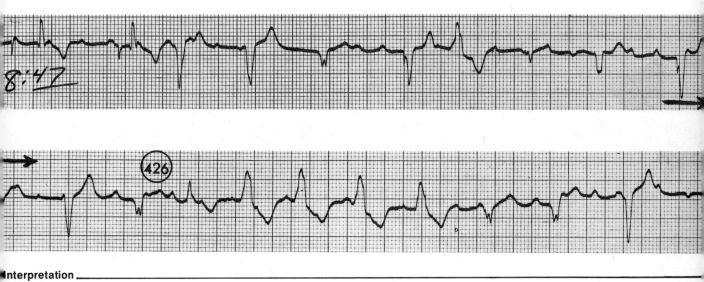

Interpretation_____

8:49 AM: The isoproterenol infusion rate was reduced to 30 drops per minute.

8:54 AM: Palpitations have disappeared.

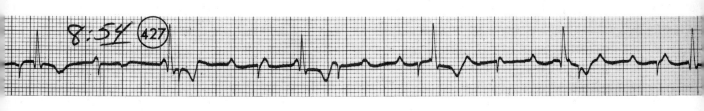

Interpretation_____

9:15 AM: Monitoring leads were attached to the patient, and the recording was made by another instrument.

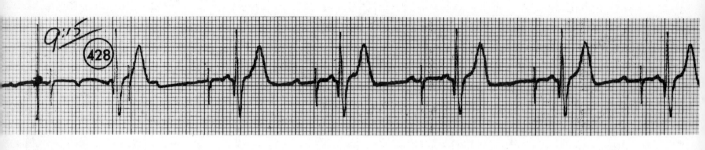

Interpretation _____

9:45 AM: The patient was taken to the operating room where an epicardial electronic pacemaker was implanted to replace the transvenous endocardial one. (This decision was made because of several previous episodes of pacemaker failure due to changing electrode position of the transvenous wire.)

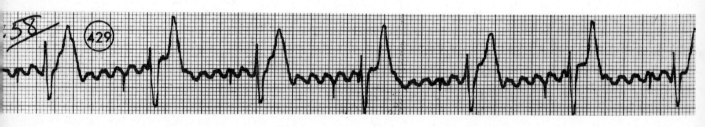

Interpretation _____

10:05 AM: An endotracheal intubation was performed. Blood pressure was maintained.

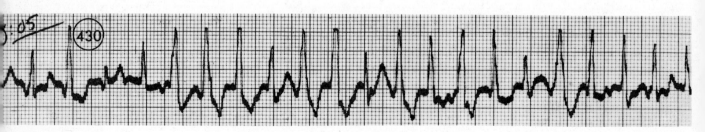

Interpretation _____

10:06 AM: Isoproterenol infusion was stopped.

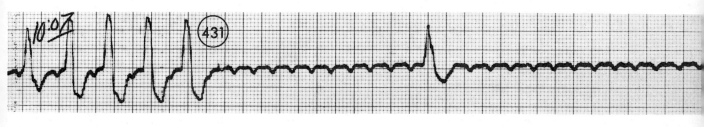

Interpretation _____

10:08 AM: Ventricular beats were stimulated by a succession of fist blows to the chest by the surgeon.

Isoproterenol infusion was restarted at 100 drops per minute momentarily, then slowed to 50 drops per minute.

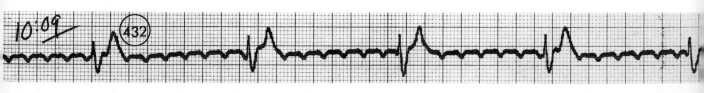

Interpretation _____

10:09 AM: Stable rhythm was maintained with isoproterenol infusion, while the surgeon proceeded with the thoracotomy and epicardial electrode placement.

10:45 AM: Wires from the epicardial electrodes were connected to the electronic pacemaker power unit. Technical problems then interfered with the electrocardiographic recording. Nevertheless, the desired information could be ascertained from this tracing.

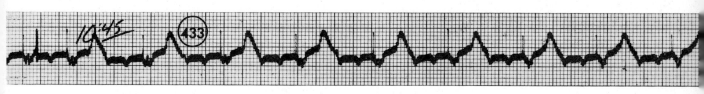

Interpretation _____

10:47 AM: Isoproterenol infusion was discontinued.

11:20 AM: The lead from the standard electrocardiogram taken in the recovery room is shown below.

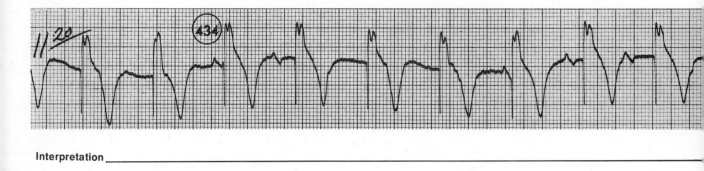

Interpretation _____

The cardiac rhythm thereafter remained entirely stable.

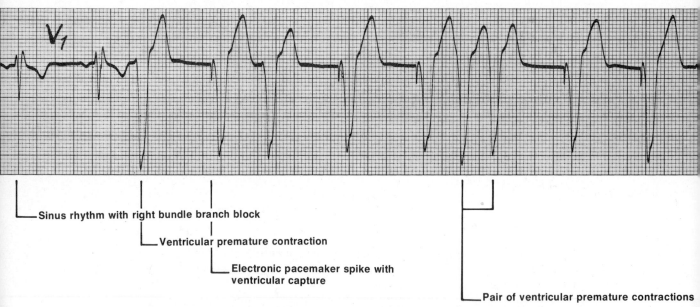

Sinus rhythm with right bundle branch block

Ventricular premature contraction

Electronic pacemaker spike with ventricular capture

Pair of ventricular premature contractions

Example of ventricular excitation induced by the electrode tip of a transvenous electronic pacemaker.

Following a ventricular premature contraction and during the compensatory pause, an electronic pacemaker spike is seen to cause a ventricular stimulation. Note that both the premature and the electronically induced contractions have similar QRS and T component forms. Both types of beats appear throughout the remainder of the tracing and continue to appear alike in form. It appears that ventricular beats are produced by impulses from the power unit, as well as by mechanical irritation from direct contact of excitable tissues of the endocardium with the tip of the electrode. On withdrawing the electrode wire a short distance, ventricular premature contractions no longer appeared, but the electronic pacemaker was still capable of stimulating the ventricles.

The combination of ventricular premature contractions with various forms of A-V block is particularly hazardous. Drugs used to suppress the excitable foci may increase the A-V block while rendering ventricular escape mechanisms ineffective. Stimulatory drugs used to counteract the A-V block, such as the adrenergic agents, will likely increase the ectopic beats, often to a dangerous level. In this dilemma, an electronic pacemaker can be used to insure a satisfactory ventricular pacemaker so that suppressor drugs can be safely used.

This therapeutic dilemma is illustrated in the following clinical experience:

An 83-year-old woman was brought to the hospital after she collapsed in her home and lost consciousness momentarily. The episode had been preceded by several days of frequent, brief periods of giddiness and weakness. Selected leads from the standard electrocardiogram obtained in the emergency room reveal a combination of rhythm disorders.

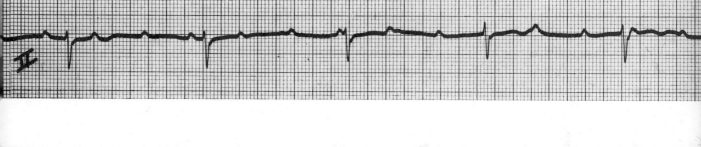

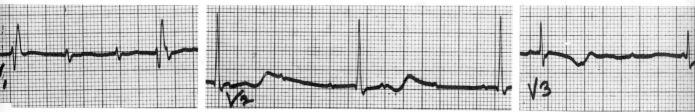

Complete A-V block

Nodal rhythm: Rate = 40/minute

Right bundle branch block

In portions of the recording, frequent ectopic beats appeared.

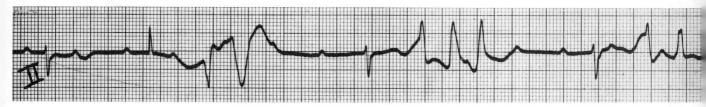

Multifocal ventricular premature contractions occurred in couplets and triplets. (Note that the second QRS complex does not display bundle branch block.)

Transient ventricular tachycardia–fibrillation were recorded in two leads.

During these episodes, the patient became restless and dazed but recovered rapidly and completely.

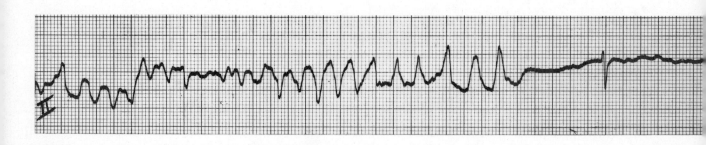

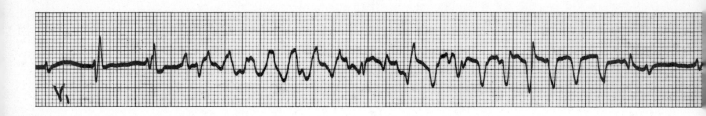

Ventricular tachycardia in an extremely disorganized pattern merged at times into ventricular fibrillation. Spontaneous recovery with resumption of complete A-V block and nodal rhythm occurred.

With combined impulse conduction depression and impulse formation excitation in the ventricles, the decision was made to begin treatment with an electronic pacemaker as an emergency measure. A transvenous electrode with an external power unit was inserted. Once this was functioning satisfactorily, ventricular ectopy was suppressed with an infusion of lidocaine. A stable cardiac rhythm was achieved.

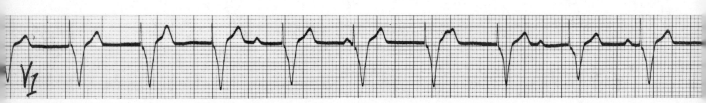

SELF-EVALUATION: STAGE 4

Each of the following electrocardiograms demonstrates compound rhythms, and two or more statements are required. Give complete interpretations.

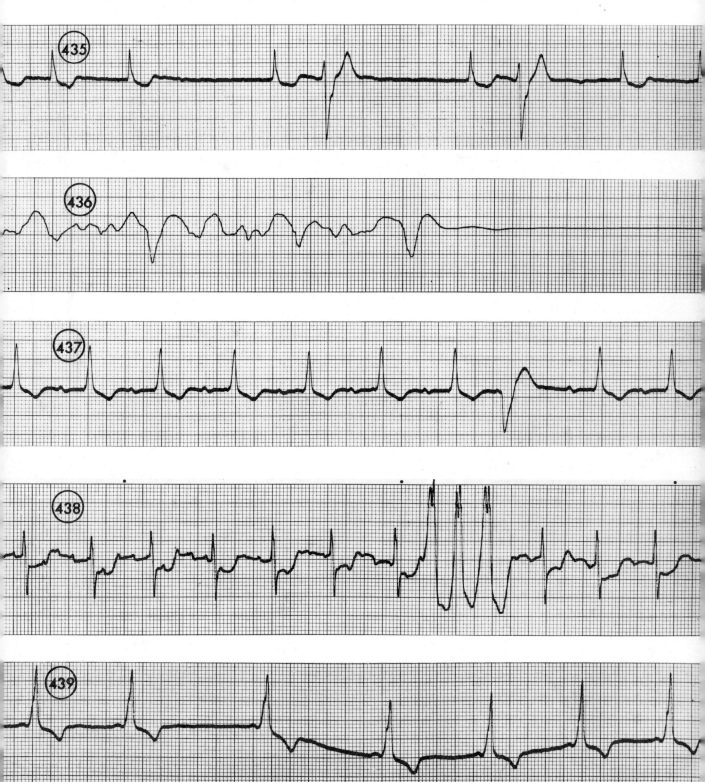

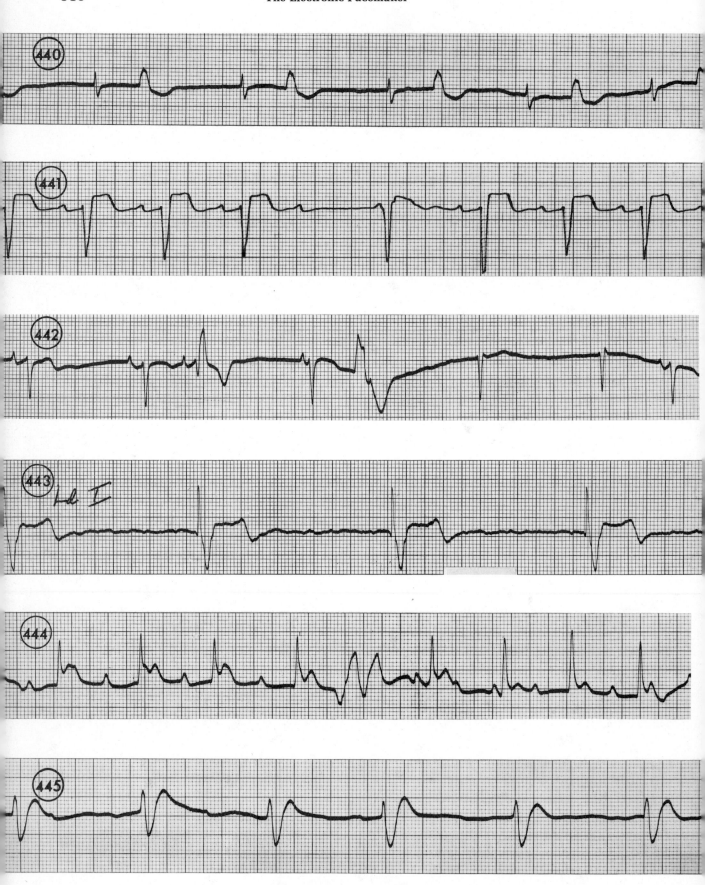

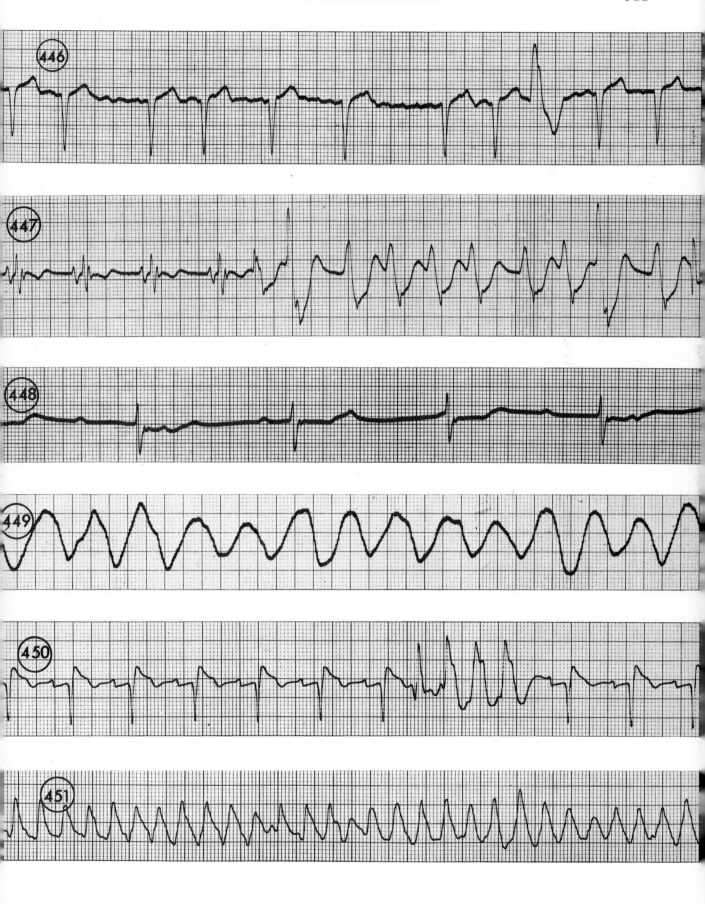

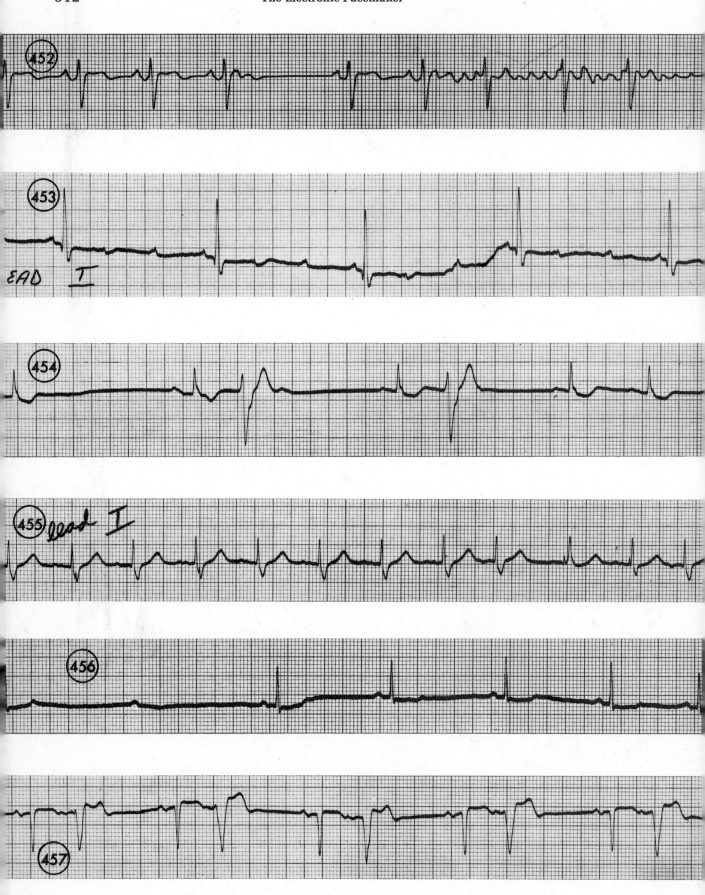

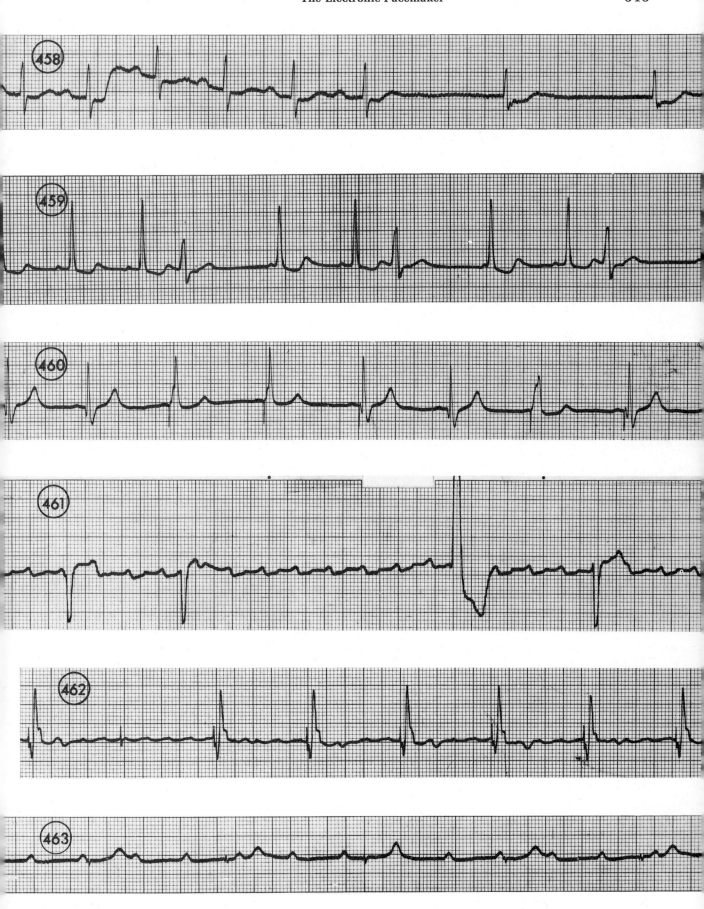

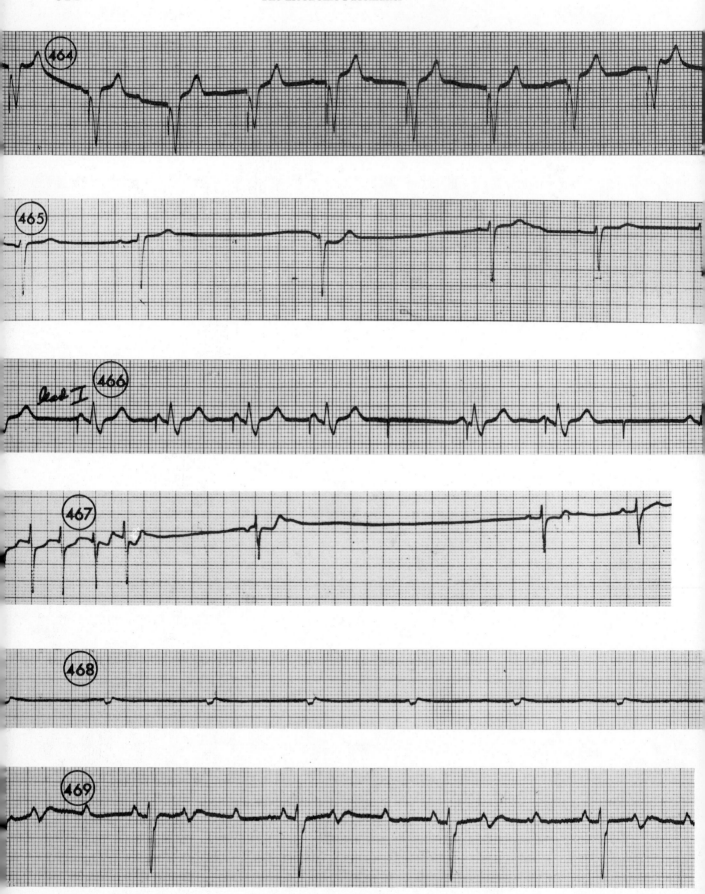

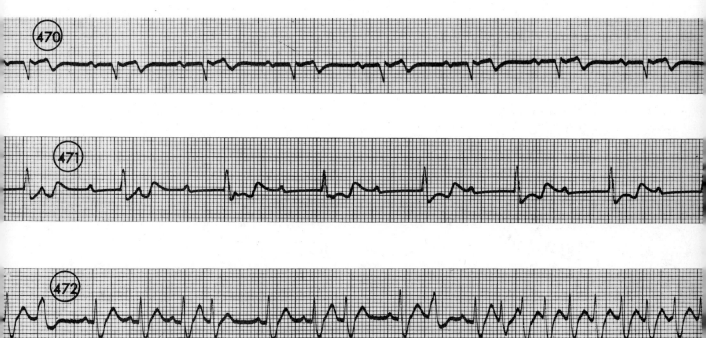

Chapter 10

THE CARDIAC DRUGS

This chapter summarizes the action of the cardiac drugs within the framework developed for the arrhythmias. It is intended as a guide for understanding the specific sites at which a drug may affect the sequences of the heart beat. It is not meant as a text in pharmacology and does not indicate the choice of drugs, dosage, route of administration, metabolism, onset and duration of action, or side effects.

Drugs may affect the heart by altering any of three functions:

1. Electrical:

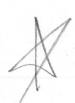

Impulse ⎡—formation
        ⎣—conduction

2. Mechanical:

Force of myocardial contraction

3. Vasomotor:

Tone of blood vessels

The cardiac drugs are arranged in this chapter according to their major actions upon **impulse formation** and **conduction.**

A. Drugs of excitation: Indicated for treatment of depression of impulse formation and conduction.
   1. Autonomic nervous system effectors
      a. adrenergic (sympathetic stimulation)
      b. anticholinergic (parasympathetic inhibition)
B. Drugs of depression: Indicated for treatment of excitation of impulse formation and conduction.
   1. Autonomic nervous system effectors
      a. antiadrenergic (sympathetic inhibition)
      b. cholinergic (parasympathetic stimulation)
   2. Direct cellular effectors
C. Digitalis: Considered in a separate class because of its complex actions on the electrical activity of the heart.

DRUGS OF EXCITATION

Sympathetic Nervous System: Stimulation

Adrenergic Agents

These agents accelerate the rate of impulse formation and conduction and are used to treat rhythms of depression. They increase the activity of automatic and conductile cells indirectly by augmentation of sympathetic nervous system effect.

Three agents of this large class are commonly used in clinical medicine. They are often referred to as the **catecholamines** because of their basic molecular structure, the catechol nucleus.

Norepinephrine (noradrenalin, Levophed) is the natural transmitter substance of the final sympathetic neuron pathways. It is produced and stored in the fiber endings and is released on stimulation of sympathetic nervous system centers in the brain or of the fibers themselves. Norepinephrine is also concentrated in the adrenal gland. On stimulation of this organ, norepinephrine is secreted into the blood stream and carried to distant sites. In this manner, the agent behaves according to a hormonal mechanism (activation of an organ by a chemical substance which has been produced in another organ and transported to it in the circulatory system).

Epinephrine is formed and stored only in the adrenal gland, and it acts exclusively as a hormone. On adrenal stimulation, both epinephrine and norepinephrine are released into the general circulation. Thus the term **adrenergic** applies to this entire class of agents.

Isoproterenol (Isuprel) is a synthetic adrenergic agent. The body has no capacity to produce it.

These adrenergic neurotransmitter substances affect the cell by activating a specific enzyme, adenyl cyclase. This, in turn, accelerates the rate of metabolic work by the cell. Thus, adrenergic stimulation has an indirect effect on cells. Some drugs to be considered later affect cellular activity directly, while others have both a direct and indirect action.

Cardiovascular Effects

1. Electrical
   a. Impulse formation

   The adrenergic agents *accelerate* the rate of impulse formation in the sinus node and in other tissues of the heart with potential pacemaker activity. These agents are used to treat rhythms of impulse formation depression such as sinus bradycardia and sinus pauses. They may also be given in complete A-V block to increase the rate of an excessively slow idionodal or idioventricular pacemaker as an emergency measure.

   Adverse effects of adrenergic agents include excessive excitation of impulse formation, which may be manifested as premature contractions and sustained tachycardia of atrial, nodal, or ventricular origin.
   b. Impulse conduction

   Adrenergic agents *accelerate* impulse conduction through the atria, A-V node, the common bundle, and the Purkinje fibers. They are given to reduce sinoatrial block, shorten the PR interval in first degree A-V block, and increase the frequency of captured ventricular beats in intermittent (or second degree) A-V block.
2. Mechanical

   Adrenergic agents generally increase the force of myocardial contraction and may benefit the failing heart. Of the three agents, isoproterenol is the most potent in this regard.

3. Vasomotor

Adrenergic stimulation modulates the tone of blood vessels by constricting or dilating them. All three agents cause dilation of the coronary arteries, but, in general, the individual drugs have dissimilar properties and will be considered separately.

a. *Norepinephrine*: Diffuse vasoconstriction is produced in skeletal muscle, skin, kidneys, liver, and the intestinal tract. The overall effect is to increase peripheral resistance to blood flow, raising the blood pressure and increasing the workload of the heart. Generalized constriction of the vascular bed produces augmentation of vagus tone by a reflex action. Thus, norepinephrine can be seen to have a dual and self-antagonistic effect on the sinus pacemaker. By its direct action, it stimulates the sinus node to fire more rapidly. By its indirect action, mediated through the parasympathetic nervous system, there is a decelerating force on impulse formation of the sinus node. Whether the pulse rate speeds up or slows down in response to norepinephrine depends upon whichever is the predominant effect in the delicate cardioregulatory balance. This is an example of the complex behavior of a pharmacologic agent on the multiple determinants of the electrical activity of the heart, a behavior which is manifested by many other cardiac drugs.

b. *Isoproterenol*: This drug causes generalized vasodilation. The total vascular space is enlarged, and the peripheral resistance to blood flow is diminished. This results in some reduction in systolic and diastolic blood pressure, with a decrease in the workload on the heart. As the coronary circulation is decreased during contraction, particularly in the left ventricle, the coronary blood flow is principally dependent upon the diastolic pressure in the aorta; with its reduction, myocardial perfusion is decreased. Isoproterenol also increases the myocardial oxygen consumption and, therefore, the metabolic cost. For these reasons, the drug may have a detrimental effect upon the failing myocardium, even though it initially increases the contractile force.

c. *Epinephrine*: In certain regions of the vascular system, epinephrine behaves similarly to norepinephrine; in other regions, it acts much like isoproterenol. Epinephrine constricts the peripheral vessels of the venous bed and the arterioles in the skin, mucosa, and splanchnic regions, as does norepinephrine. The arterioles of skeletal muscle are dilated by both epinephrine and isoproterenol. Epinephrine has more prominent metabolic effects than the other catecholamines, producing greater elevation of blood sugar, free fatty acids, and tissue oxygen consumption. The overall effect of epinephrine on heart rate and blood pressure is less predictable than that of the previously described catecholamine agents.

Graphic Summary of the Effects of Cardiac Drugs

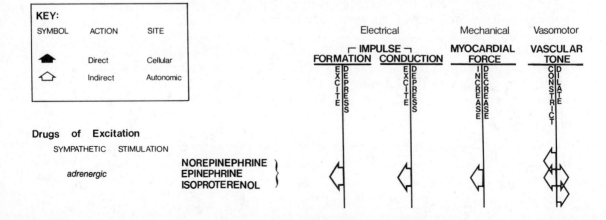

Adrenergic Responses

Autonomic regulation of smooth muscle (including blood vessels) and secretory glands is controlled by the sympathetic nervous system, which has both stimulatory and inhibitory effects. These two adrenergic responses are designated alpha (α) and beta (β). Although this system of terminology was introduced several decades ago, it has only recently come into common use because of the development of clinically useful drugs which selectively block one or the other of these responses.

The term **alpha** refers to a response to adrenergic stimulation which produces *contraction of smooth muscle and activation of secretory glands*. In blood vessels, this represents a constrictor action. A **beta** response to adrenergic stimulation is an *inhibition of contraction and secretion*. Dilation is the beta response of the vasculature to adrenergic stimulation.

The tone of blood vessels is generally controlled by the interaction of these two counterbalancing adrenergic forces of vasoconstriction and vasodilation. From the previous text, it can be appreciated that norepinephrine has an alpha effect on the vascular bed, while isoproterenol has a beta effect. Epinephrine produces either an alpha or a beta response, depending upon the specific area.

On applying this terminology to the heart, adrenergic agents which have a beta effect increase the force of myocardial contraction and accelerate pacemaker activity and conduction velocity. Opposing or inhibitory responses on these functions by adrenergic agents, that is, alpha responses, have not been clearly delineated in the heart.

All of the adrenergic agents discussed here—norepinephrine, isoproterenol, and epinephrine—have a beta effect on the heart. This nomenclature becomes pertinent in later consideration of drugs which selectively block beta responses.

Parasympathetic Nervous System: Inhibition

Agents which decrease parasympathetic tone result in a shift in autonomic forces favoring a stronger sympathetic influence. Pharmacologic suppression of the vagus nerve has an effect on certain electrical events in the heart which is similar to that of stimulation of sympathetic fibers.

Anticholinergic Agents

Atropine is considered here as a model for those drugs which inhibit the parasympathetic nervous system by antagonizing the effect of acetylcholine. The influence of atropine on the heart is confined almost entirely to its electrical activity.

Cardiovascular Effects
1. Electrical
   a. Impulse formation

   Atropine results in *acceleration* of impulse formation in the sinus node. It is used in the treatment of rhythms of pacemaker depression, such as sinus bradycardia, sinus pauses, and sinus arrest. In complete A-V block, atropine may increase the rate of a nodal escape pacemaker. Vagal blocking drugs are unlikely to affect an idioventricular pacemaker, since few, if any, vagal fibers are distributed to the ventricles.

   b. Impulse conduction

   Atropine *accelerates* conduction velocity in atrial tissues. It may decrease or abolish sinoatrial block. The inhibition of vagal tone in the A-V node by atropine increases the rate of impulse transmission to the ventricles. This may lessen the PR interval in first degree A-V block or decrease the frequency of conduction failure in second degree A-V block.

2. Mechanical

The force of myocardial contraction is not directly affected by the action of atropine and other parasympathetic agents.

3. Vasomotor

Since parasympathetic fibers do not generally innervate the blood vessels, drugs which inhibit parasympathetic impulses do not significantly alter vascular tone at ordinary clinical doses. At toxic levels, diffuse vasodilation accompanied by a fall in blood pressure may result because of the depressive effects on the vasomotor center of the central nervous system.

In summary, the major cardiac action of atropine is to block the normal inhibitory influence of the vagus nerve, resulting in sympathetic overbalance and acceleration of impulse formation and conduction in the sinus node, the atria, and the A-V node.

Graphic Summary of the Effects of Cardiac Drugs

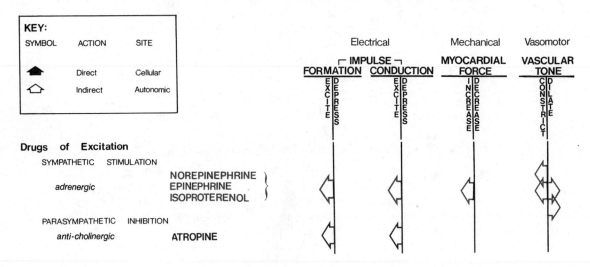

DRUGS OF DEPRESSION

These agents decrease impulse formation rate and/or conduction velocity and are used to treat rhythms of excitation. Their effects are produced by inhibition of the sympathetic nervous system, stimulation of the parasympathetic nervous system, or direct depression on impulse-forming and conducting functions of cardiac cells.

Sympathetic Nervous System: Inhibition

Antiadrenergic Agents

These drugs oppose the action of adrenergic substances, thereby lessening sympathetic tone. Their effect may be one of several mechanisms. **Propranolol** (Inderal) has both a direct inhibitory effect on automaticity and conductility of cardiac tissues and an indirect adrenergic beta blocking effect on sympathetic neurotransmission.

Cardiovascular Effects

1. Electrical
   a. Impulse formation

   The sinus rhythm is usually slowed with propranolol; this effect is most pronounced in individuals with high sympathetic tone (e.g., during anxiety states, during exercise, in congestive heart failure). Individuals on propranolol may have a subnormal rise in the pulse rate as a response to exercise. The drug also suppresses ectopic impulse formation and is used to control ectopic beats and tachycardia of both atrial and ventricular origin.

   b. Impulse conduction

   Propranolol reduces the velocity of conduction, particularly in the A-V node. This property can be used to advantage to slow the ventricular rate response to atrial flutter and fibrillation by increasing the physiological A-V block, thereby decreasing transmitted impulses.

   When propranolol is given to suppress excitation of ectopic pacemakers, it may also produce or intensify A-V block, particularly if there is already some dysfunction in the A-V node transmission. This condition is especially hazardous because lower centers of automaticity which are potential pacemakers in severe A-V block are also inhibited.

   Propranolol has proved useful in the treatment of pre-excitation syndrome. It may prevent or interrupt paroxysmal supraventricular tachycardias by inhibiting conduction in anomalous circuits near the A-V node or by blocking re-entry impulses.

2. Mechanical

   Propranolol has little influence on the force of myocardial contraction under normal conditions. However, it counteracts the effects of sympathetic stimulation on cardiac myofibrils during vigorous exercise or in congestive heart failure. For this reason, propranolol is usually contraindicated for control of arrhythmias in the presence of myocardial insufficiency.

3. Vasomotor

   Propranolol has no important action on blood vessels by itself, but it neutralizes the vasodilating properties of isoproterenol.

   Other beta-adrenergic blocking agents are currently being studied which may offer potent suppressing action on automaticity without diminishing the contractile force of myocardial fibers. One such promising drug is **bretylium,** which actually enhances the strength of cardiac muscle. This agent has been found particularly useful for ventricular tachycardia, persistent or recurrent, which other methods of treatment have failed to control. Availability of this drug or those like it for general clinical use awaits further investigation.

   Most types of drugs used in the treatment of systemic hypertension have antiadrenergic activity. Reserpine and other Rauwolfia alkaloids reduce the concentration of stored norepinephrine in sympathetic nerve endings, while guanethidine (Ismelin) blocks the release of norepinephrine. Methyldopa (Aldomet) and the various monoamine oxidase (MAO) inhibitors block certain metabolic steps in the synthesis of the adrenergic neurotransmitter substances. These antihypertensive drugs modify the response to many of the cardiac drugs, and rational therapy requires a sound knowledge of these pharmacological interactions.

Graphic Summary of the Effects of Cardiac Drugs

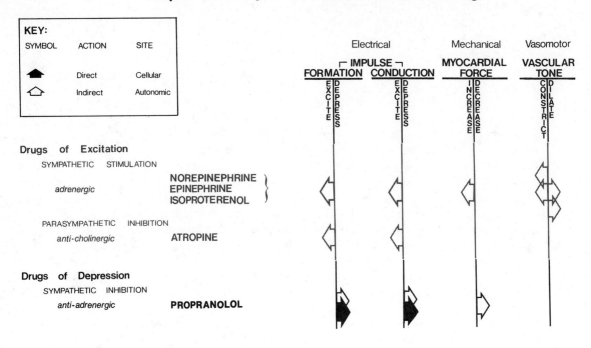

Parasympathetic Nervous System: Stimulation

Cholinergic Agents

Edrophonium (Tensilon): Agents which enhance acetylcholine effect act on the heart in a manner similar to the vagotonic maneuvers, such as carotid pressure. Tensilon,* in particular, has a rapid onset and short duration of action. Side effects from it are usually minimal, although agents in this class with prolonged action may produce symptomatic disturbances of autonomic functions. Patients with underlying asthmalike conditions are most susceptible to the bronchospastic effects of these parasympathetic stimulating drugs.

Tensilon is often effective in converting atrial tachycardia and A-V nodal tachycardia to a sinus rhythm. In atrial flutter and atrial fibrillation, the ventricular rate can usually be transiently reduced by increased resistance of impulse transmission through the A-V node. As a diagnostic procedure, Tensilon administration may clarify various forms of supraventricular tachycardia by slowing the ventricular rate and exposing atrial activity for greater visibility. Clinical experience has not revealed problematic alteration of myocardial contractility or blood pressure, although induction of sudden and serious degrees of bradycardia has been observed.

Several drugs in this class are frequently used in the treatment of noncardiac disorders because of their stimulating action on intestinal and urinary bladder contraction. Bethanechol (Myocholine or Urecholine) is a generally familiar example. Bradycardia or conduction defects may be induced or exaggerated by these agents.

---

*Because of prevailing usage, the proprietary name of this drug will be given rather than the generic.

Graphic Summary of the Effects of Cardiac Drugs

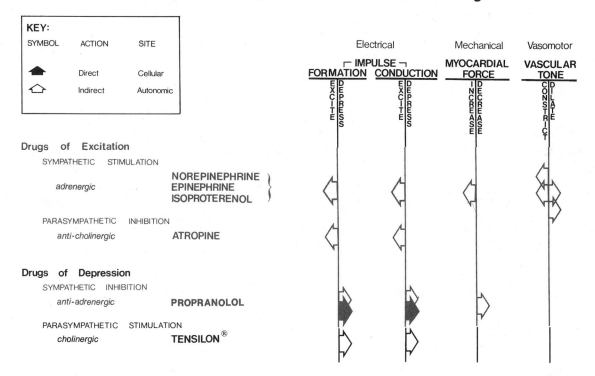

The Cardiac Cell

Quinidine and Procainamide (Pronestyl)

Quinidine and procainamide are considered together because of their similar pharmacological properties on the heart. Their fundamental action is *direct* on the **cardiac cell,** producing *suppression* of cellular activity by inhibiting the movement of sodium and potassium across the cell membrane. They also have an *indirect* action upon the autonomic nervous system, causing *inhibition* of *parasympathetic* tone. At functional sites under parasympathetic control, the direct action opposes the indirect action, so that the net effect on electrical activity depends upon the relative influence of the agents on these counterbalancing forces.

Cardiovascular Effects

1. Electrical

   a. Impulse formation

      Direct action: quinidine and procainamide suppress spontaneous pace-maker activity in the sinus node, atria, A-V junctional tissue, and ventricles. They also decrease the responsiveness of these tissues to stimuli.

      Indirect action: these agents have anticholinergic properties. By inhibiting vagal tone, thus releasing the parasympathetic brake, they tend to accelerate impulse formation in the sinus node, atria, and the A-V junctional tissue.

      These opposing actions often result in no change in the rate of impulse formation in the sinus node, but they sometimes produce a more rapid rate.

The overall effect in rhythms of atrial and A-V nodal excitation generally favors suppression. In most cases, atrial and nodal premature contractions can be controlled with relatively small doses of quinidine and procainamide, while much larger amounts are usually required to convert sustained arrhythmias, such as atrial tachycardia, flutter, and fibrillation, to a sinus rhythm. Sinus and atrial arrest are expressions of the toxicity of these agents.

Both quinidine and procainamide can be effective in suppressing premature contractions and tachycardia originating in the ventricles where there is little or no parasympathetic innervation. They also inhibit potential escape pacemakers in both A-V junctional and ventricular sites; this effect has a high degree of risk in the presence of A-V nodal or multiple conduction bundle block.

A prevailing opinion among clinicians is that quinidine is more effective for rhythms of atrial excitation, while procainamide is more effective in treating ventricular excitation. However, this impression has not been clearly established by experimental evidence. In practice, quinidine is usually chosen as an oral preparation and procainamide for parenteral use, particularly when a drug with rapid action is indicated.

b. Impulse conduction

Direct effect: quinidine and procainamide decrease the velocity of impulse conduction in the atria, A-V node, Purkinje fibers, and the ventricles by their direct action on cardiac cells.

Indirect effect: similar to the indirect action described with impulse formation, these agents have an atropinelike action on impulse conduction. A tendency for acceleration in the above mentioned tissues is created.

These conteracting influences of a single drug operate in complex relationships. The net effect depends upon the dominating action of the drug and is often unpredictable, particularly in the presence of disorders of cardiac impulse conduction. The shift of balance is usually in favor of acceleration in the A-V node (predominating anticholinergic effect), which may produce clinically significant problems in rhythms of atrial excitation. For example, quinidine given to reduce the atrial rate in atrial flutter could, in addition, increase the frequency of atrial impulses transmitted through the A-V node to the ventricles, thereby sharply increasing the ventricular rate.

Quinidine and procainamide are often given in the pre-excitation syndrome to prevent or control arrhythmias by blocking anomalous A-V pathways or re-entry circuits. These benefits, as might be expected from drugs with such complex behavior, are quite uncertain.

In the ventricles, where there is no parasympathetic blocking effect opposing the direct depressant effect of quinidine and procainamide, conduction velocity is delayed in the conduction pathways and muscle mass. Significant prolongation of the QRS complex by either drug is considered an important sign of toxicity.

2. Mechanical

The force of myocardial contraction is diminished by quinidine and procainamide. This negative inotropic effect is more pronounced at ordinary dose levels when the myocardium is already depressed by disease.

3. Vasomotor

Quinidine and procainamide produce general dilation of peripheral blood vessels, especially at high doses, and some reduction in blood pressure commonly results. This can become clinically important when myocardial insufficiency is also present.

Lidocaine (Xylocaine)

Lidocaine suppresses automaticity in cardiac tissues, mostly in the ventricles. It is usually effective in decreasing the frequency of or eliminating ventricular premature contractions, the most commonly observed arrhythmia in acute myocardial infarction. Ventricular tachycardia is frequently abolished with lidocaine.

Lidocaine does not affect the heart rate in sinus rhythms when given in ordinary therapeutic amounts. It is generally of no value in treating rhythms of atrial or A-V nodal excitation. Lidocaine does not usually cause significant changes in the velocity of impulse propagation unless there is also some pathology in the conduction pathways. Except in very high doses, lidocaine has a negligible effect on myocardial performance and peripheral vascular tone.

The wide margin of safety with its rapid onset of action and brief duration, as well as its efficacy in controlling ventricular tachyarrhythmias, has led to its extensive use in the Cardiac Care Unit. Certain central nervous system aberrations, such as depressed mentation, twitching, and seizures, which may be manifest at high drug levels, are an important noncardiac form of toxicity.

Diphenylhydantoin (Dilantin*)

Cardiovascular Effects
1. Electrical
   a. Impulse formation

   Dilantin has a *direct* suppressing action on automaticity throughout the heart. It also appears to have some depressing effect on the hypothalamus, inhibiting sympathetic impulses at a central nervous system level, thereby producing *indirect* suppression of impulse formation.

   Dilantin generally causes no change in the sinus rate, although sinus bradycardia and arrest have been produced by large doses administered rapidly. It is most useful in controlling rhythms of ventricular excitation, premature contractions, and tachycardia, while atrial tachyarrhythmias respond less well. The drug is particularly efficacious in both atrial and ventricular excitation when ectopic rhythms are produced by digitalis. The attempts to convert atrial flutter or fibrillation to a sinus rhythm with Dilantin are usually unsuccessful, although prevention of paroxysms of these arrhythmias in persons susceptible to them may be achieved.
   b. Impulse conduction

   Dilantin has a direct accelerating effect on conduction in the atria and usually in the A-V node. At the latter site, this agent tends to reverse relatively mild degrees of **A-V block** caused by digitalis or other direct suppressor drugs. For this reason, Dilantin is often an appropriate choice to control digitalis toxicity manifested by both excitation of ectopic impulse formation and retardation of A-V node conduction velocity. However, this agent is dangerous in any form of complete A-V block because of the suppression of potential ectopic pacemakers distal to the block.
2. Mechanical

   Dilantin has little effect on normal cardiac contractility at ordinary doses, but it may further compromise myocardial function in congestive heart failure.
3. Vasomotor

   Dilantin may produce hypotension through vasodilation if given too rapidly and at high dose levels.

---

*Because of prevailing usage, the proprietary name of this drug will be given rather than the generic.

Graphic Summary of the Effects of Cardiac Drugs

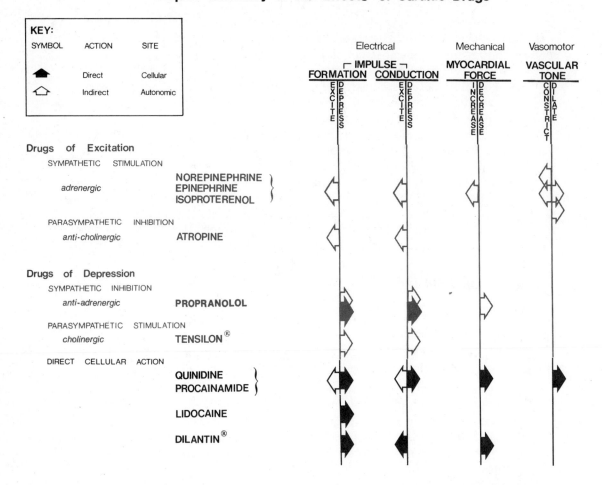

DIGITALIS

Digitalis is presented separately because of its complex pharmacological actions.

I. *Mechanical:* The primary clinical value of digitalis is to restore the efficiency of myocardial contraction in the failing heart. It acts directly upon the myofibrils and is independent of beta-adrenergic stimulation.

II. *Vasomotor:* Digitalis has a mild direct vasoconstrictive influence in the normal individual. However, in the patient with congestive heart failure, a condition associated with excessive adrenergic tone and generalized vasoconstriction, digitalis may indirectly relieve the increased vascular tone by improving myocardial contraction.

III. *Electrical:* Digitalis has a direct effect on automaticity and conductivity in the various cardiac tissues. In addition, digitalis enhances vagal tone, thus having indirect properties which modify the direct effects. These intricate properties of digitalis have both therapeutic and toxic potential and will be considered at individual functioning levels.

Impulse Formation

1. Sinus Node
   a. *Direct effect:* Inhibitory. Digitalis directly depresses the pacemaker activity of automatic cells in the sinus node.
   b. *Indirect effect:* Inhibitory. Digitalis increases parasympathetic tone on the sinus node via the vagus nerve.

   These combined effects tend to cause slight slowing of the rate of sinus impulse formation. Sinus arrhythmia, sinus bradycardia, and sinus pause or arrest can be produced or exaggerated by digitalis, especially in individuals with pre-existing strong vagal tone or with intrinsic disease affecting the sinus node.

2. Atria
   a. *Direct effect:* stimulatory. Digitalis increases the automaticity of latent atrial pacemaker tissue by its direct action upon cells. When the effective tissue levels of digitalis become great enough, this excitatory action produces atrial tachycardia, a common form of digitalis toxicity.
   b. *Indirect effect:* inhibitory. By increasing vagal impulses on atrial tissue, digitalis in therapeutic doses suppresses atrial automaticity. By this mechanism, it is often possible to abolish spontaneous atrial ectopic beats and atrial tachycardia. Paroxysmal atrial tachycardia can frequently be controlled by administration of digitalis. Occasionally atrial flutter and, rarely, atrial fibrillation are converted to normal sinus rhythm with digitalis.

   In summary, this dual action of digitalis on atrial cells is determined by *direct excitation* plus *indirect depression* by vagal stimulation. The net effect depends upon the effective tissue levels of the drug, as well as tissue sensitivity. This intricate relationship has important therapeutic implications and must be considered in every patient with atrial tachycardia who takes digitalis. Atrial tachycardia is an arrhythmia which may be *either* controlled *or* caused by the same pharmacologic agent. The paradox presents a common clinical dilemma.

3. Atrioventricular Junctional Tissue

   Digitalis has an *excitatory* action by its *direct* effect on A-V junctional cells and an *inhibitory* action by *indirect* vagotonic effect, similar to those effects, described for atrial tissue. Spontaneous A-V nodal rhythms, however, are much less common than those originating in the atria. For this reason, nodal premature contractions and nodal tachycardia in a patient taking digitalis are most likely an expression of digitalis toxicity.

4. Ventricles
   a. *Direct effect:* stimulatory. Enhanced ventricular automaticity represents one of the most frequent and early signs of digitalis toxicity. As the effective drug level and tissue sensitivity increase, ventricular premature contractions become more frequent and tend to originate from multiple foci. Ventricular bigeminy, especially with bidirectional complexes, is a sign of severe toxicity. Further increases of digitalis levels are likely to produce ventricular tachycardia and fibrillation.
   b. *Indirect effect:* inhibitory. Under certain conditions, digitalis may depress automaticity within ventricular tissues. This inhibitory action is *not* produced through vagal reflexes, since parasympathetic innervation to the ventricles is negligible. As ventricular ectopic rhythms can be generated by metabolic abnormalities in the failing myocardium, the suppressive effect of digitalis operates through improved contractile function and metabolism.

   The treatment of ventricular premature contractions often involves the perplexing problem of too little or too much digitalis. Unfortunately, the margin between the therapeutic and toxic dose is small, and extracardiac factors, such as interaction with other drugs, electrolyte balance, and oxygenation, have an important role.

Impulse Conduction

Conduction velocity is generally slowed by digitalis. This occurs partly by direct changes in cellular membrane electrical potential of conductile fibers, partly by increased tone of the vagus nerve, and by inhibition of adrenergic stimulation.

1. Sinus Node

   Digitalis may induce sinoatrial block or, when already present, may intensify its severity.

2. Atria

   The most significant effect of digitalis on atrial conduction occurs with atrial flutter. By prolonging the refractory period of atrial fibers, digitalis impedes impulses from propagating through the atria. At extreme rapid impulse formation rates, this delay may be enough that an impulse reaches portions of the atria which are still in a refractory state from the previous conducted impulses. Thus digitalis tends to produce a heterogeneous electrical state in which atrial flutter is converted to atrial fibrillation.

3. Atrioventricular Node

   Digitalis delays the transmission time of impulses in the A-V node by both direct cellular and indirect autonomic actions. In addition, the drug prolongs the refractory period of this tissue, which is normally longer than that of any other cardiac tissue. These effects of digitalis are extremely important in clinical practice and have both therapeutic and toxic significance.

   a. *Therapeutic:* Digitalis can be used to slow the ventricular rate response in certain rhythms of supraventricular excitation by reducing the frequency of impulse transmission through the A-V node to the ventricles. Atrial flutter and fibrillation are often associated with a rapid ventricular rate response, and the decreased A-V conduction produced by digitalis may slow ventricular contractions to a more efficient rate. Control of the ventricular rate in atrial fibrillation is the most commonly encountered indication for digitalis, with the exception of treatment of myocardial failure.

      Digitalis retards impulse conduction in aberrant A-V nodal pathways or re-entry beats in the pre-excitation syndrome, thereby reducing the tendency for paroxysmal tachycardias in that condition. These desired results, however, are frequently not attained with digitalis.

   b. *Toxic:* Digitalis may also induce or intensify defects in the transmission of impulses through the A-V node. Some prolongation of the PR interval commonly occurs, but it is not usually of clinical significance. First degree A-V block may be increased in severity or some blocked beats (second degree A-V block) produced. The intensification of second degree A-V block by digitalis may lead to serious bradycardia and even to complete A-V block.

      Complete A-V block in atrial flutter and fibrillation may be a manifestation of digitalis toxicity. It is identified by the regularity of ventricular contractions in the presence of irregular atrial activity. If, in treating atrial fibrillation with digitalis, the pulse becomes regular, complete A-V block should be suspected. A similar finding with a different underlying mechanism might also occur in which the digitalis produces a regular A-V nodal or ventricular tachycardia.

4. Ventricles

The conduction of impulses in Purkinje fibers and ventricular muscle is retarded by digitalis. This is usually of no clinical significance but may become so during states of ventricular excitation. In digitalis toxicity, the combined effects of increasing automaticity plus decreased conduction velocity predisposes to recurring ventricular tachycardia with an increased tendency for transition to ventricular fibrillation.

Graphic Summary of the Effects of Cardiac Drugs

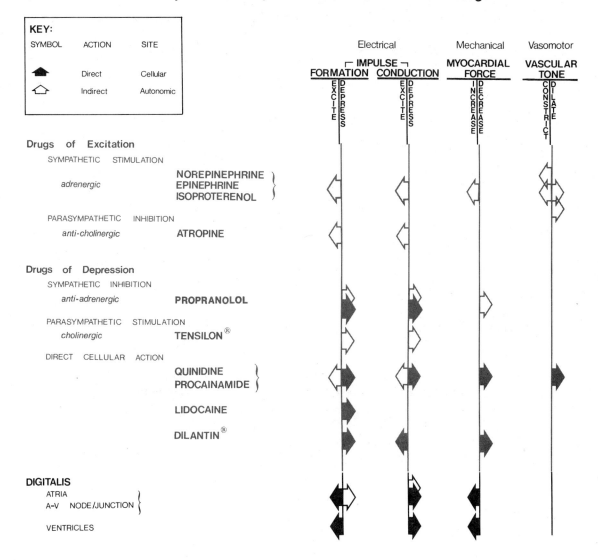

Interaction of Drugs

The effective tissue level of digitalis is modified by a great number of variables which decrease its pharmacological potency or contribute to the various forms of digitalis toxicity. In this regard, certain drugs interact with digitalis, often in complex ways.

The adrenergic agents potentiate the effect of digitalis and may exaggerate the autoexcitation in cardiac tissues. Propranolol further depresses the digitalis-induced conduction deceleration and increases the possibility of impulse conduction defects, particularly those involving the A-V node. Quinidine and procainamide, like propranolol, counteract ectopic tachyarrhythmias of digitalis toxicity, but their mixed direct and indirect action produces complex, often unpredictable effects on conduction velocity, particularly in the A-V node.

Reduction in tissue potassium intensifies the effect of digitalis on the electrical activity of the heart. Hypokalemia is most often produced by certain diuretic agents and is one of the most important contributing causes of digitalis toxicity. It may be expressed as either impulse formation excitation or conduction velocity depression. These untoward sequelae are independent of the action of digitalis on myocardial contraction and may be counterbalanced by restoring body potassium without diminishing contractile force.

Graphic Summary of the Effects of Cardiac Drugs

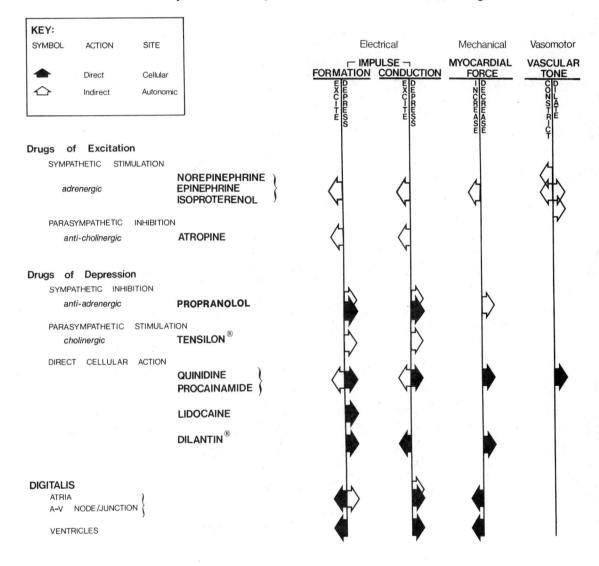

KEY:

SYMBOL	ACTION	SITE
(filled)	Direct	Cellular
(open)	Indirect	Autonomic

Electrical — **IMPULSE** — FORMATION / CONDUCTION (EXCITE / DEPRESS)

Mechanical — **MYOCARDIAL FORCE** (INCREASE / DECREASE)

Vasomotor — **VASCULAR TONE** (CONSTRICT / DILATE)

Drugs of Excitation

SYMPATHETIC STIMULATION

adrenergic — **NOREPINEPHRINE / EPINEPHRINE / ISOPROTERENOL**

PARASYMPATHETIC INHIBITION

anti-cholinergic — **ATROPINE**

Drugs of Depression

SYMPATHETIC INHIBITION

anti-adrenergic — **PROPRANOLOL**

PARASYMPATHETIC STIMULATION

cholinergic — **TENSILON®**

DIRECT CELLULAR ACTION

QUINIDINE / PROCAINAMIDE

LIDOCAINE

DILANTIN®

DIGITALIS

ATRIA

A–V NODE/JUNCTION

VENTRICLES

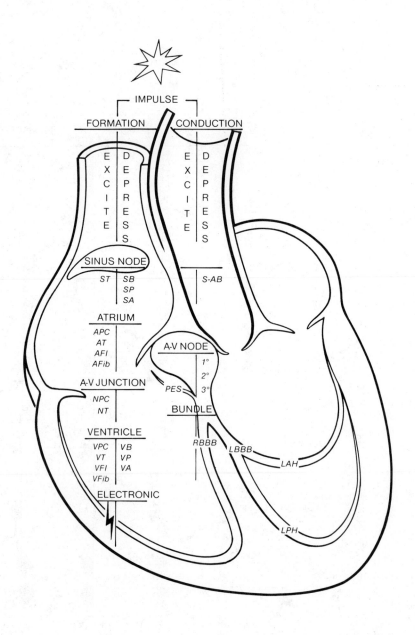

GLOSSARY*

aberration: deviation of impulse conduction from normal pathways, characterized by altered configuration of the representative electrocardiographic figure. (L. *ab-*, from; *errāre*, to stray.)

Adams-Stokes syndrome (or attacks): also referred to as Stokes-Adams syndrome. Syncope due to pathological slowing of the heart rate. Named after Robert Adams and William Stokes, who published case histories in a Dublin medical journal in 1827 and 1846, respectively.

adrenergic: having the effect of stimulating the peripheral sympathetic nerves.

antegrade: impulse conduction in the normal (or forward) direction, usually referring to the A-V node. (Synonym: anterograde.) (L. *ante*, before.)

anterograde: (Synonym: antegrade.)

antiadrenergic: having an inhibitory effect on the peripheral sympathetic nerve activity. (G. *anti*, against.)

anticholinergic: having an inhibitory effect on parasympathetic nerve activity.

arrest: cessation of contractile activity of the heart, referring to either atrial or ventricular arrest. Cardiac arrest is a less specific entity and usually implies sudden circulatory failure due either to cessation of the heart beat or to ventricular fibrillation.

arrhythmia: variation from the normal electrical rate and sequences of cardiac activity. This term in the broadest sense has come to include abnormalities of impulse formation and conduction. (Synonym: dysrhythmia.) (Gr. *a-*, without; *rhuthmos*, rhythm.)

artifact: in electrocardiography, an inscription caused by extraneous mechanical or electrical interference rather than by the electrical activity of the heart.

asystole: absence of cardiac contractions, referring to the entire heart or to a pair of chambers, such as ventricular asystole. (Gr. *a-*, without; *sustolē*, contraction.)

atrial arrest: cessation of atrial contractions. (L. *ad*, to; *restāre*, to stop.)

atrial fibrillation: turbulent, uncoordinated activity of the atria, represented by continuous, irregular deviations from the baseline of the electrocardiogram.

atrial flutter: rapid and distinct atrial depolarization (usually greater than 300 per minute) from an atrial pacemaker.

atrial premature contraction: contraction initiated within the atria, occurring early in the normal cardiac cycle and resetting the sinus pacemaker cadence.

---

*A.S. = Anglo-Saxon
Gr. = Greek
L. = Latin

atrial tachycardia: repetitive rapid contractions arising from an ectopic focus in the atria.

atrioventricular block: a conduction defect in the A-V node or the major conduction bundles. First degree (1°) A-V b.: excessive slowing of conduction time of sinus impulses as they pass through the A-V conduction pathway; Second degree (2°) A-V b.: intermittent failure of impulses originating in the sinus node to transverse completely the A-V conduction pathway; Third degree (3°) A-V b.: complete failure of all impulses to penetrate the A-V conduction pathway; Retrograde A-V b.: failure of impulses originating in the ventricles to penetrate the A-V conduction pathway and enter the atria.

atrioventricular dissociation: independent beating of the atria and ventricles, each under control of separate pacemakers.

atrioventricular node: specialized conducting fibers concentrated at the base of the atrial septum just above the ventricular septum, through which impulses pass between atria and ventricles.

atrium: contractile chamber of the heart. Right a. receives venous blood from the superior and inferior vena cava and ejects it into the right ventricle; left a. receives blood from the pulmonary veins and ejects it into the left ventricle. (L. *ātrium,* the court or central hall of a Roman house.)

auricles: muscular pouches projecting from the right and left atrial walls. While these structures comprise only a small portion of the atrial mass, the terms auricular fibrillation and flutter have long been used synonymously with atrial fibrillation and flutter. (L. *auricula,* little ear.)

automaticity: property of self-excitatory cardiac cells in which spontaneous depolarization occurs. (Gr. *autos,* self; *-matos,* willing.)

autonomic nervous system: division of the central nervous system which extends outward to various peripheral organs, blood vessels, and glands concerned with involuntary regulation, including the automatic, conductile, and contractile elements of the heart. Composed of two subdivisions: the sympathetic and parasympathetic systems.

beat: one complete electrical and mechanical cardiac cycle.

bigeminy: paired cardiac contraction beats, each from a separate pacemaker in a recurring pattern. When sinus beats alternate with ectopic beats, the rhythm is designated according to the ectopic pacemaker, e.g., atrial or ventricular bigeminy. (L. *bi-,* two; *geminus,* twin.)

biphasic: In electrocardiography, an inscription both above and below the baseline. (Synonym: diphasic.)

block: delay or obstruction of impulse conduction.

bradycardia: deceleration of the cardiac rate below arbitrarily defined limits. Sinus b.: impulse formation less than 60 per minute; nodal b.: impulse formation less than 40 per minute; ventricular b.: impulse formation less than 20 per minute. (Gr. *bradus,* slow; *kardia,* heart.)

bundle: a tract of impulse conducting fibers. (See common bundle.) (Synonym: fascicle.)

bundle of His: Demonstrated in 1893 in man and numerous animals by Wilhelm His, Jr., professor of clinical medicine in Berlin. (Synonym: common bundle.)

cadence: established rhythmicity of cardiac impulse formation.

capture: depolarization of a cardiac chamber by a stimulus, usually referring to intermittent ventricular activation by a supraventricular pacemaker in A-V dissociation, or to chamber activation by an electronic pacemaker.

cardiac arrest: 1. cessation of contractile activity of the heart. 2. a general term used to describe sudden collapse from ineffective contractions of the heart; includes ventricular arrest or fibrillation.

cholinergic: having the effect of stimulating the parasympathetic nerves or simulating their activity.

chronotropic: causing change in rate of impulse formation. Positive: increases frequency of impulse formation; negative: decreases frequency of impulse formation. (Gr. *khronos*, time; *tropos*, turn, change.)

common bundle: fibers leading from the A-V node to branches in the ventricles. (Synonym: bundle of His.) Right b. branch: fibers from the common bundle which are distributed to the endocardial surface of the right ventricle; left b. branch: fibers from the common bundle which divide into an anterior (or superior) and a posterior (or inferior) branch and are distributed to the endocardial surface of the left ventricle.

compensatory pause: in sinus rhythm, a delay in ventricular systole following a premature contraction which does not interfere with the sinus cadence but does eliminate a sinus conducted beat. The interval between R waves of the normal beats preceding and following the premature contraction is twice that of the normal R-R interval.

complete A-V block: absence of impulse conduction between atria and ventricles. (Synonym: complete heart block.)

concealed conduction: incomplete penetration of a propagating impulse, giving no directly observable electrocardiographic deflection, but having an effect upon formation or conduction of subsequent impulses.

conduction: transmission of a depolarizing impulse through tissue. (L. *com-*, together; *dūcere*, to lead.)

contraction: coordinated shortening of cardiac muscle fibers resulting in a decrease in the chamber volume. (L. *com-*, together; *trahere*, to draw.)

coupling: a time relationship occurring between paired beats, referring to a constant interval between a normal beat and a subsequent premature contraction.

deflection: deviation of an electrocardiographic line from the baseline. Positive d.: above the baseline; negative d.: below the baseline.

delta wave: deformity of the initial portion of the QRS complex in the pre-excitation syndrome. (Gr. *delta*, letter in Greek alphabet with triangular shape.)

depolarization: process of activation of automatic, conductile, and contractile elements from the resting or polarized state. (L. *dē-*, from.)

depression: refers to any inhibitory effect on the heart which decelerates impulse formation rate or conduction velocity.

diphasic: (Synonym: biphasic.)

dissociation: separation of normally related cardiac events, applied to independent beating of the atria and ventricles. [L. *dis-*, (reversal); *sociāre*, to join.)

dromotropic: causing change in velocity of conducted impulses. Positive: increases conduction velocity; negative: decreases conduction velocity. (Gr. *dromos*, running; *tropos*, turn, change.)

dysrhythmia: abnormal rhythm of the heart, generally used synonymously with *arrhythmia*. (Gr. *dus-*, faulty, diseased.)

ectopic: impulse originating in cardiac tissue outside the sinus node. (Gr. *ex-*, out of; *topos*, place.)

electrocardiogram: a recording of the electrical activity of the heart by a series of deflections which represent certain components of the cardiac cycle.

electrocardiograph: an instrument for recording the electrical activity of the heart; basically a modified galvanometer.

electrode: an electrical conducting device or terminal which completes an electrical circuit between transmitting and receiving media.

endocardium: the inner layer of connective tissue of the heart. (Gr. *endon*, within.)

epicardium: the outer layer of connective tissue of the heart. (Gr. *epi*, over.)

escape beat: contraction originating outside the sinus node in which the ectopic pacemaker is released by depression of formation or conduction of sinus impulses.

excitability: the capacity to respond to a stimulation. (L. *ex-*, out; *cīre*, to put into motion.)

excitation: refers to any stimulating effect on the heart which accelerates impulse formation rate or conduction velocity.

exit block: failure of conduction of an impulse from its origin to adjacent tissue, as in sinoatrial block.

extrasystole: a premature beat arising from an ectopic site. (Synonym: premature contraction.) (L. *extra*, outside or additional; Gr. *sustole*, contraction.)

fascicle: (Synonym: bundle.) (L. *fascis*, bundle.)

fibrillation: continuous disorganized electrical and contractile activity of cardiac chambers. (L. *fibrilla*, small fiber or fibril.)

flutter: extremely rapid impulse formation with coordinated activity of paired cardiac chambers. (A.S. *flot*, the sea; to float, fluctuate, or quiver.)

focus: a site within cardiac tissue with the capacity for impulse formation. [L. *focus*, fireplace, hearth (the center of the home).]

fusion beat: a cardiac contraction produced by two merging depolarizing waves from impulses arriving from separate sites.

idio-: prefix used with ectopic rhythms, implying self-generated impulse formation, e.g., idionodal, idioventricular. (Gr. *idios*, personal, peculiar, separate.)

infarction: area of tissue necrosis following cessation of the blood supply.

inotropic: causing change in contractile strength of muscle. Positive i.: increases contractile strength; negative i.: decreases contractile strength. (Gr. *is, inos*, fiber; *trepein*, to turn or influence.)

interference dissociation: a form of A-V dissociation in which an accelerated ventricular rhythm renders the A-V node refractory to supraventricular impulses.

interpolated: refers to ectopic premature contractions which do not prevent formation of the subsequent normal beat, which thus appears as an extra beat between two normal uninterrupted beats. (L. *inter-*, between; *polīre*, to adorn.)

isorhythmic A-V dissociation: form of A-V dissociation in which the atria and ventricles beat at identical, or nearly identical, rates. (Gr. *isos*, equal.)

joule: a unit of energy equal to one watt-second. After James Prescott Joule, a British physicist (1818-1889).

junctional: refers to tissue with potential for automaticity located adjacent to the A-V node and the common bundle. Probable origin of nodal rhythms. (Synonym: A-V junctional.)

lead: arrangement of electrical conductors through which electrical activity from the body is brought to a recording device; or, the recording from such a set of conductors.

Mobitz phenomenon: form of second degree A-V block consisting of intermittent blocked sinus beats with constant PR intervals of conducted beats.* Named after Walter Mobitz of Germany, who proposed a system of classification of intermittent A-V block in 1924.

multifocal: refers to ectopic beats originating from two or more impulse forming sites. (L. *multus*, much, many.)

myocardium: the muscle mass of the heart. (Gr. *mus*, muscle.)

nodal premature contraction: a premature contraction originating in the A-V junctional tissue. (L. *nōdus*, knob, knot.)

nodal rhythm: series of contractions initiated in the A-V junctional tissue at a rate of 40 to 60 per minute. (Synonym: idionodal rhythm; A-V junctional rhythm.)

---

*Also known as Type II second degree A-V block.

nodal tachycardia: rhythm originating in the A-V junctional tissue at a rate faster than 60 per minute. (Synonym: accelerated nodal rhythm.)

noncompensatory pause: delay in ventricular systole following a premature contraction which resets the dominant sinus cadence. In contrast with a compensatory pause, there is no elimination of a normal cardiac cycle.

oscilloscope: an instrument which forms a continuous visual image on the screen of a cathode ray tube from electrical currents of an external source. (L. *ōscillare,* to swing; Gr. *skopein,* to examine.)

pacemaker: 1. cell or group of cells which depolarize spontaneously, forming impulses which propagate and initiate cardiac contraction. 2. electronic pulse generator: a. demand pacemaker: electronic pacemaker which is sensitive to spontaneous cardiac contractions which momentarily delay the electronic pulsation; b. fixed pacemaker: electronic pacemaker which operates continuously regardless of spontaneous cardiac activity; c. synchronous pacemaker whose rate of impulses to the ventricles is governed by the rate of atrial contractions.

parasympathetic nervous system: fibers of the autonomic nervous system derived from the brain stem and lower spinal cord. 1. motor: generally has an inhibiting effect on blood vessel tone, causing dilation, and on cardiac impulse formation rate and conduction velocity, causing deceleration. 2. sensory: relays responses from the heart and major arteries to the central nervous system. Both motor (efferent) and sensory (afferent) fibers of the cardiac parasympathetic nervous system are contained in the vagus nerve.

parasystole: contractions initiated by an ectopic pacemaker at regular intervals, unrelated to the dominant rhythm. (Gr. *para,* beside.)

paroxysmal: refers to recurring episodes of cardiac arrhythmias with sudden onset and cessation. [Gr. *para* (intensifier), beside; *oxunein,* to sharpen, goad.]

polarity: difference in electrical energy between the inner and outer surface of the cell membrane, known as the transmembrane potential.

P-P interval: duration of one complete cardiac cycle.

pre-excitation syndrome: a clinical entity in which anomalous conductile pathways between atria and ventricles short-circuit the A-V node. (Synonym: Wolff-Parkinson-White or WPW syndrome.)

PR interval: segment of the electrocardiographic cycle measured from the beginning of the P wave to the beginning of the QRS complex.

P wave: electrocardiographic representation of atrial depolarization.

Purkinje system (or network): conductile fibers in the subendocardial tissues of the ventricles. Described in 1839 by Johannes Purkinje, a Bohemian physiologist and pioneer in microscopic anatomy.

Q wave: first negative deflection of the ventricular depolarization complex on the electrocardiogram.

re-entry: a phenomenon wherein a depolarizing front enters the myocardium, which contains areas having unequal conduction velocities. A contraction is produced from the normal front, followed by a contraction produced from an impulse emerging from the slower conducting area. A postulated mechanism for premature contractions.

refractory period: an interval during repolarization of automatic, conductile, and contractile tissue during which there is a decreased degree of excitability for subsequent depolarizing stimuli. 1. absolute r.p.: initial phase of repolarization in which tissue will not respond to stimuli, however intense. 2. relative r.p.: later phase of repolarization in which the tissue can respond to stimuli of greater than normal intensity. (L. *refractus,* broken off.)

repolarization: process of restoration to the normal resting electrical polarity following depolarization.

retrograde: impulse conduction in reverse or backward direction, usually referring to the A-V node. (L. retrō, backward.)

R-R interval: distance between corresponding points of two consecutive R waves, representing the duration of one cardiac cycle.

R wave: first positive deflection of the ventricular depolarization complex on the electrocardiogram.

septum: fibrous and muscular partition which separates the right cardiac chambers from the left. (L. sēptum, partition, from *saepes*, hedge.)

sinoatrial block: a form of exit block wherein impulses formed in the sinus node fail to emerge from it.

sinus node: group of specialized myocardial cells located in the right atrial tissue with automatic activity. This activity results in impulse formation which is ordinarily more rapid than that of other cardiac automatic centers, so that the sinus node is the normal pacemaker of the heart. (Synonym: sinoatrial node.) [L. *sinus*, a curve (suggested by the shape of the sinus node).]

sinus arrest: cessation of automaticity in the sinus node.

sinus arrhythmia: an exaggeration of the normal phasic variation in the rate of sinus impulse formation associated with ventilatory activity.

sinus bradycardia: excessive slowing of impulse formation in the sinus node to below 60 per minute.

sinus irregularity: erratic variations in the cadence of sinus impulse formation unrelated to ventilatory cycles.

sinus pause: momentary cessation of automaticity in the sinus node.

sinus rhythm: natural cardiac rhythm directed by pacemaker activity of the sinus node, normally at 60 to 100 per minute.

sinus syndrome: markedly abnormal variability of sinus node impulse formation rate, characterized by periods of rapid and slow pacemaker activity. (Synonym: sinoatrial syndrome, bradycardia-tachycardia, sluggish sinus node syndrome, sick sinus syndrome.)

sinus tachycardia: impulse formation in the sinus node exceeding 100 per minute.

Stokes-Adams syndrome: see Adams-Stokes syndrome.

supraventricular: refers to a site above or proximal to the ventricles, e.g., sinus node, atria, and A-V node. (L. suprā, above.)

S wave: negative deflection in the electrocardiogram occurring after the R wave of the ventricular depolarizing complex.

sympathetic nervous system: fibers of the autonomic nervous system derived from the thoracolumbar spinal cord. These generally have a stimulating effect on blood vessel tone (constriction), cardiac impulse formation rate and conduction velocity (acceleration), and myocardial contractility (increased force).

tachyarrhythmia: abnormally accelerated heart beat from any focus of automaticity.

tachycardia: acceleration of the cardiac rate above defined limits. Sinus t.: impulse formation faster than 100 per minute; nodal t.: impulse formation faster than 60 per minute; ventricular t.: impulse formation faster than 50 per minute. (Gr. *takhus*, swift.)

threshold: the minimal intensity of stimulation required to cause a response in automatic, conductile, and contractile tissue.

transthoracic: inserted through the chest wall; refers to a method of placing an electronic pacemaker wire electrode onto the heart.

transvenous: inserted through a vein; refers to a method of implanting an electronic pacemaker wire-electrode into the heart.

trigeminy: recurring pattern of three beats, wherein the second and third beats of each group consist of premature contractions. (Gr. *tri-*, three; *geminus*, twin.)

T wave: electrocardiographic representation of ventricular repolarization.

unifocal: refers to ectopic beats originating from a single site. (L. ūnus, one.)

U wave: electrocardiographic representation of after-potentials which normally follow ventricular repolarization.

vagotonic: influence which increases the tone of the vagus nerve.

vagus nerve: the tenth cranial nerve; either of paired nerves of the parasympathetic nervous system with multiple branches to various visceral organs, including the heart, and containing motor and sensory fibers. [L. *vagus*, wandering (referring to its diffuse branching).]

vasovagal reflex: parasympathetic stimulation initiated by sensory impulses from the thoracic aorta and its larger branches, which are transmitted centrally to the cranial nerve nuclei and are relayed peripherally by an effector impulse in the vagus nerve, causing slowing of the sinus rate and A-V conduction and generalized vasodilation. (L. *vās*, vessel.)

ventricle: contractile chamber of the heart. Right v.: receives venous blood from the right atrium and ejects it into the pulmonary artery; left v.: major muscular chamber of the heart which receives arterial blood from the left atrium and ejects it into the aorta. (L. *ventriculus*, a swollen part, diminutive of *venter*, belly or abdomen.)

ventricular arrest: cessation of ventricular contractions. (Synonym: ventricular standstill.)

ventricular bradycardia: slowing of an idioventricular rate to less than 20 per minute.

ventricular fibrillation: multifocal and grossly asynchronous contractions of the ventricles resulting in continuous uncoordinated twitching and cessation of circulatory flow.

ventricular flutter: extremely rapid ventricular rhythm producing an electrocardiographic pattern in which QRS complexes merge into T waves without discernible separation.

ventricular premature contraction: beat occurring early in the normal cardiac cycle which originates from the ventricle, characterized by aberration of the QRS complex (prolonged and distorted) and the T wave form.

ventricular rhythm: sustained impulse formation from a ventricular focus which paces the ventricles at a rate of 20 to 50 per minute. (Synonym: idioventricular rhythm.)

ventricular tachycardia: rhythm resulting from an accelerated firing of an automatic focus or foci within the ventricle faster than 50 per minute. (Synonym: accelerated ventricular rhythm.)

vulnerable period: interval during repolarization in which the tissue is hypersensitive to stimulation, and subthreshold stimuli may produce electrical instability. Such stimuli applied during this period have a tendency to induce sustained rhythms of excitation, e.g., tachycardia, flutter, or fibrillation. (L. *vulnus*, wound.)

wandering pacemaker: impulse formation shifting from site to site within the sinus node, atria, and A-V junctional tissue, causing variation in cadence, in P wave contour, and in PR intervals.

watt-second: a unit of electrical energy, expressing the amount of current exerted over time; equal to one joule.

Wenckebach phenomenon: form of second degree A-V block consisting of progressive lengthening of PR intervals in consecutive cardiac cycles until interrupted by a blocked sinus beat. Also known as Type I second degree A-V block. Named after Karel Wenckebach of Holland, who described the forms of intermittent A-V block in 1906.

Wolff-Parkinson-White syndrome: (Synonym: WPW or pre-excitation syndrome.) Named after Louis Wolff, John Parkinson, and Paul D. White, who reported eleven cases in 1930.

ABBREVIATIONS IN COMMON USE

AFib	atrial fibrillation
AFl	atrial flutter
APC	atrial premature contraction
AT	atrial tachycardia
A-V	atrioventricular
BBB	bundle branch block
CA-VB	complete atrioventricular block
CP	carotid pressure
ECG	electrocardiogram
EKG	electrocardiogram
EPM	electronic pacemaker
LAH	left anterior hemiblock
LBBB	left bundle branch block
LPH	left posterior hemiblock
MI	myocardial infarction
NPC	nodal premature contraction
NSR	normal sinus rhythm
NT	nodal tachycardia
PAT	paroxysmal atrial tachycardia
PES	pre-excitation syndrome
RBBB	right bundle branch block
SA	sinus arrest
S-A	sinoatrial
S-AB	sinoatrial block
SB	sinus bradycardia
SP	sinus pause
ST	sinus tachycardia
SVT	supraventricular tachycardia
VA	ventricular arrest
VB	ventricular bradycardia
VFib	ventricular fibrillation
VFl	ventricular flutter
VP	ventricular pause
VPC	ventricular premature contraction
VT	ventricular tachycardia
WPW	Wolff-Parkinson-White syndrome

THE CARDIAC RHYTHM RULER

A transparent, heavy plastic version of this ruler in colors and index card size (3″ × 4″) is available for one dollar.

ECG COMPONENT SYMBOLS

Dry transfer sheets of press-on type containing more than 800 symbols can be obtained for five dollars. These figures are useful for annotating electrocardiographic records. The following symbols are included:

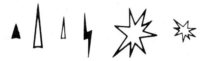

Postal address:

THE CARDIAC RHYTHMS
Box 413
Tarrytown, New York 10591

ANSWER SECTION

This section provides answers to all electrocardiograms which require a reader response and which are identified by a circled number.

Read Before Proceeding:

1. Interpretations given follow the descriptive method. Alternate terminology may be preferred when more consistent with that used at your institution.

2. Abbreviations used are listed on page 340.

3. Cardiac rates are expressed in beats per minute. They have been determined using the three beat ruler where feasible, beginning with the first cardiac cycle on the left unless otherwise indicated.

4. Specific electrocardiographic events are located by the distance in millimeters measured from the left-hand edge. A cardiac cycle is measured to the onset of that particular cycle (not necessarily at the maximum deflection) for consistency in identification.

5. Your measurements may vary somewhat from those provided. This is partially the result of distortions in reproduction inherent in commercial printing. However, these variations should be of minor degree and of no importance.

Good luck.

1. Good monitoring lead.
2. Poor monitoring lead. R amplitude too low. Move LA electrode or reverse polarity.
3. Good monitoring lead.
4. Poor monitoring lead. R amplitude too low. Move LA electrode or reverse polarity.
5. Good monitoring lead.
6. Poor monitoring lead. T amplitude too high. Move LA electrode or reverse polarity.
7. Good monitoring lead.
8. Poor monitoring lead. R amplitude too low and T amplitude too high. Move LA electrode or reverse polarity.
9. Poor monitoring lead. P and T wave amplitude too high. Move LA electrode.
10. Fastest = 115; slowest = 62.

11. Rates per minute: 78, 80, 81, 84, 86, 88, 88, 87, 85, 79.
12. Rates per minute: 82, 53, 58, 63, 75, 63, 53.
13. Rates per minute: 87, 80, 62, 75, 78, 84, 85, 84, 73.
14. Fastest = 88; slowest = 58.
15. Fastest = 82; slowest = 49.
16. Fastest = 92; slowest = 46.
17. Fastest = 93; slowest = 46.
18. Fastest = 82; slowest = 48.
19. Fastest = 72; slowest = 48.
20. Rate = 71; rate = 58.
21. Rate = 70; rate = 56.
22. Rate = 90.
23. Rate = 90; rate = 52.

24. Rate = 83.
25. Rate = 164.
26. Rate = 80.
27. Rate = 104.
28. Rate = 167.
29. Rate = 82.
30. Rate = 113.
31. Rate = 85.
32. Rate = 100.
33. Rate = 78.
34. Rate = 158.
35. Rate = 132; rate = 76.
36. Rate = 123.
37. Rate = 83.
38. Rate: ruler = 126; grid = 130; scan = 6 × 20 = 120.
39. Rate: ruler = 122; grid = 125; scan = 6 × 20 = 120.
40. Rate: ruler = 133; grid = 140; scan = 7 × 20 = 140.
41. Rate: ruler = 128; grid = 130; scan = 120.
42. Rate: ruler = 167; grid = 160; scan = 190.
43. Rate: ruler = 130; grid = 140; scan = 120.
44. Rate: ruler = 38; grid = 37; scan = 40.
45. Rate: ruler = 42; grid = 40; scan = 40.
46. Rate = 47.
47. Rate = 61 to 43.
48. Rate = 47.
49. Rate = 43.
50. Rate: shortest interval = 40; longest interval = 20.
51. Rate = 70; rate = 40.
52. Initial rate = 111; depressed rate = 71.
53. Initial rate = 45; depressed rate = 28.
54. Initial rate = 128; depressed rate = 80.
55. Initial rate = 65; depressed rate = 39.
56. Initial rate = 91; depressed rate = 27.
57. Basic rate = 61; delayed rate = 32.
58. Basic rate = 72; delayed rate = 39.
59. Basic rate = 63; delayed rate = 18. (Calculated rate: 17 large squares × 0.20 second = 3.40 seconds interval. Sixty seconds per minute divided by 3.40 = 18 per minute).
60. Rate = 45.
61. Ventricular inactivity = 6.60 seconds (33 large squares × 0.20 seconds).
62. Rate = 40.
63. Rate = 76.
64. Rate = 37.
65. Rate = 69; S-A block at 140 mm.
66. Rate = 81.
67. Rates: 57, 54, 51, 51.
68. Rates: 80, 67.
69. NSR, rate = 69; ectopic beats = 2 APC's.
70. Basic rhythm = NSR, rate = 88; ectopic beats = 3 APC's.
71. Rate = 88.
72. Basic rhythm = NSR, rate = 85; ectopic beats = 2 APC's.
73. Coupling rates: 106, 127, 107.
74. Sinus rate = 54; atrial rate = 120.
75. APC's at 16, 53, 89, 125, 160 mm.
76. APC's at 27, 80, 137 mm.

77. Basic rhythm = sinus; ectopic beats = 4 APC's; sinus/atrial ratio 1:1; interpretation; atrial bigeminy.
78. Basic rhythm = sinus; ectopic beats = 6 APC's; sinus/atrial ratio 1:1; interpretation: atrial bigeminy.
79. Basic rhythm = sinus; ectopic beats = 4 APC's; sinus/atrial ratio 1:1; interpretation: atrial bigeminy, transient.
80. Sinus rate = 47; ectopic rate = 88.
81. Sinus rate = 45; ectopic rate = 73.
82. Blocked APC at 45.5 mm.
83. Blocked APC at 78, 114 mm.
84. Blocked APC's at 66, 158 mm.
85. Blocked APC's at 42, 158 mm.
86. Rate = 142.
87. Atrial rate = 109, regular; sinus rate = 50, not regular.
88. Atrial rate = 135, regular; sinus rate = 82, not regular.
89. Rate = 220.
90. Rate = 62.
91. Atrial rate = 282; ventricular rate = 141; A/V ratio = 2:1.
92. Atrial rate = 126; ventricular rate = 63; A/V ratio = 2:1.
93. Atrial rate = 220; ventricular rate = 110; A/V ratio = 2:1.
94. Atrial tachycardia with 2:1 A-V block.
95. Atrial tachycardia: rate = 135; dominant A/V ratio 1:1, 3:1 at 59 mm., 2:1 at 127 mm., and 1:1 at 156 mm.
96. Atrial tachycardia with 2:1 A-V ratio.
97. Atrial rate = 344; ventricular rate = 172.
98. Atrial rate = 207; ventricular rate = 144.
99. 5.52 seconds.
100. Ventricular rate = 155; A-V conduction: constant.
101. Atrial rate = 292; A-V ratio = 2:1.
102. Atrial rate = 280; ventricular rate = 70; A-V conduction: constant; A-V ratio = 4:1.
103. Atrial rate = 240; ventricular rate = 31 to 54; A-V conduction: variable.
104. Atrial rate = 320; ventricular rate = 70 to 120; A-V conduction: variable.
105. Atrial rate = 264; ventricular rate = 70 to 130; A-V conduction: variable.
106. Atrial rate = 320; ventricular rate = 80 (average); A-V conduction: variable.
107. Atrial rate = 276; ventricular rate = 69; A-V conduction: constant; A-V ratio = 4:1.
108. Atrial rate = 310; ventricular rate = 110 (average); A-V conduction: variable.
109. Atrial rate = 325; ventricular rate = 120 (average); A-V conduction: variable; note alternating 3:1 and 2:1 A-V ratios.
110. APC's at 12, 93, 174 mm.
111. APC at 50 mm.
112. Rate: three second marks, 3.0 beats × 20 = 60.
113. Rate: three beat ruler = 60-132. Three second marks, 4.0 beats × 20 = 80.
114. Rate: three beat ruler = 75 (average).

Three second marks, 4.0 beats × 20 = 80.

115. Rate: three beat ruler = 80. Three second marks, 4.0 beats × 20 = 80.

116. Rates: sinus rhythm = 77; atrial fibrillation = 50 (average).

117. Rate = 110.

118. Rate = 65.

119. Rate = 40.

120. Rate = 146; rate = 43.

121. Rate = 80; rate = 39.

122. Rate = 50; rate = 20.

123. Rate = 126.

124. Rate = 67.

125. Rate = 140.

126. Rate = 104.

127. Rate = 88.

128. Rate = 39.

129. Rate = 96.

130. Rate = 84.

131. Ventricular rate = 130.

132. Atrial rate = 340; ventricular rate = 170.

133. Atrial rate = 325; ventricular rate = 115.

134. Atrial flutter, variable A-V block, and moderate ventricular rate = 70 (average).

135. Atrial fibrillation, average ventricular rate = 90.

136. Sinus tachycardia with two APC's, rate = 100.

137. Normal sinus rhythm with three APC's, rate = 76.

138. Atrial fibrillation with transitions to atrial flutter and rapid ventricular rate response at 115.

139. Sinus tachycardia, rate = 140. Artifact at 95 mm.

140. Atrial fibrillation with moderate ventricular rate = 75 (average).

141. Sinus rhythm with atrial bigeminy, rate = 98 (average).

142. Sinus bradycardia, rate = 48.

143. Normal sinus rhythm with blocked APC's in bigeminal pattern, rate = 80.

144. Normal sinus rhythm, rate = 83. Sinus pause, rate to 23, induced by carotid pressure, followed by transient sinus bradycardia.

145. Atrial fibrillation, rapid ventricular rate response = 132 (average).

146. Normal sinus rhythm, rate = 61, with APC at 65 mm.

147. Atrial fibrillation with rapid ventricular rate response = 110 (average) *to* sinus bradycardia, rate = 58.

148. Atrial fibrillation with moderate ventricular rate response = 60 (average).

149. Atrial tachycardia, rate = 129, to sinus rhythm, rate = 80 for two cardiac cycles, *to* atrial tachycardia.

150. Sinus bradycardia, rate = 42.

151. Atrial tachycardia with 2:1 A-V block; atrial rate = 138; ventricular rate = 69.

152. Wandering atrial pacemaker, rate = 60 (average).

153. Sinus tachycardia, rate = 114.

154. Atrial tachycardia, rate = 210, to sinus tachycardia, rate = 125.

155. Sinus bradycardia, rate = 47.

156. Atrial flutter, variable A-V conduction, ventricular rate response of 70 to 140.

157. Atrial flutter with transition *to* atrial fibrillation, rapid ventricular rate response = 110.

158. Sinus arrhythmia, rate = 50 to 82.

159. Atrial flutter with variable A-V conduction and moderate ventricular rate response = 65 (average).

160. NSR, rate = 65; APC's at 78 and 114 mm. Blocked APC at 149 mm.

161. Atrial flutter with variable A-V conduction and moderate ventricular rate response = 90 (average).

162. Sinus tachycardia, rate = 117, with sinus pause at 135 mm. or possibly blocked APC at 127 mm., atrial escape beat at 142 mm.; *to* atrial fibrillation at 155 mm., to sinus beat at 180 mm.

163. Normal sinus rhythm, rate = 84, and development of baseline artifact (60-cycle disturbance, probably due to disconnection of right leg electrode). Note that the rhythm pattern is generally discernible throughout this electrical interference. Find R spike with calipers.

164. Sinus rhythm with atrial bigeminy, rate = 69.

165. Sinus bradycardia, rate = 32 (average).

166. Normal sinus rhythm, rate = 80. APC at 113 mm.

167. Atrial fibrillation, ventricular rate response = 40 to 132.

168. Atrial fibrillation with rapid ventricular rate = 105 (average).

169. PR interval = 0.13 second.

170. PR interval = 0.18 second.

171. PR interval = 0.14 second.

172. PR interval = 0.18 second.

173. Rhythm: sinus, rate = 93; PR interval = 0.08 second.

174. Rate = 84.

175. Rate = 76; PR interval = 0.10 second.

176. Rate = 83; PR interval = 0.10 second.

177. Rate = 97.

178. Rate = 75; PR interval = 0.35 second.

179. Rate = 63; PR interval = 0.28 second.

180. Rate = 125; PR interval = 0.22 second.

181. Rate = 31; PR interval = 0.38 second.

182. Rate = 83; PR interval = 0.23 second.

183. Rate = 85; PR interval = 0.23 second.

184. Rate = 70; PR interval = 0.44 second.

185. Rate = 80; PR interval = 0.25 second.

186. Rate = 71; PR interval = 0.31 second.

187. Rate = 107; PR interval = 0.23 second.

188. Rate = 114.

189. Rate = 65; PR interval = 0.44 second.

190. Rate = 65; PR interval = 0.26 second.

191. Rate = 72; PR interval = 0.23 second.

192. Atrial rate = 76; ventricular rate = 38.

193. Blocked sinus beats occur at 33, 95, 174 mm.; PR interval = 0.13 second; ratio = 5:4.

194. Atrioventricular ratio = 2:1.

195. Second degree A-V block: A/V ratio = 2:1; ventricular rate = 31.

196. Second degree A-V block: A/V ratio of

central group = 4:3; prolonged PR interval (0.24 second) of conducted sinus beats; sinus rate = 57.

197. Second degree A-V block: A/V ratio = 2:1. Sinus rhythm (rate = 114) and prolonged PR intervals of conducted sinus beats (0.28 second).

198. Atrial rate = 108; ventricular rate = 36; A/V ratio = 3:1; PR interval = 0.16 second.

199. Atrial rate = 108; ventricular rate = 36; A/V ratio = 3:1; PR interval = 0.14 second.

200. Rate = 66; PR interval = 0.20 second.

201. Sinus rhythm with blocked sinus beats and absent ventricular action.

202. Sinus rhythm with no A-V conduction to sinus tachycardia with 2:1 A-V block.

203. Sinus rate = 106.

204. PR intervals: 0.32, 0.38, 0.38, 0.40, 0.45, sinus block at 169 mm.; 0.32.

205. PR intervals: 0.28, 0.34, 0.38, sinus block at 55 mm.; 0.22, 0.28, 0.34, 0.40, sinus block at 133 mm.; 0.22, 0.28, 0.36. Ratio = 5:4 in central group.

206. PR intervals: 0.20, 0.34, sinus block at 24 mm.; 0.22, 0.34, sinus block at 60 mm.; 0.20, 0.34, sinus block at 94 mm.; 0.20, 0.34, sinus block at 130 mm.; 0.20, 0.34, sinus block at 165 mm.; 0.20, 0.34. Ratios = 3:2, 3:2, 3:2, 3:2, 3:2.

207. PR intervals: 0.23, 0.26, 0.28, 0.28, 0.30, 0.36, 0.38, sinus block at 108 mm.; 0.23, 035, sinus block at 155 mm.; 0.24, 0.34. Ratios=8:7, 3:2.

208. Sinus block at 91 mm.; PR interval: 0.12, sinus block at 121 mm.; 0.12, sinus block at 150 mm.; 0.12, sinus block at 180 mm. Ratios = 2:1, 2:1, 2:1, 2:1.

209. PR intervals: 0.18, 0.28, sinus block at 38 mm.; 0.18, 0.28, sinus block at 87 mm.; 0.16, 0.30, sinus block at 136 mm.; 0.18, 0.28, sinus block at 185 mm. Ratios = 3:2, 3:2, 3:2, 3:2.

210. PR intervals: shortest = 0.18 second; longest = 0.24 second. A/V ratio = 9:8.

211. PR intervals: shortest = 0.22 second; longest = 0.36 second. A/V ratio = 8:7.

212. PR intervals: shortest = 0.26 second; longest = 0.38 second. A/V ratio = 5:4.

213. Prolongation of PR interval begins at 102 mm.; blocked sinus beat at 127 mm.

214. Rate = 174; A/V ratio = 1:1.

215. PR interval = 0.26 second.

216. Blocked sinus beats at 57, 153 mm.

217. Atrial/ventricular ratio = 2:1.

218. Sinus rate = 40, 39.

219. Ventricular rate = 79, 49, 50; standardization marker at 144 mm.

220. Rate = 37.

221. Rate = 46, 39.

222. Rate = 40, 28.

223. Rate = 62.

224. Sinus rate = 96; A-V nodal rate = 39; no; interpretation: complete A-V block with A-V nodal rhythm.

225. Sinus rate = 111; A-V nodal rate = 54; no; complete A-V block with nodal rhythm.

226. Sinus rate = 96; A-V nodal rate = 39; no; complete A-V block with nodal rhythm.

227. Atrial rate = 180; nodal rate = 79. Atrial/ventricular activity, unrelated; interpretation: complete A-V block with nodal rhythm.

228. Atrial rate = 108; ventricular rate = 57. Atrial/ventricular activity, unrelated; interpretation: complete A-V block with nodal rhythm.

229. Atrial rate = 59; ventricular rate = 37. Atrial/ventricular activity, unrelated; interpretation: complete A-V block with nodal rhythm.

230. Atrial rate = 52; ventricular rate = 37. Atrial/ventricular activity, unrelated; interpretation: complete A-V block with nodal rhythm.

231. Nodal rate = 154.

232. Sinus rate = 74.

233. Nodal tachycardia, rate = 192. Sinus tachycardia, rate = 114.

234. Atrial rate = 65; nodal rate = 66.

235. Tachycardia: rate = 190; sinus tachycardia: rate = 126.

236. Atrial tachycardia (or flutter) with 2:1 A/V ratio. Atrial rate = 352; ventricular rate = 176.

237. Second degree A-V block with 2:1 A/V ratio: atrial rate = 76; ventricular rate = 38.

238. Second degree A-V block of Wenckebach type with 2:1 and 3:1 A/V ratios; PR intervals = 0.24 to 0.50 second. Atrial rate = 96; ventricular rate = 58-64.

239. Second degree A-V block of Wenckebach type with 5:4 and 4:3 A/V ratios: PR intervals = 0.36 to 0.60 second. Atrial rate = 70; ventricular rate = 60 (average).

240. Second degree A-V block of Wenckebach type: PR intervals = 0.28 to 0.42 second.

241. First degree A-V block; sinus rate = 69; PR interval = 0.34 second.

242. Sinus irregularity with nodal escape beat at 132 mm. Rate = 60 (average).

243. Advanced second degree A-V block (3:1 A/V ratio). Atrial rate = 84; ventricular rate = 28.

244. Second degree A-V block (Wenckebach) 5:4 A/V ratio; PR intervals: 0.24 to 0.34 second. Atrial rate = 75; ventricular rate = 60.

245. Sinus bradycardia with NPC at 182 mm. Rate = 43.

246. Atrial tachycardia. (Possibly sinus tachycardia although strict regularity suggests atrial rhythm.) Rate = 144.

247. Normal sinus rhythm with NPC at 60 mm. Rate = 75.

248. Normal sinus rhythm (rate = 91) to nodal escape rhythm (rate = 56).

249. Second degree A-V block; variable A/V ratio, sinus rate = 86 with nodal escape beat at 126 mm.

250. Atrial tachycardia with intermittent A-V conduction and Wenckebach phenomenon (4:3 and 3:2 A/V ratios); PR interval: 0.14 to 0.30 second. Atrial rate = 195; ventricular rate = 132.

251. Normal sinus rhythm to transient pre-excitation rhythm (4 beats) at 50 mm. Rate = 98.

252. First degree A-V block; PR interval = 0.28 second. Rate = 94.

253. Second degree A-V block (advanced) with

3:1 A/V ratio. Atrial rate = 108; ventricular rate = 36.

254. Sinus tachycardia with second degree A-V block of Wenckebach type (3:2 A/V ratio); PR intervals: 0.22 to 0.26 second. Atrial rate = 112; ventricular rate = 60 − 107.

255. Second degree A-V block with Wenckebach phenomenon (4:3 A/V ratio); PR intervals: 0.26 to 0.36 second. Atrial rate = 65; ventricular rate = 34 − 64.

256. Sinus rhythm with sinus slowing and blocked sinus beat at 102 mm. Initial rate = 70.

257. Complete A-V block with nodal rhythm. Atrial rate = 60; ventricular rate = 37.

258. Second degree A-V block of Wenckebach type; PR intervals: 0.30 to 0.48 second. Ventricular rate = 50 (average).

259. Sinus rhythm with pre-excitation phenomenon. Rate = 87.

260. Accelerated nodal rhythm. Rate = 96.

261. Supraventricular tachycardia. Rate = 185.

262. Second degree A-V block (Wenckebach) with 3:2 and 2:1 A-V ratios. Note two forms of ventricular conduction (patterns).

263. Normal sinus rhythm. Rate = 100.

264. Second degree A-V block of Wenckebach type with 3:2 A/V ratio in central group. Nodal escape beat at 155 mm. Atrial rate = 70; ventricular rate = 57.

265. Accelerated nodal rhythm. Rate = 72.

266. First degree A-V block; PR interval = 0.28 second. Rate = 97.

267. Nodal rhythm, variable rate = 47 to 94.

268. Sinus bradycardia with nodal escape beat at 121 mm. Rate = 44.

269. Atrial fibrillation. Rate = 60 (average).

270. Sinus bradycardia (rate = 46) with progressive sinus slowing to nodal escape rhythm (rate = 30) (note retrograde P waves).

271. Complete A-V block with nodal rhythm. Atrial rate = 100; ventricular rate = 69.

272. A-V dissociation with accelerated nodal rhythm at 95/minute.

273. Sinus bradycardia (rate = 55) with progressive sinus slowing to sinus pause and nodal escape beat at 125 mm.

274. Nodal rhythm. Rate = 45.

275. Complete A-V block with nodal rhythm. Atrial rate = 110; ventricular rate = 50.

276. Second degree A-V block (2:1 A/V ratio). Atrial rate = 104; ventricular rate = 52.

277. Sinus bradycardia (rate = 38) to nodal rhythm (rate = 37).

278. Second degree A-V block (Wenckebach 3:2); PR intervals: 0.24 to 0.40 second. Atrial rate = 87; ventricular rate = 62.

279. Sinus bradycardia (rate = 27) with nodal escape beat at 115 mm.

280. Sinus rhythm (rate = 76) with sinus slowing (or sinus arrest) to nodal rhythm (rate = 69).

281. First degree A-V block (PR interval = 0.32 second). Rate = 86.

282. Rate = 107. PR interval = 0.12 second; QRS interval = 0.13 second.

283. Sinus rate = 106; ventricular rate = 36; QRS duration = 0.12 second.

284. Sinus tachycardia: QRS = 0.08 second; APC: QRS = 0.13 second.

285. APC with RBBB at 77 mm.

286. Beats with RBBB at 6, 30, 78, 105, 138 mm.

287. PR intervals and QRS durations: 0.20, 0.11, 0.20, 0.11, 0.26, 0.14; blocked sinus beat; 0.20, 0.11; 0.23, 0.14; 0.27, 0.14.

288. PR intervals and QRS durations: 0.29, 0.14, 0.31, 0.14, 0.33, 0.14; blocked sinus beat at 70 mm.: 0.20, 0.11.

289. Right bundle branch block at 1, 52, 131, 182 mm.

290. QRS duration = 0.14 second. QRS duration = 0.10 second.

291. QRS duration = 0.18 second.

292. Sinus arrest. Ventricular rhythm, rate = 50; QRS duration = 0.18 second (end point of QRS uncertain).

293. Sinus arrest. Ventricular rate = 41; QRS duration = 0.12 second.

294. Sinus arrest. Ventricular rate = 30; QRS duration = 0.36 second (end portion of QRS uncertain).

295. Sinus arrest. Ventricular rate = 25; QRS duration = 0.18 second.

296. Sinus rate = 75; ventricular rate = 29; QRS duration = 0.20 second.

297. Sinus rate = 34; ventricular rate = 42; QRS duration = 0.20 second.

298. Complete A-V block. Sinus rate = 102; ventricular rate = 32; QRS duration = 0.12 second.

299. Complete A-V block. Sinus rate = 128; ventricular rate = 43; QRS duration = 0.20 second.

300. Complete A-V block. Sinus rate = 96; ventricular rate = 57; QRS duration = 0.13 second.

301. VPC at 109 mm.

302. VPC at 10 mm. (pause = 1.04 seconds); VPC at 88 mm. (pause = 1.04 seconds); VPC at 166 mm. (pause = 1.04 seconds).

303. VPC at 54 mm. (pause = 1.24 seconds); VPC at 119 mm. (pause = 1.16 seconds); VPC at 180 mm.

304. VPC's at 55, 138 mm.

305. VPC at 62 mm.

306. APC's at 52, 163 mm. VPC's at 13, 88, 125 mm.

307. VPC's at 30, 96, 162 mm.

308. VPC's at 37, 139 mm.

309. VPC at 62 mm. (pause = 1.20 seconds).

310. VPC at 12 mm. (pause = 0.58 second); P at 102 mm., VPC at 104 mm. (pause = 0.56 second); P at 180 mm., VPC at 182 mm. (pause = 0.58 second).

311. VPC at 39 mm. (pause = 0.92 second); VPC at 101 mm. (pause = 0.94 second); VPC at 163 mm. (pause = 0.96 second).

312. Sinus rhythm, rate = 62; two VPC's, unifocal.

313. Sinus rhythm, rate = 76; four VPC's, unifocal.

314. Sinus rhythm, rate = 74; two VPC's, unifocal.

315. Sinus tachycardia, rate = 115.

316. Sinus bradycardia with ventricular bigeminy *to* marked sinus slowing with nodal escape beat at 139 mm. having aberrant ventricular conduction *to* paired ventricular premature contractions.

317. Atrial fibrillation, rate = 80. Two multifocal VPC's at 69 mm. and 105 mm., variable coupling intervals.

318. Normal sinus rhythm, rate =61. Unifocal VPC's in couplet at 78 mm. and 93 mm. and VPC from a second focus at 146 mm.

319. Normal sinus rhythm, rate = 75. Multifocal VPC's at 16 and 194 mm. and nodal escape beat at 42 mm.

320. Normal sinus rhythm, rate = 90. VPC's = 4, unifocal; coupling interval: 0.40 second, constant. (This is *not* ventricular trigeminy—see glossary definition.)

321. Sinus rhythm with ventricular bigeminy (main stem VPC's or NPC's with aberrant ventricular conduction). Note retrograde P wave at 25 mm.; this figure does *not* occur half way between sinus beats and is therefore not of sinus origin.

322. Normal sinus rhythm; rate = 80. VPC's = 4, unifocal; two VPC's occur as couplet. Coupling interval: 0.42 to 0.46 second, slightly variable.

323. Normal sinus rhythm with frequent unifocal VPC's having variable coupling intervals (0.58, 0.56, 0.62 second).

324. Normal sinus rhythm with unifocal VPC's having markedly variable coupling intervals (0.40 and 0.75 second).

325. Normal sinus rhythm, rate = 80; two VPC;s, unifocal; fixed coupling intervals.

326. Atrial fibrillation, rate = 73. One VPC.

327. Normal sinus rhythm, rate = 71; two VPC's, probably unifocal with varying ventricular conduction; fixed coupling intervals.

328. Sinus tachycardia, rate = 108. Ten VPC's, unifocal, three couplets, one triplet; fixed coupling intervals of VPC's which follow sinus beats.

329. Normal sinus rhythm, rate = 72; three VPC's (two unifocal at 44 mm. and 170 mm.); one fusion beat at 109 mm.; variable coupling intervals.

330. Sinus bradycardia, rate = 59; PR interval = 0.16 second; Ventricular rhythm, rate =61; PR interval, none.

331. Rate = 71. Rate = 144.

332. Sinus tachycardia (rate = 106) and transient ventricular tachycardia (rate = 180 to 250).

333. Sinus rhythm, rate = 130. Ventricular rhythm, rate = 132.

334. Sinus rhythm, rate = 90. Ventricular rhythm, rate = 187.

335. Sinus rhythm, rate = 106. Ventricular rhythm, rate = 180.

336. Sinus rhythm, rate = indeterminate. VPC's at 15 mm. and 45 mm. Ventricular rhythm, rate = 170.

337. Rate = 144.

338. Ventricular rhythm; rate = 156.

339. Rate = 200.

340. Regular ventricular tachycardia; rate = 130.

341. Irregular ventricular tachycardia; rate = 178.

342. Irregular ventricular tachycardia; rate = 195.

343. Irregular ventricular tachycardia, rate = 190; to ventricular rhythm, rate = 52.

344. Regular ventricular tachycardia; rate = 184.

345. Regular accelerated ventricular rhythm; rate = 76.

346. Regular accelerated ventricular rhythm; rate = 81.

347. Ventricular flutter; rate = 210.

348. Ventricular flutter; rate = 315.

349. VPC's at 51, 60, 138 mm.

350. Rate = 170. Rate = 74.

351. Rate = 39, 20.

352. Rate = 132, 36, 21.

353. Rate = 49, 32, *to* electrical standstill; QRS duration = 0.24 second.

354. Rate = 18, 130, 18.

355. Rate = 19, 24. Multifocal ventricular beats.

356. A/V ratio = 3:1; QRS interval = 0.12 second.

357. A/V ratio = 2:1; QRS interval = 0.15 second.

358. Rate = 79; QRS interval = 0.20 second.

359. Rate = 48.

360. Sinus rate = 31 (at center of tracing). Ventricular bradycardia, rate = 32.

361. Complete A-V block: sinus rhythm (rate = 96) and nodal rhythm (rate = 45) with right bundle branch block.

362. Ventricular fibrillation.

363. Ventricular rhythm, rate = 47.

364. Sinus rhythm (rate = 90) with frequent unifocal VPC's (mainstem with left branch block) and variable coupling intervals.

365. Sinus rhythm *to* sinus arrest and nodal escape rhythm, then sinus rhythm; ventricular bigeminy throughout with unifocal VPC's.

366. Second degree A-V block (2:1) and intraventricular conduction defect.

367. Ventricular fibrillation.

368. A-V dissociation: sinus tachycardia and nodal rhythm with right bundle branch block; VPC at 178 mm.

369. Normal sinus rhythm; unifocal VPC's.

370. Normal sinus rhythm; four APC's with one manifesting right bundle branch block.

371. Sinus tachycardia, sinus arrest (or long pause) with failure of escape mechanism and ventricular asystole.

372. Normal sinus rhythm; nodal (or mainstem ventricular) premature contractions with right bundle branch block in bigeminal pattern.

373. Normal sinus rhythm; episode of ventricular tachycardia.

374. Normal sinus rhythm with ventricular bigeminy.

375. Ventricular tachycardia (slightly varying upstroke suggests dissociated atrial activity).

376. Ventricular bradycardia.

377. Sinus bradycardia; PNC with right bundle branch block, followed by sinus slowing (or arrest) and nodal rhythm.

378. Ventricular tachycardia *to* ventricular fibrillation.

379. Ventricular tachycardia with marked intraventricular conduction delay.

380. Ventricular tachycardia *to* ventricular fibrillation.

381. Ventricular rhythm, sinus arrest (or possibly retrograde A-V conduction).

382. Atrial fibrillation with moderate ventricular rate response and unifocal VPC's having fixed coupling intervals.

383. Normal sinus rhythm with intermittent right bundle branch block and ventricular bigeminy.

384. Sinus tachycardia with unifocal VPC's, having short coupling intervals, some of which occur in couplets.

385. Ventricular fibrillation.

386. Normal sinus rhythm, unifocal VPC's.

387. Second degree A-V block of Wenckebach type.

388. Ventricular rhythm, sinus arrest.

389. Ventricular fibrillation.

390. Atrial flutter with advanced A-V conduction block and multifocal VPC's.

391. Atrial flutter with 2:1 conduction; one VPC at 95 mm.

392. Atrial fibrillation with moderate ventricular rate response.

393. Atrial tachycardia (or flutter) at 260 beats per minute with variable A-V block.

394. Sinus tachycardia with unifocal VPC's.

395. Ventricular fibrillation.

396. Normal sinus rhythm with unifocal VPC's, some of which occur in couplets.

397. Atrial fibrillation with rapid ventricular rate response. (Since QRS durations are at upper limits of normal, ventricular tachycardia may be present.)

398. Ventricular rhythm with multifocal beats. Supraventricular rhythm may be atrial fibrillation.

399. Rate = 74.

400. Rate = 82.

401. Rate = 83.

402. Rate = 80.

403. Rate = 70.

404. Rate = 74.

405. Rate = 70.

406. Sinus rate = 96. EPM rate = 81.

407. Complete A-V block. Sinus rate = 72. EPM rate = 76.

408. Complete A-V block: sinus rate = 71, EPM rate = 68.

409. Complete A-V block: atrial tachycardia rate = 250, EPM rate = 90.

410. Complete A-V block: atrial fibrillation, EPM rate = 64.

411. EPM rate = 61; ventricular rate = 30.

412. Complete A-V block; EPM rate = 70. Capture failure at 70 mm.

413. EPM rate = 74; sinus rate = 77.

414. Spontaneous beats with RBBB (origin not positively identified).

415. EPM rate = 72; sinus rate = 66, 75, 73, 72, 70, 68.

416. EPM rate = 71; note delay in EPM cadence after each VPC.

417. EPM rhythm (rate = 74), demand mode *to* sinus tachycardia (rate = 108).

418. EPM rhythm (rate = 77), demand mode *to* NSR with right bundle branch block (rate = 83).

419. EPM rhythm (rate = 62), demand mode *to* NSR (rate = 75).

420. Sinus pacemaker stimulation at 145 mm.

421. EPM impulses at 71, 91, 110, 165 mm.

422. EPM rate = 126.

423. Complete A-V block: sinus rhythm (rate = 86); electronic pacemaker rhythm (rate = 69) with frequent failure of ventricular capture and long period of ventricular asystole (5.8 seconds).

424. Complete A-V block: sinus tachycardia (rate = 120), EPM (rate variable due to frequent resetting by spontaneous beats) with complete failure of ventricular capture and nodal pacemaker (rate = 29) with RBBB.

425. Complete A-V block: sinus tachycardia (rate = 155), EPM activity with no ventricular capture (rate variable), nodal rhythm (rate = 53).

426. Complete A-V block: intermittent atrial tachycardia (rate = 120, irregular), accelerated ventricular rhythm of multifocal beats (rate = 90, average).

427. Complete A-V block: sinus tachycardia (rate = 166), nodal rhythm (rate = 41), EPM impulses with complete lack of ventricular capture. The sensor turn-off mechanism is not operating (EPM impulses formed immediately after some nodal beats).

428. Sinus bradycardia (rate = 45) with RBBB and frequent blocked APC's. EPM impulses with failure of ventricular capture and sensor turn-off mechanism.

429. Complete A-V block: atrial flutter with nodal rhythm (rate = 53) with RBBB. (Regular ventricular rate in presence of variable F-R intervals indicates absence of A-V conduction and independent pacemakers.) Nonstimulating EPM impulses.

430. Irregular atrial tachycardia or flutter with A-V dissociation and nodal tachycardia (rate = 170), and variable aberrant ventricular conduction.

431. Atrial flutter with A-V dissociation (variable F-R intervals) and nodal tachycardia (rate = 135), and aberrantly conducted ventricular beats to marked bradycardia.

432. Atrial flutter, possibly with complete A-V block, and nodal rhythm (rate = 35) with RBBB.

433. Complete A-V block: atrial flutter with EPM rhythm (rate = 71) and complete ventricular capture. Distortion at 8 mm. produced by stopping recorder momentarily.

434. Complete A-V block: sinus rhythm and

EPM rhythm (rate = 75) with complete ventricular capture.

435. Atrial fibrillation with slow ventricular rate response. Unifocal ventricular premature contractions.

436. Ventricular fibrillation *to* ventricular arrest.

437. First degree A-V block (moderate severity); VPC at 142 mm.

438. Atrial flutter, variable A-V conduction, moderate ventricular rate response; episode of ventricular tachycardia.

439. Sinus bradycardia with pre-excitation phenomenon.

440. Fine atrial fibrillation with slow ventricular rate response and ventricular bigeminy.

441. Second degree A-V block: prolonged PR intervals of conducted sinus beats, occasional blocked sinus beat and nodal escape beat.

442. Sinus bradycardia with APC having RBBB at 51 mm. *to* temporary sinus arrest and nodal escape rhythm; VPC at 101 mm.

443. Complete A-V block: atrial fibrillation, nodal rhythm with right bundle branch block.

444. Complete A-V block: sinus tachycardia, accelerated nodal rhythm, VPC's in couplet.

445. Complete A-V block: sinus bradycardia, ventricular rhythm.

446. Atrial fibrillation, moderate ventricular rate response, VPC.

447. Normal sinus rhythm with right bundle branch block *to* ventricular tachycardia.

448. Complete A-V block: sinus bradycardia, slow nodal rhythm.

449. Ventricular fibrillation.

450. Normal sinus rhythm, episode of ventricular tachycardia.

451. Ventricular flutter.

452. Normal sinus rhythm, blocked APC at 64 mm. *to* atrial flutter with variable A-V conduction and moderate ventricular rate response.

453. Advanced second degree A-V block: sinus tachycardia, 3:1 A/V ratio, right bundle branch block.

454. Sinus bradycardia, unifocal VPC's at 68 and 125 mm., *to* normal sinus rhythm.

455. Normal sinus rhythm with right bundle branch block, APC at 134 mm. followed by sinus

beat without RBBB. Electronic pacemaker, demand mode, at 156 mm. and 174 mm. without cardiac stimulation (occurring during sinus conducted beats).

456. Second degree A-V block: sinus bradycardia with blocked sinus beat at 36 mm.

457. Sinus rhythm with atrial bigeminy and aberrant ventricular conduction of premature beats.

458. First degree A-V block *to* sinus arrest and nodal escape rhythm.

459. Normal sinus rhythm; unifocal VPC's with fixed coupling intervals, each followed by a nodal escape beat.

460. Normal sinus rhythm with RBBB. Periods of sinus slowing and intermittent appearance of EPM rhythm, demand mode.

461. Atrial flutter (or tachycardia) with advanced A-V block; ventricular escape beat.

462. Complete (or third degree) A-V block: atrial flutter; electronic pacemaker rhythm with occasional failure of ventricular capture.

463. Complete A-V block: sinus tachycardia; slow nodal rhythm.

464. Complete A-V block: sinus rhythm; electronic pacemaker rhythm with complete ventricular capture.

465. Sinus bradycardia with first degree A-V block and periods of sinus slowing with nodal escape beats.

466. Sinus irregularity with RBBB; electronic pacemaker impulses of demand mode with complete failure of cardiac stimulation.

467. Atrial tachycardia *to* atrial escape beat *to* atrial standstill *to* sinus bradycardia.

468. Sinus rhythm with ventricular asystole.

469. Advanced second degree A-V block: sinus tachycardia; 3:1 A/V ratio; intraventricular conduction defect.

470. Second degree A-V block: sinus tachycardia; 2:1 A/V ratio, prolonged PR intervals of conducted beats.

471. Complete A-V block: sinus tachycardia; nodal rhythm.

472. Sinus tachycardia with RBBB; APC's at 59 mm. and 96 mm.; VPC's at 15 mm. and 122 mm. (unifocal with fixed coupling intervals); *to* atrial tachycardia with variable A-V conduction.

INDEX

Note: Page numbers in *italics* refer to illustrations.